DIET AND DRUGS
IN ATHEROSCLEROSIS

Diet and Drugs
in Atherosclerosis

*European Atherosclerosis
Group Meeting*

Lugano, Switzerland

Editors

Giorgio Noseda, M.D.
*Reparto di Medicina
Ospedale della Beata Vergine
Mendrisio, Switzerland*

Barry Lewis, M.D.
*Department of Chemical Pathology
and Metabolic Disorders
St. Thomas's Hospital Medical
School
London, England*

Rodolfo Paoletti, M.D.
*Istituto di Farmacologia
e di Farmacognosia
Universita di Milano
Milan, Italy*

Raven Press ▪ New York

Raven Press, 1140 Avenue of the Americas, New York, New York 10036

Made in the United States of America

Great care has been taken to maintain the accuracy of the information contained in the volume. However, Raven Press cannot be held responsible for errors or for any consequences arising from the use of the information contained herein.

Materials appearing in this book prepared by individuals as part of their official duties as U.S. Government employees are not covered by the above-mentioned copyright.

Library of Congress Cataloging in Publication Data

Main entry under title:

Diet and drugs in atherosclerosis.

Includes index.
1. Atherosclerosis–Nutritional aspects–Congresses. 2. Atherosclerosis–Chemotherapy--Congresses. 3. Probucol–Congresses. I. Noseda, Giorgio. II. Lewis, Barry. III. Paoletti, Rodolfo. IV. European Atherosclerosis Group. (DNLM: 1. Arteriosclerosis--Drug therapy–Congresses. 2. Diet, Atherogenic--Congresses. WG550 D565 1979)
RC692.D53   616.1'36   80-19855
ISBN 0-89004-491-0

Preface

The etiology of atherosclerosis is multifactorial, and elevated serum cholesterol represents one of the major risk factors associated with development of coronary heart disease. In many industrialized countries, this condition is one of the most common causes of death.

Nutritional factors have been recognized as representing important contributions to the development of hyperlipidemia. There is now increasing firm evidence, derived from experimental models, that development, progression, and regression of atherosclerosis in various arterial segments are affected by dietary measures. Consequently, dietary changes have become the cornerstone of therapeutic regimens in clinical practice and represent the first step in the management of hyperlipidemia.

In addition to a fat-modified, low cholesterol diet, new regimens such as soya protein and high fiber diets have been tested and have yielded promising results. However, the reduction of high cholesterol levels as a result of dietary measures alone is often insufficient, and drug treatment may be necessary. On the other hand, current therapeutic measures to treat hypercholesterolemia are unsatisfactory and new hypocholesterolemic drugs are required.

Important advances have been achieved recently in the diagnosis and treatment of plasma lipid disorders, a complex area for pharmacological and clinical investigation.

In keeping with this progress, the European Atherosclerosis Group held a meeting in Lugano, Switzerland, in September 1979. Part of the proceedings are included in this volume.

We express our gratitude to all distinguished contributors and to Drs. Claudia Fragiacomo and Vittoria Patrini for technical assistance.

We expect that this volume will update the information of many clinicians and biologists in this important area.

Giorgio Noseda
Barry Lewis
Rodolfo Paoletti

Contents

Probucol

Summaries*

---

*Eng = English summaries, Fr = French summaries, Ger = German summaries, It = Italian summaries, Port = Portuguese summaries, Sp = Spanish summaries.

Contributors

P. Amodeo
Centro per la Lotta alle Malattie
    Dismetaboliche e all'Arteriosclerosi
Istituto di Terapia Medica Sistematic
Università di Roma
00161 Rome, Italy

A. Anastasi
Diabetes and Lipid Research Laboratory
St. Bartholomew's Hospital
London EC 1, England

F. Angelico
Centro per la Lotta alle Malattie
    Dismetaboliche e all'Arteriosclerosi
Istituto di Terapia Medica Sistematic
Università di Roma
00161 Rome, Italy

L. Angelucci
Institute of Pharmacology and Pharmacognosy
University of Rome
00161 Rome, Italy

J. F. Ascaso
Department of Internal Medicine
University of Murcia
Murcia, Spain

P. Avogaro
Regional General Hospital
Unit for Atherosclerosis
National Council for Research
30100 Venice, Italy

G. Baggio
Department of Internal Medicine
Division of Gerontology and Metabolic Diseases
University of Padua
35100 Padova, Italy

M. R. Baiocchi
Department of Internal Medicine
Division of Gerontology and Metabolic Diseases
University of Padua
35100 Padova, Italy

R. Bakir
Department of Plasma and Tissue Lipoproteins
UER Medecine Paris VII
Villemin and
Internal Medicine Service
Hôpital Saint-Louis
75010 Paris, France

G. Baldo
Department of Internal Medicine
Division of Gerontology and Metabolic Diseases
University of Padua
35100 Padova, Italy

S. D. Barnard
Health and Consumer Products Department
The Dow Chemical Company
Indianapolis, Indiana 46268

B. Barros
Department of Cardiology
Almada Medical Center
Almada, Portugal

J. L. Beaumont
Unité de Recherches sur l'Athérosclérose
I.N.S.E.R.M. U. 32
Hôpital Henry-Mondor
94010 Créteil, France

V. Beaumont
Unité de Recherches sur l'Athérosclérose
I.N.S.E.R.M. U32
Hôpital Henry-Mondor
F 94010 Créteil, France

V. Bertelé
Istituto di Richerche Farmacologiche "Mario
    Negri"
20157 Milan, Italy

D. J. Betteridge
Diabetes and Lipid Research Laboratory
St. Bartholomew's Hospital
London EC1, London

M. Bihari-Varga
Second Department of Pathology
Semmelweis Medical University
Budapest, 1091 Ulloi ut 93, Hungary

G. Bittolo Bon
Regional General Hospital
Unit for Atherosclerosis
National Council for Researches
30100 Venice, Italy

C. Borgogelli
Centro per la Lotta alle Malattie
Dismetaboliche e all'Arteriosclerosi
Istituto di Terapia Medica Sistematic
Università di Roma
00161 Rome, Italy

B. Brusoni
De Gasperis Division
Ospedale Ca' Granda
20100 Milan, Italy

J. C. Buxtorf
Unité de Recherches sur l'Athérosclérose
I.N.S.E.R.M. U. 32
Hôpital Henry-Mondor
94010 Creteil, France

A. Cantafora
Istituto Superiore di Sanità
Rome, Italy

G. Cappello
Istituto di Clinica Medica Generale
dell'Universita
34129 Trieste, Italy

R. Carmena
Department of Internal Medicine
University of Murcia
Murcia, Spain

M. Carragata
Department of Cardiology
Almada Medical Center
Almada, Portugal

A. Castro Ribeiro
Serviço de Patalogia Médica
Faculdade de Medicina do Porto
Porto, Portugal

G. Catenazzo
Vergani Medical Division and Center E. Grossi
Paoletti
Ospedale Ca' Granda
20100 Milan, Italy

L. Cattin
Istituto di Clinica Medica Generale
dell'Universita
34129 Trieste, Italy

G. Cazzolato
Regional General Hospital
Unit for Atherosclerosis
National Council for Researches
30100 Venice, Italy

B. Chanu
Department of Plasma and Tissue Lipoproteins
UER Medecine Paris VII
Villemin and
Service de Medecine Interne
Hôpital Saint-Louis
75010 Paris, France

P. Cŏk
Istituto di Clinica Medica Generale
dell'Universita
34129 Trieste, Italy

G. Crepaldi
Department of Internal Medicine
Division of Gerontology and Metabolic Diseases
University of Padua
35100 Padova, Italy

E. Csonka
Second Department of Pathology
Semmelweis Medical University
Budapest, 1091 Ulloi ut 93, Hungary

P. G. Da Col
Istituto di Clinica Medica Generale
dell'Università
34129 Trieste, Italy

G. d'Atri
LPB Cinisello Balsamo
Milan, Italy

G. de Gaetano
Istituto di Richerche Farmacologiche "Mario
Negri"
20157 Milan, Italy

J. L. De Gennes
Service d'Endocrinologie et Metabolisme
Groupe Hospitalier Pitié-Salpêtrière
75013 Paris, France

G. C. Descovich
Istituto di Clinica Medica II
Università di Bologna
Bologna, Italy

M. Diaz Curiel
Unidad Metabolica
Fundacion Jiménez Díaz
Madrid 3, Spain

G. Di Minno
Istituto di Richerche Farmacologiche "Mario Negri"
20157 Milan, Italy

I. Dionisio
Department of Cardiology
Almada Medical Center
Almada, Portugal

C. Ehnholm
Second Departmant of Medicine
University of Helsinki and
Central Public Health Laboratory
00290 Helsinki 29, Finland

E. Farinaro
Semeiotica Medica
Second Faculty of Medicine
University of Naples
Naples, Italy

S. Felix
Department of Cardiology
Almada Medical Center
Almada, Portugal

R. Fellin
Department of Internal Medicine
Division of Gerontology and Metabolic Diseases
University of Padua
35100 Padova, Italy

G. Fiorini
Vergani Medical Division and Center E. Grossi Paoletti
Ospedae Ca' Granda
20100 Milan, Italy

M. Fonda
Istituto di Clinica Medica Generale dell'Universita
34129 Trieste, Italy

C. Fragiacomo
Ospedale Beata Vergine
6850 Mendrision, Switzerland

Sz. Füzesi
Second Department of Pathology
Semmelweis Medical University
Budapest, Hungary

E. Galimberti
LPB Cinisello Balsamo
Milan, Italy

J. Galton
Diabetes and Lipid Research Laboratory
St. Bartholomew's Hospital
London EC1, England

P. Gomarasca
LPB Cinisello Balsamo
Milan, Italy

A. Gouveia
Department of Cardiology
Almada Medical Center
Almada, Portugal

J. Goy-Leoper
Department of Plasma and Tissue Lipoproteins
UER Medecine Paris VII
Villemin and
Service de Medecine Interne
Hôpital Saint-Louis
75010 Paris, France

A. Gustafson
University Hospital
Lund, Sweden

J. Hársing
Second Department of Pathology
Semmelweis Medical University
Budapest, Hungary

H. D. Holler
Department of Medical Research
Boehringer Mannheim GmbH
6800 Mannheim 31, West Germany

J. K. Huttunen
Second Department of Medicine
University of Helsinki and
Central Public Health Laboratory
00290 Helsinki 29, Finland

R. Infante
Liver Research Unit
I.N.S.E.R.M. U.9
75571 Paris Cedex 12, France

C. Iovine
Semeiotica Medica
Second Faculty of Medicine
University of Naples
Naples, Italy

B. Jacotot
Unité de Recherches sur l'Athérosclérose
I.N.S.E.R.M. U.32
Hôpital Henry-Mondor
94010 Creteil, France

H. Jellinek
Second Department of Pathology
Semmelweis Medical University
Budapest, 1091 Ulloi ut 93, Hungary

M. Jirsa
First Medical Department
Faculty of General Medicine
Charles University
Prague, Czechoslovakia

M. Jost
Geriatric Clinic Kantonsspital Basel
Swiss Federal Research Station for Animal
  Production Grangeneuve
Unit of Social and Preventive Medicine
University of Basel
CH-4031 Basel, Switzerland

J. Kaliman
Atherosclerosis Research Group
Department of Medical Physiology
Atherosclerosis and Thrombosis Research
  Commission
Austrian Academy of Sciences and
Department of Cardiology
Second Department of Internal Medicine
University of Vienna
Vienna, Austria

M. Keller
Lipid Research Laboratory and Institute for
  Clinical and Experimental Cancer Research
University of Bern
Bern, Switzerland

K. Klein
Atherosclerosis Research Group
Department of Medical Physiology
Atherosclerosis and Thrombosis Research
  Commission
Austrian Academy of Sciences and
Department of Cardiology
Second Department of Internal Medicine
University of Vienna
Vienna, Austria

D. M. Klurfeld
Wistar Institute of Anatomy and Biology
Philadelphia, Pennsylvania 19104

V. Kordač
First Medical Department
Faculty of General Medicine
Charles University
Prague, Czechoslovakia

G. M. Kostner
Institute of Medical Biochemistry
University of Graz
A-8010 Graz, Austria

D. Kritchevsky
Wistar Institute of Anatomy and Biology
Philadelphia, Pennsylvania 19104

L. Kučerová
First Medical Department
Faculty of General Medicine
Charles University
Prague, Czechoslovakia

T. Kumlin
Second Department of Medicine
University of Helsinki and
Central Public Health Laboratory
00290 Helsinki 29, Finland

F. Lamenza
Semeiotica Medica
Second Faculty of Medicine
University of Naples
Naples, Italy

P. D. Lang
Department of Medical Research
Boehringer Mannheim GmbH
6800 Mannheim 31, West Germany

J. LeBeau
Health and Consumer Products Department
The Dow Chemical Company
Indianapolis, Indiana 46268

S. Lenzi
Istituto di Clinica Medica II
Università di Bologna
Bologna, Italy

B. Lewis
Department of Chemical Pathology and
  Metabolic Disorders
St. Thomas's Hospital Medical School
London SE1 7EH, England

R. Lugli
Institute of Clinical Medicine
University of Modena
41100 Modena, Italy

F. Maccari
Department of Biology
Sigma-Tau S.p.A.
Research Laboratories
Pomezia, Rome, Italy

M. Mancini

Semeiotica Medica
Second Faculty of Medicine
University of Naples
Naples, Italy

G. Mannino

Cattedra di Analisi Numerica
Università di Modena
Modena, Italy

O. Mantero

Vergani Medical Division and Center E. Grossi
    Paoletti
Ospedale Ca' Granda
20100 Milan, Italy

E. Manzato

Department of Internal Medicine
Division of Gerontology and Metabolic Diseases
University of Padua
35100 Padova, Italy

Z. Mareček

First Medical Department
Faculty of General Medicine
Charles University
Prague, Czechoslovakia

S. Martini

Department of Internal Medicine
Division of Gerontology and Metabolic Diseases
University of Padua
35100 Padova, Italy

B. Martz

Health and Consumer Products Department
The Dow Chemical Company
Indianapolis, Indiana 46268

S. Mattila

Second Department of Medicine
University of Helsinki and
Central Public Health Laboratory
00290 Helsinki 29, Finland

D. McCaughan

Department of Medicine
Veterans Administration Hospital
The Peter Brigham Hospital and
    Harvard Medical School
Boston, Massachusetts 02130

H. Micheli

Division de Diabétologie
Département de Médecine
Hôpital Cantonal
Geneva, Switzerland

T. A. Miettinen

Second Department of Medicine
University of Helsinki and
Central Public Health Laboratory
00290 Helsinki 29, Finland

M. Moczar

Laboratoire de Biochimie du Tissu Conjonctif
Faculté de Médecine
Université Paris-Val de Marne
94010 Creteil, France

J. A. Molello

Health and Consumer Products Department
The Dow Chemical Company
Indianapolis, Indiana 46268

U. Montaguti

Istituto di Clinica Medica II
Università di Bologna
Bologna, Italy

A. Montali

Centro per la Lotta alle Malattie
    Dismetaboliche e all'Arteriosclerosi
Istituto di Terapia Medica Sistematic
Università di Roma
00161 Rome, Italy

R. Mordasini

Lipid Research Laboratory and
Institute for Clinical and Experimental Cancer
    Research
University of Bern
Bern, Switzerland

W. D. Müller

Institute of Medical Biochemistry
University of Graz and
Universitätskinderklinik
A-8010 Graz, Austria

S. Muntoni

Center for Metabolic Diseases and
    Atherosclerosis
Regional General Hospital "Ospedali Riuniti"
09100 Cagliari, Italy

V. Naukkarinen

Second Department of Medicine
University of Helsinki and
Central Public Health Laboratory
00290 Helsinki 29, Finland

A. Noronha

Department of Cardiology
Almada Medical Center
Almada, Portugal

G. Noseda

Department of Medicine
Ospedale Beata Vergine
6850 Mendrisio, Switzerland

A. Oberhänsli

Geriatric Clinic Kantonsspital Basel
Swiss Federal Research Station for Animal
  Production Grangeneuve
Unit of Social and Preventive Medicine
University of Basel
CH-4031 Basel, Switzerland

S. Otto

Institute of Medical Biochemistry
University of Graz and
Universitätskinderklinik
A-8010 Graz, Austria

A. Pereira Viana

Serviço de Patologia Médica
Faculdade de Medicina do Porto
Porto, Portugal

D. Petit

Liver Research Unit
I.N.S.E.R.M. U.9
75571 Paris Cedex, 12, France

D. Pometta

Division de Diabétologie
Département de Médecine
Hôpital Cantonal
Geneva, Switzerland

A. Postiglione

Semeiotica Medica
Second Faculty of Medicine
University of Naples
Naples, Italy

G. B. Quinci

Regional General Hospital
Unit for Atherosclerosis
National Council for Researches
30100 Venice, Italy

M. T. Ramacci

Department of Biology
Sigma-Tau S.p.A.
Research Laboratories
Pomezia, Rome, Italy

A. Rapado

Unidad Metabolica Fundacion Jiménez Díaz
Madrid-3, Spain

J. Renais

Centre de Recherches Cardiologiques de
  l'Association Calude Bernard
Hôpital Boucicaut
75015 Paris, France

G. Ricci

Centro per la Lotta alle Malattie
  Dismetaboliche e all'Arterosclerosi
Istituto di Terapia Medica Sistematica
Università di Roma
00161 Rome, Italy

W. F. Riesen

Lipid Research Laboratory and Institute for
  Clinical and Experimental Cancer Research
University of Bern
Bern, Switzerland

G. Ritzel

Geriatric Clinic Kantonsspital Basel
Swiss Federal Research Station for Animal
  Production Grangeneuve
Unit of Social and Preventive Medicine
University of Basel
CH-4031 Basel, Switzerland

H. Rosegger

Universitätskinderklinik
A-8010 Graz, Austria

J. Rouffy

Service de Medecine Interne
Hôpital Saint-Louis
75010 Paris, France

P. Rubba

Semeiotica Medica
Second Faculty of Medicine
University of Naples
Naples, Italy

R. Salati

Institute of Clinical Medicine
University of Modena
41100 Modena, Italy

G. Salvioli

Institute of Clinical Medicine
University of Modena
41100 Modena, Italy

J. P. Sauvanet

Department of Plasma and Tissue Lipoproteins
UER Medicine Paris VII and
Internal Medicine Service
Hôpital Saint-Louis
75010 Paris, France

L. Scebat
Centre de Recherches Cardiologiques de
  l'Association Claude Bernard
Hôpital Boucicaut
75015 Paris, France

H. Schneeberger
Geriatric Clinic Kantonsspital Basel
Swiss Federal Research Station for Animal
  Production Grangeneuve
Unit of Social and Preventive Medicine
University of Basel
CH-4031 Basel, Switzerland

K. Silberbauer
Atherosclerosis Research Group
Department of Medical Physiology
Atherosclerosis and Thrombosis Research
  Commission
Austrian Academy of Sciences and
Department of Internal Medicine
University of Vienna
Vienna, Austria

H. Sinzinger
Atherosclerosis Research Group
Department of Medical Physiology
Atherosclerosis and Thrombosis Research
  Commission
Austrian Academy of Sciences and
Department of Cardiology
Second Department of Internal Medicine
University of Vienna
Vienna, Austria

C. R. Sirtori
Center E. Grossi Paoletti and Chemotherapy
  Chair
University of Milan
Milan, Italy

H. B. Stähelin
Geriatric Clinic Kantonsspital Basel
Swiss Federal Research Station for Animal
  Production Grangeneuve
Unit of Social and Preventive Medicine
University of Basel
CH-4031 Basel, Switzerland

S. Stefanović
Clinica A of Internal Medicine
University Medical Faculty
Belgrade, Yugoslavia

H. Taylor
Health and Consumer Products Department
The Dow Chemical Company
Indianapolis, Indiana 46268

R. Tedeschi
Health and Consumer Products Department
The Dow Chemical Company
Indianapolis, Indiana 46268

J. Truffert
Service d'Endocrinologie et Métabolisme
Groupe Hospitalier Pitié-Salpêtrière
75013 Paris, France

S. Vergari
Centro per la Lotta alle Malattie
  Dismetaboliche e all'Arteriosclerosi
Istituto di Terapia Medica Sistematica
Università di Roma
00160 Rome, Italy

S. Villa
Istituto di Richerche Farmacologiche "Mario
  Negri"
20157 Milan, Italy

J. Vollmar
Department of Medical Research
Boehringer Mannheim GmbH
6800 Mannheim 31, West Germany

L. Vučić
Clinica A of Internal Medicine
University Medical Faculty
Belgrade, Yugoslavia

M. Wanner
Geriatric Clinic Kantonsspital Basel
Swiss Federal Research Station for Animal
  Production Grangeneuve
Unit of Social and Preventive Medicine
University of Basel
CH-4031 Basel, Switzerland

Diet and Drugs in Atherosclerosis,
edited by G. Noseda, B. Lewis, and R. Paoletti.
Raven Press, New York © 1980.

The LDL Theory and the HDL Hypothesis

Barry Lewis

*Department of Chemical Pathology and Metabolic Disorders, St. Thomas's Hospital,
Medical School, London, SE 1 7EH England*

Not a few lay writings in the past year and even some academic publications might give the impression of a counterreformation in the field of atherosclerosis research in Europe (51). This chapter is a brief review of the quality of the evidence causally linking two of the lipoproteins of plasma with ischemic heart disease (IHD): low density lipoprotein (LDL) and high density lipoprotein (HDL).

The dictionary definition of an hypothesis is a formulation that provides a basis for investigation but which need not be based on data. Clearly, most hypotheses are rejected as experimental data accumulate, a few evolving to theories supported by a consistent body of evidence. Despite the empirical basis of much medical practice, it is obvious that tenable theories are required for sound practice in both treatment and prevention. This chapter examines the theoretical basis for the clinical management of lipoprotein disorders in heart disease prevention. What is the logical status today of the relationships between LDL and HDL and IHD?

LIPOPROTEIN METABOLISM

Very low density lipoprotein (VLDL) (26) carrying triglyceride and cholesterol, is secreted into plasma by the splanchnic organs (5) and, chiefly from animal data (18), by the liver. Much of triglyceride is cleared by lipoprotein lipase as the VLDL passes through the capillaries of peripheral tissue. The process yields fatty acids, which largely enter the cells, especially of adipose tissue and muscle, leaving two products within the circulation. One product is a series of smaller lipoproteins (IDL), which are in part converted to LDL (3,22,41). LDL is triglyceride-poor but contains some 60 to 70% of circulating cholesterol in adult man. The other product comprises some of the surface components of VLDL, including polar lipids and apolipoproteins; these transfer to HDL. LDL is metabolized within the cells, chiefly in peripheral tissues, providing much or all of their cholesterol requirements. This is mediated by high affinity receptors (15), well documented in surviving peripheral cell lines, which promote the internalization of LDL and release of its contained cholesterol following hydrolysis in secondary lysosomes. That this process occurs *in vivo* is suggested by the effect on LDL metabolism in man of modifying its apoprotein to prevent its recognition by the receptor (48). This substantially decreases its fractional rate of catabolism. Hence VLDL and LDL provide for the centrifugal transport of lipids from liver and gut to the periphery. It is possible that some LDL is catabolized in the liver, and that LDL loses some cholesterol ester as it passes through the liver (44); this cholesteryl ester may transfer to VLDL and thus recycle (43).

We have been investigating the splanchnic and peripheral metabolism of these lipoproteins in man by measurement of arteriovenous differences of concentration and of radioactivity during infusion of labeled lipoproteins (49). These affirm that VLDL, specifically its least dense subclass (Sf 100 to 400), is secreted in the splanchnic bed but not catabolized in this site. Conversely, IDL particles of Sf 12 to 60 are extracted from plasma in the splanchnic territory; of the structural protein of these extracted particles, apoB, approximately 55% reappears in hepatic venous blood in the form of LDL. By contrast, a nonsignificant proportion of IDL is converted to LDL in the peripheral tissues, as assessed by arterial-inferior vena caval differences in radioactivity.

Hence the splanchnic territory is the major site for IDL-LDL conversion in man. Parenchymal liver cells have high affinity receptors for IDL (9). There is a hepatic lipase which, unlike lipoprotein lipase, shows selective affinity for IDL, hydrolyzing its triglyceride more rapidly than that of VLDL of Sf 100 to 400 (34).

The origin, catabolism, and metabolic role of HDL are the subjects of extensive current research. A cohesive picture is beginning to emerge but is less well defined than that of VLDL, IDL, and LDL. Nascent HDL particles containing apoE, apoAI, and apoC are secreted by the liver (17). Discoidal HDL particles are consistently demonstrable in human hepatic vein blood (50). This class of lipoprotein appears to undergo considerable remodeling in the circulation. Furthermore, apoAI and apoAII synthesized in the intestinal mucosa enter plasma as components of chylomicrons and rapidly transfer to HDL (21). HDL acquires further polar lipids and apoC from chylomicrons and VLDL as these lipoproteins undergo catabolism by lipoprotein lipase (12).

There is growing evidence that HDL may play a role in the centripetal transport of cholesterol, destined for excretion or catabolism by the liver. Free cholesterol has been shown to transfer from cultured cells, including arterial smooth muscle cells, to HDL *in vitro* (6,6a). The mass of exchangeable tissue determined by isotope dilution is inversely proportional to plasma HDL-cholesterol concentration (31). The specific activity of cholesterol in plasma lipoprotein has been followed in obese subjects injected with labeled cholesterol and then placed on a reducing diet (33). Mobilization of tissue cholesterol was shown by a rise in specific activity of cholesterol in HDL but not in other lipoprotein fractions, implying a role for HDL as an acceptor for tissue cholesterol. A minor subclass of HDL, HDL-I, has the property of competing with LDL for high affinity cell surface lipoprotein receptors on fibroblast and smooth muscle cells (29). This fraction of HDL could act to reduce internalization of LDL by peripheral cells, and hence to reduce uptake of circulating cholesterol. However, there is another effect of HDL on the receptor mechanism, potentially of opposite effect on cholesterol transport; lipoprotein receptor activity is increased in cells incubated with HDL (32).

Evidence that HDL cholesterol is taken up and metabolized by the liver is limited. Hepatocytes possess cell surface receptors for HDL. Injection of lipoproteins complexed with labeled cholesterol into a subject with a bile fistula has shown preferential utilization of HDL free cholesterol as a precursor for bile acids and biliary cholesterol (39). An alternative or additional role for HDL in centripetal transport of cholesterol is possible. This envisages free cholesterol transferring to HDL from peripheral tissues and undergoing esterification by LCAT. The cholesteryl ester is then seen as undergoing mass transfer to VLDL, a process mediated by the well-documented circulating exchange protein (8). This would permit hepatic uptake of the cholesteryl ester, since VLDL remnant particles are taken up by the liver via a high affinity receptor mechanism. Hence there is considerable indirect evidence for the hypothesized role of HDL in centripetal transport of cholesterol.

EVIDENCE OF ASSOCIATION

There is strong and mostly noncontroversial evidence of associations between IHD and plasma lipoprotein abnormalities. Among the many case-control studies, two carried out to a common protocol on substantial numbers have confirmed the significantly higher mean levels of total VLDL and LDL cholesterol and lower levels of HDL cholesterol in IHD patients (7,28). Prospective surveys similarly attest to the predictive association of high levels of total or LDL cholesterol and low levels of HDL cholesterol with IHD risk (16,30). These are continuous graded relationships, albeit not linear; hence the association of these risk factors with IHD shows dose-response characteristics, as would be expected of a causal relationship.

Further evidence is obtainable from comparisons of populations that differ widely in IHD mortality rates (24). In one such study of four carefully screened normal population samples (27) (in London, Uppsala, Geneva, and Naples, named in decreasing order of national IHD mortality), plasma LDL cholesterol and VLDL triglyceride levels were highest at all ages in London and Uppsala and lowest in Naples. However, these population samples had almost identical frequency distributions and means of HDL cholesterol concentration. The environmental factors influencing IHD risk and determining levels of VLDL and LDL were without effect on HDL, the concentration of which appeared to be independent of these variables. This is in no way incompatible with the evidence of an inverse association between HDL-cholesterol level and IHD risk, from prospective and case-control studies within populations; it indicates that the regional variation in IHD mortality referred to cannot be accounted for by HDL-mediated risk.

One form of case-control study which received recent attention is the comparison of quantitative scoring of atherosclerosis seen on coronary angiography with plasma lipoprotein analyses. Inverse relationships with HDL levels and direct ones with LDL have been reported (19,23). Recently, we have noted a strong inverse relationship between the extent of coronary disease and the distribution of cholesterol between the two major subclasses of HDL: the higher the HDL_2/HDL_3 ratio, the lower the atherosclerosis score.

Striking though the epidemiological evidence is, embodying association, prediction of risk, and dose-response relationship between lipoprotein levels and IHD, such evidence is best analyzed in the context of experimental data, and of the availability of plausible mechanisms by which such associations could reasonably be interpreted as causal.

MECHANISMS

LDL transports approximately 70% of circulating cholesterol in man. The demonstration by a variety of means that LDL is present in the arterial intima suggested that cholesterol might enter the vessel wall in this form. *In vivo* and postmortem studies have shown positive correlations between immunoreactive apo-LDL in human arteries and plasma levels of cholesterol or LDL (36). More recently, methods have been developed for estimating the net flux rate of LDL from plasma into human arterial intima in surgical patients. A positive correlation exists between this flux and plasma LDL cholesterol concentration (35). Hence high LDL concentrations in plasma appear to be a determinant of the rate at which the major cholesterol-bearing lipoprotein enters the arterial intima. This is a plausible basis for the association between hypercholesterolemia and cholesterol accumulation in the vessel wall. It may also account for the smooth muscle cell proliferation, which is so striking a feature of atheromatous plaques: LDL from primates with diet-induced hyperlipidemia is mitogenic for arterial smooth muscle cells and fibroblasts (13). In fact, this effect is specifically attributable to a subclass of LDL (38).

EXPERIMENTAL EVIDENCE

Experimental production of atherosclerosis-like lesions by diet-induced or diet- and drug-induced hyperlipidemia has been carried out in most laboratory species (52). The causal implication of such studies is greatly enhanced by the recent demonstration in primates that restoration of more normal lipid levels (by dietary means or drugs) leads to partial regression of the arterial lesions (1). Regression of such lesions, first documented by Armstrong and colleagues, have been observed in nine laboratories.

A natural experiment, the mutant gene for familial hypercholesterolemia,

illustrates the effect on IHD risk of a single, well-defined lesion of LDL catabolism in man. The risk is 10 to 12-fold greater in male heterozygotes than in
the general population (42,47). The occurrence of IHD as part of the natural
history of this common metabolic disorder is evidence of the influence of LDL
concentration on the risk of heart disease. The arterial pathology in heterozygotes
is typical atherosclerosis (37).

A comparable but less well-defined heritable disorder in which HDL cholesterol levels are elevated has been reported (2). The effect on IHD risk is in
striking contrast: not only is it not elevated, but reports suggest that IHD is
underrepresented in affected relatives (14). Xanthomas do not develop in this
disorder.

Numerous controlled trials of plasma cholesterol reduction by diet or drugs
have been reported; the results have been variable (40). One was the randomized
controlled trial by Dorr et al. (11) in which hypercholesterolemic subjects were
effectively treated with the bile acid sequentrant colestipol. This trial, like all
others (positive and negative), is open to criticism, (46) but it had two desirable
characteristics. One was the use of hyperlipidemic subjects, unlike most earlier
trials; the other was the substantial reduction in cholesterol levels obtained in
the intervention groups. The cholesterol reduction was followed by a major
decrease in fatal and nonfatal IHD in male subjects and a moderate fall in
total mortality.

It is relevant to discuss the magnitude of cholesterol reduction which consti-
tutes a reasonable test of the view that high levels of cholesterol and LDL

TABLE 1. *Cholesterol reduction and outcome of clinical trials*

Outcome	Cholesterol reduction (%)	Design	Intervention
−	6	2°	Coronary drug project (clofibrate)
−	13	2°	MRC (diet)
±	10	2°	Coronary drug project (nicotinate)
±	11	1°	Anticoronary club (diet)
±	12	1°	Los Angeles (diet)
±	11	2°	Newcastle (clofibrate)
±	13	2°	Edinburgh (clofibrate)
+	13	1°,2°	Colestipol
+	16	2°	Clofibrate + nicotinate
+	9	1°	WHO (clofibrate)
+	15	1°	Krasno et al. (clofibrate)
+	18	2°	Leren (diet)
+	21	1°	Turpeinen et al. (diet)
+	21	Regression	Barndt and Blankenhorn (diet, medication)

are causally associated with IHD. This in turn leads to a discussion of normal ranges of lipids and lipoproteins in plasma. So varied are observed ranges in normal subjects from different communities that this source of normative data alone is prone to difficulties of interpretation (27). A recent workshop devoted to this problem proposed optimal mean cholesterol levels in adults to be 4.5 mmoles/liter (180 mg/100 ml), with an upper limit of 5.5 mmoles/liter (220 mg/100 ml) (4).

By such criteria, lipid reduction in all published trials has been far from adequate. It is of interest to attempt to rank the published controlled trials of lipid reduction by the magnitude of the fall in serum cholesterol level. Clearly, the outcome is influenced by a number of features of trial design. Scrutiny of such a listing suggests that the chance of a positive outcome is greater in trials in which the fall in serum cholesterol level is substantial (Table 1).

Experimental data have yet to be produced concerning the effect on atherosclerosis of manipulation of plasma HDL concentrations. Despite the problems of experimental design, the prospect of performing such studies in laboratory animals is reasonable. In the absence of such information, caution is required in predicting the effects of altering HDL concentrations on the natural history of human IHD.

THE QUALITY OF PROOF

Although the evidence is strong, rigorous proof is lacking that reduction of LDL levels will prevent or lead to regression of human atherosclerosis (25,45). A necessary precondition is that the risks of such intervention should be shown to be very low. There are abundant precedents in preventive medicine for action on the basis of incomplete data. Cigarette smoking is a clear example. Although self-selected quitters have a lower risk of several diseases than continuing smokers (10), such evidence falls short of a randomized controlled trial; yet the medical profession is virtually unanimous on the need to discourage smoking. Treatment of obesity, hyperglycemia, and mild hypertension are further examples of normal clinical practice without rigorous proof.

By such standards, there is no need to apologize for the quality of evidence relating high LDL concentrations to IHD risk. The evidence concerning HDL is at an earlier stage. For the present, we should regard the protective effect of HDL as an hypothesis; but there is now a strong theoretical basis for the treatment of hypercholesterolemia due to elevated LDL concentration.

REFERENCES

1. Armstrong, M. L., and Megan, B. M. (1972): *Cir. Res.,* 30:675.
2. Avogaro, P., and Cazzolato, G. (1975): *Atherosclerosis,* 22:63.
3. Berman, M., Hall, M. III., Levy, R., Eisenberg, S., Bilheimer, D. W., Phair, R. D., and Goebel, R. H. (1978): *J. Lipid Res.,* 19:38.
4. Blackburn, H., Lewis, B., Wissler, R., Wynder, E. L., et al. (1979): *Prev. Med.,* 8:609.

5. Boberg, J., Carlson, L. A., Freyschuss, U., Lassers, B. W., and Wahlquist, M. (1972): *Eur. J. Clin. Invest.,* 2:454.
6. Bondjers, G., and Bjorkerud, G. (1975): *Eur. J. Clin. Invest.,* 9:51.
6a. Bondjers, G., Olsson, G., Nyman, L. L., and Bjorkerud, A. (1977): In: *Atherosclerosis IV,* edited by G. Schettler, Y. Gotto, Y. Mata, and G. Klose. Springer, Berlin.
7. Carlson, L. A., and Ericsson, M. (1975): *Atherosclerosis,* 21:435.
8. Chajek, T., and Fielding, C. J. (1978): *Proc. Nat. Acad. Sci., USA,* 75:3445.
9. Cooper, A. D. (1977): *Biochem. Biophys. Acta,* 488:464.
10. Doll, R., and Peto, R., (1976): *Br. Med. J.,* 2:1525.
11. Dorr, A. E., Gunderson, K., Schneider, J. C., Spencer, T. W., and Martin, W. B. (1978): *J. Chron. Dis.,* 31:(1978).
12. Eisenberg, S. (1978): *J. Lipid Res.,* 19:229.
13. Fischer-Dzoga, K., and Wissler, R. W. (1976): *Atherosclerosis,* 24:515.
14. Glueck, C. J., Gartside, P., Fallot, R. W., et al. (1976): *J. Lab. Clin. Med.,* 88:941.
15. Goldstein, J. L., Anderson, R. G. W., and Brown, M. S. (1979): *Nature,* 279:679.
16. Gordon, T., Castelli, W. P., Hjortland, M. C., Kannel, W. B., et al. (1977): *JAMA,* 235:497.
17. Hamilton, R. L. (1980): In: *Atherosclerosis V,* edited by A. M. Gotto, L. Smith, and B. Allen, p. 174. Springer, Berlin.
18. Hamilton, R. L. (1972): *Adv. Exp. Med. Biol.,* 26:7.
19. Hammett, F., Saltissi, S., Miller, N. E., Rao, S., Van Zeller, H., Coltart, J. and Lewis, B. (1979): *Circulation (abstr.),* 59:11–167.
20. Hammond, E. C., and Garfinkel, L. (1969): *Arch. Environ. Health,* 19:167.
21. Havel, R. J. (1978): In: *High Density Lipoproteins and Atherosclerosis,* edited by A. M. Gotto, Jr., N. E. Miller, and M. F. Oliver, p. 21. Elsevier, Amsterdam.
22. Janus, E. D., Nicoll, A., Wootton, R., Turner, P. R., Magill, P. J., and Lewis, B. (1980): *Eur. J. Clin. Invest. (in press).*
23. Jenkins, P. J., Harper, R. W., and Nestel, P. J. (1978): *Br. Med. J.,* 2:388.
24. Keys, A. (1980): *Seven Countries: Death and Coronary Heart Disease in Ten Years.* Harvard University Press, Cambridge.
25. Lewis, B. (1978): *J. Roy. Soc. Med.,* 71:809.
26. Lewis, B. (1976): *The Hyperlipidaemias: Clinical and Laboratory Practice.* Blackwell, Oxford.
27. Lewis, B., Chait, A., Sigurdsson, G., Mancini, M. et al. (1978): *Eur. J. Clin. Invest.,* 8:165.
28. Lewis, B., Chait, A., Oakley, C. M., et al. (1974): *Br. Med. J.,* 3:489.
29. Mahley, R. W., Weisgraber, K. H., Bersot, J. P., and Innerarity, T. L. (1978): In: *High Density Lipoproteins,* edited by A. M. Gotto, N. E. Miller, and M. F. Oliver, p. 149. Elsevier, Amsterdam.
30. Miller, N. E., Førde, O. H., and Thelle, D. S. (1977): *Lancet,* i:965.
31. Miller, N. E., Nestel, P. J., and Clifton-Bligh, P. (1976): *Atherosclerosis,* 23:535.
32. Miller, N. E., and Yin, A. (1978): *Biochim. Biophys. Acta,* 530:145.
33. Nestel, P. J., and Miller, N. E. (1978): In: *High Density Lipoproteins and Atherosclerosis,* edited by A. M. Gotto, N. E. Miller, and M. F. Oliver, p. 51. Elsevier, Amsterdam.
34. Nicoll, A., Janus, E., Sigurdsson, G., and Lewis, B. (1977): *Circulation (abstr.),* 56:111:23.
35. Niehaus, C. E., Nicoll, A., Coltart, D. J., Lewis, B., et al. (1977): *Lancet,* iii:469.
36. Onitiri, A. C., Lewis, B., Bentall, H., Jamieson, C., et al. (1976): *Atherosclerosis,* 23:513.
37. Roberts, W. C., Ferrans, V. J., Levy, R. I., and Fredrickson, D. S. (1973): *Am. J. Cardiol.,* 31:557.
38. Scanu, A. (1980): In: *Atherosclerosis V,* edited by A. M. Gotto, L. Smith, and B. Allen, p. 607. Springer, Berlin.
39. Schwartz, C. C., Halloran, L. G., Vlahcevic, Z. R., Gregory, D. H., and Swell, L. (1978): *Science,* 200:62.
40. Shaper, A. G. (1975): *Postgrad. Med. J.,* 52:464.
41. Sigurdsson, G., Nicoll, A., and Lewis, B. (1975): *J. Clin. Invest.,* 56:1481.
42. Slack, J. (1969): *Lancet,* ii:1380.
43. Sniderman, A., and Teng, B. (1980): In: *Atherosclerosis V,* edited by A. M. Gotto, L. Smith, and B. Allen, p. 596. Springer, Berlin.
44. Sniderman, A., Thomas, D., Marpole, D., and Teng, B. (1978): *J. Clin. Invest.,* 61:867.
45. Stamler, J. (1978): *Circulation,* 58:3.
46. Stone, N. (1978): *J. Chron. Dis.,* 31.
47. Stone, N. J., Levy, R. I., Fredrickson, D. S., and Kerter, J. (1974): *Circulation,* 49:476.

48. Thompson, G. R., Soutar, A. K., Knight, B. L., Gavigan, S., Myant, N. B., and Shepherd, J. (1980): *Clin. Sci. (abstr.) (in press).*
49. Turner, P. R., Coltart, J., Hazzard, W. R., Bacchus, R., Nicoll, A., Miller, N. E., and Lewis, B. (1979): *Eur. J. Clin. Invest. (abstr.),* 9:3:26.
50. Turner, P., Miller, N., Chrystie, I., Coltart, J., Mistry, P., Nicoll, A., and Lewis, B. (1979): *Lancet,* i:645.
51. Werkö, L. (1979): *Acta Med. Scand.,* 206:435.
52. Wissler, R. W. (1968): In: *Progress in Bichemical Pharmacology 4,* edited by C. J. Maras, A. Howard and R. Paoletti, p. 378.

Diet and Drugs in Atherosclerosis,
edited by G. Noseda, B. Lewis, and R. Paoletti.
Raven Press, New York © 1980.

Dietary Protein in Atherosclerosis

David Kritchevsky

The Wistar Institute of Anatomy and Biology, Philadelphia, Pennsylvania 19104

The earliest experiments designed to test the effect of protein in atherosclerosis were carried out by Ignatowski (5), who fed rabbits diets rich in animal protein and observed anemia, cirrhosis, and aortic atherosclerosis. Ignatowski hypothesized that the active component in the diet was animal protein, but the report by Anitschkow (1) that cholesterol *per se* was atherogenic led most observers to conclude that the cholesterol content of the Ignatowski diet led to the observed atherosclerosis, and little attention was paid to dietary protein. Newburgh and Clarkson (14) showed that powdered beef was atherogenic for rabbits, and the time required for appearance of atheromata was a function of the protein level. Thus a diet in which powdered beef supplied 27% of protein caused atherosclerosis in 11 months; one in which powdered beef supplied 36% of protein required 2 to 3 months for appearance of atherosclerotic lesions.

Meeker and Kesten (10,11) fed rabbits diets containing casein or soy protein with or without added cholesterol. In the absence of cholesterol, the casein diet resulted in average atherosclerosis of 0.75 (0 to 3 scale), whereas no lesions were seen on either soybean or control diets. When the diet contained 60 mg/day cholesterol, average atherosclerosis was basal, 0.89; soy, 0.33; and casein, 2.07.

Middleton et al. (12) fed squirrel monkeys diets containing 25% butter, 0.5% cholesterol, and either 9 or 25% protein and found that both coronary and aortic atherosclerosis were 2 to 5 times more severe in the animals fed the high protein diet. Strong and McGill (16) made a similar observation in regard to sudanophilia in baboons.

Our work showed that, regardless of protein level, casein was more cholesteremic than soy protein in rats fed cholesterol and cholic acid (13). Experiments using conventional or germ-free chickens showed that the casein effect persisted even in the absence of intestinal microflora (7).

The early work discussed above involved the feeding of a limited number of proteins. Hamilton and Carroll (4) showed that protein of animal origin was more cholesteremic for rabbits than protein of vegetable origin. They also showed a wide range of activity within both protein types.

Comparison of the atherogenic effects of casein and soy protein in rabbits fed a semipurified, cholesterol-free diet confirmed the atherogenic effect of casein

TABLE 1. Influence of protein and fiber on rabbit atherosclerosis

Group[a]	No.	Serum lipids (mg/dl)		Liver lipids (g/100 g)		Atheroma[b]	
		Cholesterol	Triglyceride	Cholesterol	Triglyceride	Arch	Thoracic
CC	8/14	402 ± 40	164 ± 45	0.81 ± 0.08	0.43 ± 0.04	1.81	1.19
SC	5/14	248 ± 44	41 ± 8	0.93 ± 0.11	0.45 ± 0.05	1.50	1.00
CW	12/14	375 ± 42	94 ± 19	0.84 ± 0.05	0.37 ± 0.03	1.17	0.88
SW	13/14	254 ± 35	66 ± 9	0.85 ± 0.05	0.39 ± 0.02	1.04	0.77
CA	10/14	193 ± 34	60 ± 8	0.73 ± 0.07	0.48 ± 0.05	0.70	0.55
SA	13/14	159 ± 20	62 ± 17	0.77 ± 0.03	0.42 ± 0.02	0.88	0.58

[a] CC, casein-cellulose; SC, soy protein-cellulose; CW, casein-wheat straw; SW, soy protein-wheat straw; CA, casein-alfalfa; SA, soy protein-alfalfa. Diets contained 40% sucrose, 25% protein, 15% fiber, 14% coconut oil, 5% salt mix, and 1% vitamin mix. Fed for 10 months.
[b] Graded on a 0 to 4 scale.

TABLE 2. *Influence of protein on atherosclerosis in rabbits[a]*

	Group			
	Beef	Casein	TVP	Beef-TVP (1:1)
No.	12/12	11/12	9/12	11/12
Serum lipids (mg/dl)				
Cholesterol	185 ± 24	200 ± 18	37 ± 4	61 ± 6
Triglyceride	59 ± 8	92 ± 10	58 ± 7	70 ± 13
Liver lipids (g/100 g)				
Cholesterol	0.77 ± 0.90	0.38 ± 0.06	0.28 ± 0.01	0.47 ± 0.04
Triglyceride	0.77 ± 0.08	0.55 ± 0.08	1.16 ± 0.39	0.72 ± 0.12
Average atherosclerosis[b]				
Arch	1.3 ± 0.2	1.3 ± 0.2	0.7 ± 0.1	0.7 ± 0.1
Thoracic	0.8 ± 0.1	0.9 ± 0.2	0.2 ± 0.1	0.4 ± 0.1

[a] Diets contained 40% carbohydrate, 25% protein, 15% cellulose, 14% beef tallow, 5% salt mix, and 1% vitamin mix. Fed for 8 months.
[b] Graded on a 0 to 4 scale.

but showed that this effect could be mediated by the type of fiber in the diet (Table 1) (9). Serum cholesterol levels were higher in the individual casein-fiber groups than in the corresponding soy protein-fiber groups. The differences in the groups fed casein-cellulose and those fed casein-wheat straw were significant ($p < 0.05$). Cholesterol levels were significantly lower in the casein-alfalfa group than in the group fed casein-wheat straw ($p < 0.01$) or casein-cellulose ($p < 0.001$). The serum cholesterol levels were significantly lower in the rabbits fed soy protein-alfalfa than in the rabbits fed soy protein-wheat straw ($p <$

TABLE 3. *Influence of protein on atherosclerosis in rabbits[a]*

	Group		
	Corn protein	Wheat gluten	Lactalbumin
No.	10/22	12/22	16/22
Serum lipids (mg/dl)			
Cholesterol	245	193	428
Triglyceride	94	103	135
Phospholipid	85	82	72
Liver lipids (g/100 g)			
Cholesterol	1.23	1.21	1.29
Triglyceride	2.14	2.82	1.69
Phospholipid	1.97	2.03	2.08
Average atherosclerosis[b]			
Arch	0.8	0.8	1.8
Thoracic	0.4	0.5	1.1

[a] Diets contained 40% sucrose, 25% protein, 15% cellulose, 14% coconut oil, 5% salt mix, and 1% vitamin mix. Fed for 8 months. Summary of two experiments.
[b] Graded on a 0 to 4 scale.

0.05). Serum triglycerides were elevated in the casein-cellulose group. Liver lipid levels were similar in all groups.

We have also studied the interaction of proteins and fats in rabbits fed this semipurified, cholesterol-free diet (6). In this experiment, the dietary fat was beef tallow and the protein was either beef, textured vegetable protein (TVP), casein or beef-TVP (1:1). As can be seen from Table 2, beef and casein are equally cholesteremic and atherogenic; TVP is significantly less atherogenic; and a 1:1 mixture of TVP with beef gives cholesterol levels slightly higher than those seen in rabbits fed TVP alone but are significantly lower than in rabbits fed casein or beef tallow. The atherogenicity of the beef-TVP (1:1) diet was identical to the TVP diet. The effects of corn protein, wheat gluten, and lactalbumin also have been compared using this type of diet (Table 3). Lactalbumin is more cholesteremic than either corn protein or wheat gluten (by 75 and 122%, respectively) and is more atherogenic than corn protein and wheat gluten (by 142 and 123%, respectively).

Differences in amino acid composition have been found when comparing casein with soy protein; one is the lysine/arginine ratio, which is about 2.0 in casein and only 0.9 in soy protein. Lysine inhibits liver arginase activity (2), which could permit more arginine to be available for synthesis of the arginine-rich apoprotein. This arginine-rich apoprotein is a component of the lipoprotein, which is most atherogenic for rabbits (15).

We have carried out experiments in which rabbits were fed a semipurified diet, which contained casein, soy protein, casein plus enough arginine to bring its lysine/arginine ratio to 0.9, or soy protein plus enough lysine to raise its lysine/arginine ratio to 2.0 (8). The results of three experiments are summarized in Table 4. Addition of lysine to soy protein raises serum cholesterol levels from 124 to 190 mg/dl. The average atherogenicity is increased by 64%. Addition of arginine to casein does not affect serum cholesterol levels but reduces atherogenicity by 24%. These differences are also reflected in the lipoprotein spectra of the four groups of rabbits (Table 5) (3). The distribution of lipoproteins in the sera of rabbits fed casein or soy protein differs in the greater concentration of VLDL and IDL in the casein group and the preponderance of HDL in the soy protein group. Addition of arginine to casein causes a drop in the concentration of VLDL plus IDL and increases LDL and HDL, respectively. The lipoprotein spectra of the sera of rabbits fed soy protein or casein plus arginine resemble each other. Conversely, addition of lysine to soy protein results in a sharp rise in concentration of VLDL plus IDL and a drop in HDL. Lipoproteins of sera of rabbits fed soy protein plus lysine resemble those of rabbits fed casein.

In summary, we find that protein of animal origin is generally more atherogenic and cholesteremic than protein of vegetable origin. This effect can be modified by the type of fiber in the diet, by adding specific amino acids to the diet, or by mixing the two types of protein. Insofar as quantity of protein is concerned, high protein diets are generally more atherogenic than their low protein counterparts.

TABLE 4. *Influence of specific amino acids on atherogenicity of casein or soy protein[a]*

	Group			
	Casein (C)	C + arginine	Soy (S)	S + lysine
No.	20/31	20/31	25/31	25/31
Serum lipids (mg/dl)				
Cholesterol	241	238	124	190
Triglycerides	105	123	66	74
Liver lipids (g/100 g)				
Cholesterol	1.33	1.36	1.30	1.25
Triglycerides	2.22	1.67	1.81	2.74
Average atherosclerosis[b]				
Arch	1.63	1.30	0.70	1.10
Thoracic	1.05	0.73	0.40	0.70

[a] All diets contained 40% sucrose, 25% protein, 15% cellulose, 14% coconut oil, 5% salt mix, and 1% vitamin mix. Fed for 8 months. Summary of three experiments.
[b] Graded on a 0 to 4 scale.

TABLE 5. *Distribution of lipoproteins in sera of rabbits fed various proteins*

	Lipoprotein class (μg/ml) (%)			
Diet	VLDL	IDL	LDL	HDL
Casein (C)	21 (2.3)	130 (14.4)	288 (31.9)	465 (51.4)
C + arginine	10 (0.9)	88 (7.8)	405 (35.8)	627 (55.5)
Soy protein (S)	9 (1.1)	62 (7.7)	242 (30.0)	494 (61.2)
S + lysine	14 (2.2)	114 (17.8)	194 (30.2)	320 (49.8)

ACKNOWLEDGMENTS

This work was supported in part by grant HL 03299 and by Research Career Award HL 0734 from the National Institutes of Health and by grants-in-aid from Miles Laboratories, ADM, the National Dairy Council, and the National Live Stock and Meat Board. The work described herein was carried out in collaboration with Dr. Jon A. Story, Dr. David M. Klurfeld, Ms. Shirley A. Tepper, and Ms. Susanne K. Czarnecki.

REFERENCES

1. Anitschkow, N. (1913): Über die Veränderungen der Kaninchenaorta bei experimentaller Cholesterinsteatose. *Beitr. Pathol. Anat. Allg. Pathol.,* 56:379–404.
2. Cittadini, D., Pietropaolo, C., DeCristofaro, D., and D'Ayjello-Caracciolo, M. (1964): In vitro effect of L-lysine on rat liver arginase. *Nature,* 203:643.
3. Czarnecki, S. K., and Kritchevsky, D. (1979): The effect of dietary proteins on lipoprotein metabolism and atherosclerosis in rabbits. *J. Am. Oil Chem. Soc.,* 56:388A.

4. Hamilton, R. M. G., and Carroll, K. K. (1976): Plasma cholesterol levels in rabbits fed low fat, low cholesterol diets. Effects of dietary proteins, carbohydrates and fibre from different sources. *Atherosclerosis,* 24:47–62.

5. Ignatowski, A. (1909): Über die Wirkung des tierischen Eiweisses auf die Aorta und die parenchymatösen Organe der Kaninchen. *Virchows Arch. Pathol. Anat. Physiol. Klin. Med.,* 198:248–270.

6. Kritchevsky, D. (1979): Vegetable protein and atherosclerosis. *J. Am. Oil. Chem. Soc.,* 56:135–146.

7. Kritchevsky, D., Kolman, R. R., Guttmacher, R. M., and Forbes, M. (1959): Influence of dietary carbohydrate and protein on serum and liver cholesterol in germ-free chickens. *Arch. Biochem. Biophys.,* 85:444–451.

8. Kritchevsky, D., Tepper, S. A., and Story, J. A. (1978): Influence of soy protein and casein on atherosclerosis in rabbits. *Fed. Proc.,* 37:747.

9. Kritchevsky, D., Tepper, S. A., Williams, D. E., and Story, J. A. (1977): Experimental atherosclerosis in rabbits fed cholesterol-free diets. 7. Interaction of animal or vegetable protein with fiber. *Atherosclerosis,* 26:397–403.

10. Meeker, D. R., and Kesten, H. D. (1940): Experimental atherosclerosis and high protein diets. *Proc. Soc. Exp. Biol. Med.,* 45:543–545.

11. Meeker, D. R., and Kesten, H. D. (1941): Effect of high protein diets on experimental atherosclerosis in rabbits. *Arch. Pathol.,* 31:147–162.

12. Middleton, C. C., Clarkson, T. B., Lofland, H. B., and Prichard, R. W. (1967): Diet and atherosclerosis of squirrel monkeys. *Arch. Pathol.,* 83:145–153.

13. Moyer, A. W., Kritchevsky, D., Logan, J. B., and Cox, H. R. (1956): Dietary protein and serum cholesterol in rats. *Proc. Soc. Exp. Biol. Med.,* 92:736–737.

14. Newburgh, L. H., and Clarkson, S. (1923): The production of atherosclerosis in rabbits by feeding diets rich in meat. *Arch. Intern. Med.,* 31:653–676.

15. Shore, B., Shore, V., Salel, A., Mason, D., and Zelis, R. (1974): An apolipoprotein preferentially enriched in cholesteryl ester-rich very low density lipoproteins. *Biochem. Biophys. Res. Commun.,* 58:1–7.

16. Strong, J. P., and McGill, H. C., Jr. (1967): Diet and experimental atherosclerosis in baboons. *Am. J. Pathol.,* 50:669–690.

Diet and Drugs in Atherosclerosis,
edited by G. Noseda, B. Lewis, and R. Paoletti.
Raven Press, New York © 1980.

Serum Lipoprotein Pattern in Rats Following Fat Load: Modifications by L-Carnitine

F. Maccari, M. T. Ramacci, and *L. Angelucci

*Sigma-Tau S.p.A., Research Laboratories Pomezia, and * Institute of Pharmacology and Pharmacognosy, University of Rome, Rome, Italy*

Carnitine, γ-trimethyl, β-hydroxybutyrobetaine (CAR), plays an important role in lipid metabolism by acting as a mobile carrier for the mitochondrial transmembrane movement of long chain fatty acids (4). Tissues deficient in CAR are unable to oxidize the long chain fatty acids. They are characterized by an increase in both the synthesis of triglycerides and the accumulation of fatty acids and long chain acyl-CoA (11). In several pathological situations, anomalous serum or tissue levels of CAR are correlated with an impairment in lipid metabolism. Some of these situations have been treated with CAR. Improvement has been found in type I lipid storage myopathy (1,7), dyslipidemia due to hemodyalisis (3), and hypertriglyceridemia due to malabsorption syndromes (8). In a number of disease conditions characterized by diabetic hyperlipidemia (2) and type IV hyperlipoproteinemia (9,10), levels of CAR have not been studied, but a marked improvement has been obtained with CAR administration.

It appeared reasonable, therefore, to study the effect of CAR on blood lipids and lipoproteins, which, to some extent, reflect lipid metabolism in tissue. CAR, D- and L-diastereoisomer, 500 mg/kg^{-1} os, was administered to unfasted rats loaded with olive oil, 30 ml/kg^{-1} os, 1 hr before. The control group received oil and solvent solution, and the blank group received solvent solution only. The triglyceride, phospholipid, and cholesterol levels and the CAR concentration in serum (free and short chain acyl-carnitines) were assayed in rats sacrificed at different times after oil load. The lipoprotein pattern was determined electrophoretically.

Figure 1 shows that 1 hr after oil administration, triglyceride, phospholipid, and cholesterol levels in the control group were higher than those in the blank group. The increase lasted until the fourth hour. L-CAR administration promptly produced a remarkable decrease in serum lipids: triglycerides, phospholipids, and cholesterol were statistically different from control values and overlapped those of the blanks. The values obtained from rats treated with D-CAR were similar to those of control groups. However, in some rats, these values were notably higher than the mean value of controls. This may indicate the possibility

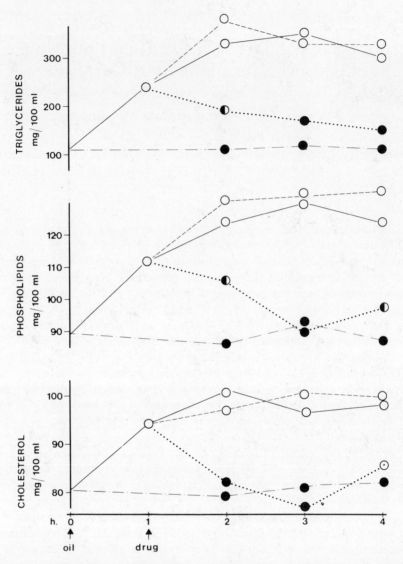

FIG. 1. Effect of L- and D-CAR, 500 mg/kg^{-1} os, on triglyceride, phospholipid, and cholesterol serum levels in rats loaded with olive oil, 30 ml/kg^{-1} os, 1 hr before. *Dash/dot line,* blank; *solid line,* control; *dotted line,* L-CAR; *dashed line,* D-CAR. *Dotted, half filled, and filled symbols, p* = 0.05, 0.01, 0.001, respectively. *N* = 10 in each group.

of competition of exogenous D-CAR with endogenous L-CAR. Competition refers to the active transport through the cell membrane via a common carrier (6).

As shown in Fig. 2, in the control group, the chylomicron and prebeta-lipoprotein fraction increased 1 hr after oil load. The difference from the blank group

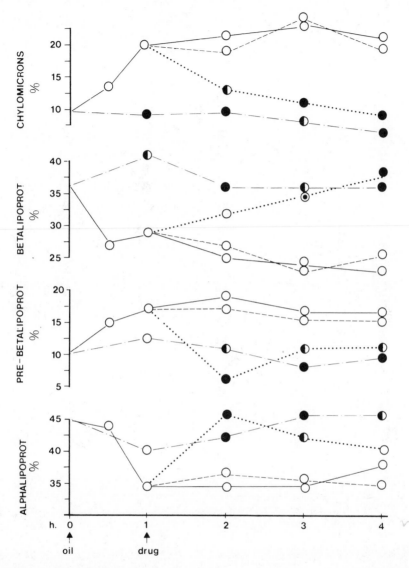

FIG. 2. Effect of L- and D-CAR, 500 mg/kg⁻¹ os, on serum lipoprotein pattern in rats loaded with olive oil, 30 ml/kg⁻¹ os, 1 hr before. *Dash/dot line,* Blank; *solid line,* control; *dotted line,* L-CAR; *dashed line,* D-CAR. *Dotted, half filled, and filled symbols, p = 0.05, 0.01, 0.001,* respectively. *N* = 10 in each group.

was significant after 1 hr. Simultaneously, the percentages of beta- and alpha-lipoproteins decreased. In rats treated with L-CAR, a significant decrease in chylomicrons and prebeta-lipoproteins was obtained; the effect was strongly evident 1 hr after drug administration and was likewise present until the fourth hour. At the same time, with the decrease of chylomicrons and prebeta fractions,

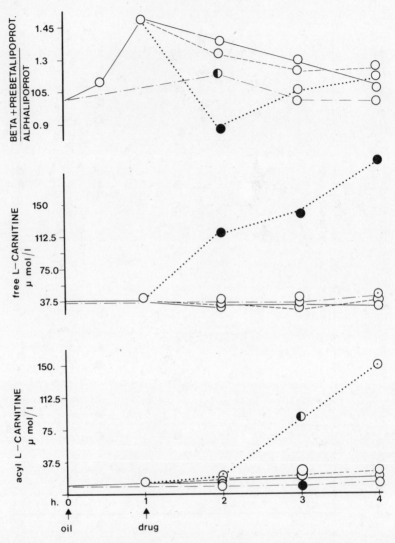

FIG. 3. Effect of L- and D-CAR, 500 mg/kg⁻¹ os, on beta- + prebeta-/alpha-lipoprotein ratio, free L-CAR and acyl L-CAR serum levels in rats loaded with olive oil, 30 ml/kg⁻¹ os, 1 hr before. *Dash/dot line,* blank; *solid line,* control; dotted line, L-CAR; *dashed line,* D-CAR. *Dotted, half filled, and filled symbols, $p = 0.05, 0.01, 0.001$, respectively. $N = 10$ in each group.*

an increase in the percentage of beta-lipoproteins as well as a remarkable increase in alpha-lipoproteins was evident. The lipoprotein pattern of L-CAR-treated rats was similar to the blank one. Also in this case, however, the unnatural dextroisomer form of CAR was completely devoid of activity.

The prebeta + beta-/alpha-lipoprotein ratio, reported in Fig. 3, shows that in L-CAR-treated rats, the ratio value was even lower than in normal animals.

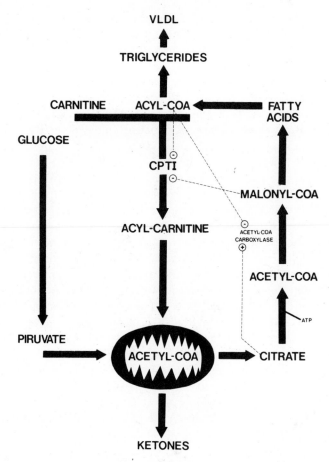

FIG. 4. Mc Garry Scheme, 1979. CPTI, palmitoyl CoA: CAR palmitoyl transferase.

This may indicate a real increase of alpha-lipoproteins because the decrease in prebeta is partially compensated for by the increase of the beta fraction.

As expected, the free L-CAR serum concentration in the control group gradually decreased to a statistically significant degree. On the other hand, plasma free L-CAR concentration increased in animals receiving exogenous L-CAR. Concomitantly, the short acyl-carnitines, the only ones considered in the present study, increased in their concentration in the treated animals slowly at first and then rapidly. Presumably, this is due to the exogenous L-CAR, since in control animals the increase in the short acyl-carnitines remained moderate throughout the experiment. The increase in free L-CAR serum levels occurred at the same time as the reduction of serum triglyceride, phospholipid, and cholesterol levels. At this time, 1 hr after oral drug administration, the acyl-CAR levels were not yet very high. As expected, D-CAR was completely ineffective.

On the basis of our results, which have been confirmed in patients fed parenterally with Intralipid® and treated with L-CAR, we propose some hypotheses.

Triglycerides, absorbed as monoglycerides and free fatty acids, can be utilized to resynthesize triglycerides at the microsomal level. Moreover, fatty acids can be oxidized through the mitochondrial beta-oxidative process. The acyl-CoA, which is the active form of free fatty acids, plays an important role in both the above mechanisms. In accordance with Mc Garry's interpretation (Fig. 4), if the acyl-CoA does not have a sufficient amount of L-CAR available, it becomes an inhibitor of the enzymatic system palmitoyl-CoA: CAR palmitoyl transferase (5). The acyl-CAR and the acyl-CoA formations, which occur, respectively, outside and inside the mitochondria, could both be blocked.

Hence in control animals, the microsomal acyl-CoA can be utilized prevalently for a resynthesis of triglycerides, giving rise to a parallel increase of chylomicrons, prebeta-lipoproteins, and so on. In treated animals, the availability of excess L-CAR facilitates the utilization of acyl-CoA in the mitochondrial beta-oxidative process, leading to a reduction in triglycerides and, consequently, triglyceride-rich lipoproteins. The effect of L-CAR on blood phospholipids and cholesterol can be interpreted as an indirect effect of the same mechanism of action.

More intricate is the interpretation of the L-CAR-induced increase of alpha-lipoprotein. It is difficult to ascribe such an increase to the known CAR action. It is tempting to speculate that L-CAR could also have an effect on blood lipoprotein-associated enzymes, particularly those involved in acyl transfer, i.e., lecitin cholesterol acyl transferase (LCAT).

Further research is needed to clarify this point; however, the unexpected increase of alpha-lipoproteins induced by L-CAR is relevant in relation to the importance of this event in decreasing the risk of vascular diseases.

ADKNOWLEDGMENT

We thank A. Arseni and P. Pessotto for their excellent technical assistance.

REFERENCES

1. Angelini, C. et al. (1976): Carnitine deficiency of skeletal muscle: Report of a treated case. *Neurology,* 26(7):633.
2. Bekaert, J., and Deltour, G. (1960): Effet de la carnitine sur l'hyperlipidémie diabétique. *Clin. Chim. Acta,* 5:177.
3. Bohmer, T. et al. (1978): Carnitine deficiency induced during intermittent haemodialysis for renal failure. *Lancet,* 1:126.
4. Friedman, S., and Fraenkel, G. (1955): Reversible enzymatic acetylation of carnitine. *Arch. Biochem. Biophys.,* 59:491.
5. Fritz, I. B. (1967): An hypothesis concerning the role of carnitine in the control of interrelations between fatty acid and carbohydrate metabolism. *Perspect. Physiol. Scand.,* 34:367.
6. Huth, P. J., Hall, P. V., and Shug, A. L. (1979): Stereospecificity and properties of carnitine transport in rat brain and kidney cortex slices. In: *FASEB "XIth International Congress of Biochemistry,"* Ottawa 1979.
7. Karpati, G. et al. (1975): The syndrome of systemic carnitine deficiency. *Neurology,* 25:16.

8. Konig, B. et al. (1978): Effect of a lipid load on blood and urinary carnitine in man. *Clin. Chim. Acta,* 88:121.
9. Maebashi, M. et al. (1978): Lipid lowering effect of carnitine in patients with type-IV hyperlipoproteinaemia. *Lancet,* 2:805.
10. Pola, P. et al. (1980): Carnitine in the therapy of dyslipidaemic patients. *Curr. Ther. Res.,* 27:(2)208.
11. Shug, A. L. et al. (1978): Changes in tissue levels of carnitine and other metabolites during myocardial ischemia and anoxia. *Arch. Biochem. Biophys.,* 187(1):25.

Diet and Drugs in Atherosclerosis,
edited by G. Noseda, B. Lewis, and R. Paoletti.
Raven Press, New York © 1980.

Objective Evaluation of the Compliance to Hypocholesterolemic Dietary Prescriptions

G. Ricci, F. Angelico, P. Amodeo, C. Borgogelli, *A. Cantafora, A. Montali, and S. Vergari

*Centro per la lotta alle malattie dismetaboliche e all'arteriosclerosi, Istituto di Terapia Medica Sistematica, Università di Roma, and *Istituto Superiore di Sanità, Rome, Italy*

The prescription of a diet low in saturated fats and cholesterol and rich in polyunsaturated fats (PUF) is the first step in the treatment of hypercholesterolemia. Persisting high cholesterol levels after prolonged dietary treatment suggest the advisability of a pharmacological approach.

In medical practice, however, it is often initiated without a careful evaluation of the results of dietary treatment. One reason for this is the difficulty encountered when establishing the level of adherence to dietary prescriptions, based mainly on subjective adherence ratings, which do not conform to truth.

To overcome these drawbacks, we have set up gas chromatographic analysis of both plasma and erythrocyte fatty acids, since changes in the fatty acid pattern represent an objective index of short- and medium-term modifications in dietary lipids (2,4,8).

Particular attention is paid to routine analysis of plasma fatty acid composition to monitor the short-term compliance of hypercholesterolemic outpatients at our center to diets varied in fatty acid composition. This technique enables the availability of objective data on changes in food consumption at each subsequent examination; where poor adherence is seen, the dietary message is changed accordingly or administered more incisively. Moreover, it is possible to identify with certainty the nonresponders, who are the only candidates for drug treatment.

The results of our investigation on a sample of outpatients at our center are reported.

MATERIAL AND METHODS

Our research was carried out in 30 dyslipidemic patients, ages 22 to 72 years (21 classified as type IIA, three as IIB, and six as IV), referred to our center since all previous dietary and pharmacological treatments had failed.

Fasting blood samples were drawn from all patients (at least 1 month after the previous drug treatment had been discontinued) for serum cholesterol, triglyceride, and lipoprotein determinations, as well as for both plasma and erythrocyte fatty acid analyses. High density lipoprotein (HDL)-cholesterol was also determined in a few subjects. A second blood collection was performed after 10 days. During this interval, a dietary investigation on weekly food consumption (expressed in terms of weight) was carried out. At second examination, a normocaloric, hypocholesterolemic diet, rich in PUF and low in saturated fats and cholesterol was prescribed (PUF diet), its fat content amounting to about 30%, the polyunsaturated/saturated (P/S) ratio being 3.4. Whole milk, butter, cheese, and olive oil were completely abolished, while a daily intake of 40 g sunflower oil was prescribed. Diets were calculated according to the food consumption tables of the National Institute for Nutrition (6).

The mean value of plasma and erythrocyte fatty acids, determined in another group of free living subjects (42 men and 48 women) aged 20 to 60 years, was taken as control parameter. This group was randomly selected from a sample of the general population living in the same Rome district, enrolled from the electoral register, and examined during the initial screening of a multifactorial, primary prevention trial of coronary heart disease (National Research Council, Special Project on Preventive Medicine, Atherosclerosis RF2) (5).

Plasma and erythrocyte fatty acid patterns were determined by gas chromatography by a previously described method (1). Cholesterol and triglyceride determinations were obtained according to Roeschlau et al. (9) and Eggstein (3), respectively. HDL-cholesterol was determined after precipitation with heparin/$MnCl_2$, as previously reported (7). Statistical evaluation of the results was obtained with the Student's t-test.

RESULTS AND DISCUSSION

The mean plasma and erythrocyte fatty acid composition showed very slight differences between the two groups (30 dyslipidemic patients and 90 free living subjects). Percentage values of polyunsaturated fatty acids were similar in both groups at entry, although dyslipidemic patients reported having been classified by their personal physicians as nonresponders. Since the fatty acid patterns were similar, the conclusion can be drawn that, in clinical practice, true nonresponders are quite rare; we are more often faced with a faulty or ignored dietary message. Confirming evidence is provided by the results of the dietary investigation through a 7-day food record, which showed a low P/S ratio (0.31 ± 0.11). During the PUF diet (P/S = 3.4), remarkable changes in plasma fatty acids were observed.

Figure 1 reports the results of a 60-day follow-up study of 18 dyslipidemic patients. The levels of miristic and palmitic acids (saturated) and palmitoleic and oleic acids (monounsaturated) dropped significantly, while linoleic acid levels remarkably increased, P/S and linoleic/oleic (L/O) ratios rising accordingly. (L/O ratio is considered the best index to evaluate fatty acid changes when administering a hypocholesterolemic diet.) At the same time, a striking mean

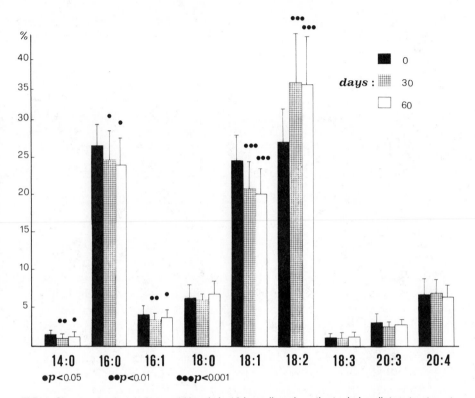

FIG. 1. Changes in plasma fatty acid levels in 18 hyperlipemic patients during dietary treatment.

reduction in total cholesterol and triglyceride levels was observed (Table 1).

In another group of 12 subjects (follow-up, 30 days) in whom HDL-cholesterol was also determined, noticeable changes in miristic and linoleic acids as well as in plasma L/O and P/S ratios were found as early as 15 days after starting the diet. No changes in HDL-cholesterol levels were noticed, whereas total cholesterol remarkably decreased. HDL-cholesterol/total cholesterol ratio (considered a far better index to estimate coronary risk) rose accordingly (Table 2).

Three main behaviors were identified by the simultaneous determination of plasma fatty acid and blood cholesterol modifications in the individual patients: (a) good adherence to the diet, with a significant increase in plasma L/O ratio and strongly reduced cholesterol levels; (b) good adherence to the diet, with a scanty reduction in cholesterol levels: we are faced with nonresponders, and drug treatment must be taken into consideration; and (c) poor adherence to dietary prescriptions, as shown by either an insufficient or an unsteady increase in plasma L/O ratio; a more penetrating dietary message must be administered to these subjects, who are too often defined as nonresponders.

ADHERENCE TO PUF DIET

TABLE 1. Changes in serum lipids and plasma fatty acids (expressed as L/O and P/S ratios) during dietary treatment in 18 hyperlipemic subjects[a]

	Days		
Serum lipid	0	30	60
Cholesterol (mg/dl) Δ %	288 ± 83.0	251 ± 64.5 −12.8%	248 ± 65.0 −13.8%
Triglycerides (mg/dl) Δ %	225 ± 135	133 ± 56.8[c] −40.8%	162 ± 132.8 −28%
Plasma L/O Δ %	1.14 ± 0.25	1.70 ± 0.60[d] +49%	1.79 ± 0.57[d] +57%
Plasma P/S Δ %	1.07 ± 0.25	1.30 ± 0.36[b] +21.4%	1.44 ± 0.37[d] +34.5

[a] Student's paired t-test.
[b] $p < 0.05$; [c] $p < 0.01$; [d] $p < 0.001$.

Table 2 shows the percentage distribution of these three different behaviors 60 days after starting the diet, good adherence meaning L/O values higher than 1.50 (mean value + SD in the control group). Furthermore, it is possible to identify two different ways of action: (a) subjects who are good responders during the first period of dietary treatment who subsequently slacken their adherence, and (b) subjects who are poor responders at the beginning who become good adherers after a prolonged time interval. This gives further support to the need for a correct and penetrating dietary message, repeatedly and constantly verified over time.

Figure 2 reports the behavior of three hypercholesterolemic patients on a PUF diet, whose follow-up lasted 150 days. In the first 2 months, the three subjects showed three different behaviors: good adherence, unresponsiveness, and poor compliance, respectively. After 60 days, patients 1 and 2 showed a gradually decreasing adherence.

Contrary to plasma fatty acids, erythrocyte fatty acids show significant changes only after the PUF diet has been observed for a prolonged period. In fact,

TABLE 2. Identification of the different behaviors 60 days after hypocholesterolemic dietary prescriptions

Classification	No.	%
Good adherers	7	38.9
Good adherers "resistant"	4	22.2
Poor adherers	7	38.9
Total	18	100

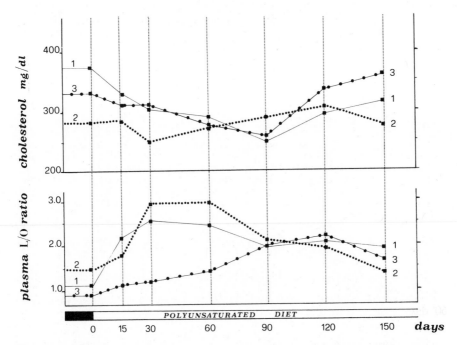

FIG. 2. Changes in serum cholesterol and plasma L/O ratio in three hypercholesterolemic patients during dietary treatment.

remarkable modifications have been noticed only 3 months after starting the diet. Erythrocyte fatty acid determination, therefore, is the best instrument to monitor long-term adherence.

SUMMARY

In summary, through the study of both plasma and erythrocyte fatty acid composition, we may obtain: (a) the objective evaluation of the subject's adherence to the PUF diet, as well as of the adequacy of changes in food consumption, at the very beginning of the dietary treatment; (b) the identification of poor and good responders; (c) the selection of true nonresponders, who are the only candidates for drug treatment; (d) the monitoring of changes in the degree of compliance; and (e) a good index of the mean adherence to a prolonged dietary treatment.

ACKNOWLEDGMENT

This work was supported in part by grant no. 78.00625.83 from the National Research Council.

REFERENCES

1. Angelico, F., Amodeo, P., Borgogelli, C., Cantafora, A., Montali, A., and Ricci, G. (1980): Red blood cell fatty acid composition in a sample of Italian middle-aged men on free diet. *Nutr. Metab. (in press).*
2. De Gennes, J. L., Truffert, J., and Lagarde, J. P. (1975): Contrôle en chromatographie en phase gazeuse du profil des acides gras en fonction de l'apport lipidique en graisses désaturées. In: *Proc. II Congreso Internacional sobre el valor biologico del aceite de oliva,* pp. 171–174.
3. Eggstein, M. (1966): Qualitative Bestimmung der Fettsäure—Ester im Blutserum. *Z. Klin. Chem.,* 4:12–21.
4. Farquhar, J. W., and Ahrens, E. H., Jr. (1963): Effects of dietary fats on human erythrocyte fatty acid pattern. *J. Clin. Invest.,* 42:675–686.
5. Menotti, A., Ricci, G., and Urbinati, G. C. (1979): Sui rapporti tra il Progetto Romano di Prevenzione della Cardiopatia Coronarica (PPCC) e la linea di ricerca RF2 del Subprogetto Aterosclerosi del Progetto Finalizzato "Medicina Preventiva" del C.N.R. *Giorn. Arterioscl.,* 2:155–166.
6. Ministero dell'Agricoltura e delle Foreste, Istituto Nazionale della Nutrizione (1978): *Tabelle di composizione degli alimenti.* I.N.N., Rome.
7. Morisi, G., Amodeo, P., Arca, M., Pacioni, F., Terzino, M., and Angelico, F. (1979): La determinazione del colesterolo-HDL; confronto tra metodiche. *Patol. Clin.,* 5:64–68.
8. Ricci, G., Amodeo, P., Arca, M., Borgogelli, C., Montali, A., Veggian, T., Vergari, S., and Angelico, F. (1980): Adherence to hypocholesterolemic dietary treatment. *Atherogenese* [Suppl. 3] *(in press).*
9. Roeschlau, J., Bernt, E., and Gruber, W. (1974): Enzymatische Bestimmung des gesamt Cholesterins im Serum. *Z. Klin. Chem. Klin. Biochem.,* 12:403–407.

Diet and Drugs in Atherosclerosis,
edited by G. Noseda, B. Lewis, and R. Paoletti.
Raven Press, New York © 1980.

Effect of Bran on Serum Lipoprotein and on Fecal Bile Acids and Neutral Sterols

Gianfranco Salvioli, Roberto Salati, and Ruggero Lugli

Institute of Clinical Medicine, University of Modena, 41100 Modena, Italy

Serum cholesterol is lower in people who have high intake of dietary fiber (29). Although some studies did not demonstrate any significant effect of the simple dietary fiber addition on lipid metabolism in man (24,28), others found a lowering effect on serum cholesterol (15,22) and triglycerides (13).

Wheat bran, the most widely consumed dietary fiber, has been found to be slightly effective as a hypocholesterolemic agent (30). These studies, however, were carried out using a limited intake of bran; therefore we studied the effects of short-term administration of high intakes of bran on cholesterol metabolism in man.

MATERIALS AND METHODS

Protocol

Eight subjects, three women and five men aged 48 to 56 years, neither suffering from metabolic or gastroenterological diseases nor receiving drugs, were fed for 40 days with a constant, eucaloric diet (35 cal/kg) containing 0.8 g cholesterol and 0.5 g Cr_2O_3 as a marker for quantitative daily fecal sterol excretion. The diets were prepared from conventional foods. Caloric intake was composed as follows: carbohydrates, 50%; protein, 20%; and lipids, 30%. After 10 days three stool and three fasting plasma samples were collected. Subsequently, 60 g bran, containing 8% crude fiber, was added in three daily doses to the diet. After 30 days, the three stool and plasma samples were repeated.

Chemical Methods

Lipoproteins [very low density lipoprotein (VLDL), low density lipoprotein (LDL), and high density lipoprotein (HDL)] were separated using rotor 50 in a Spinco L 50 Ultracentrifuge and the precipitation of LDL with heparin and manganese chloride. Lipids (cholesterol and triglycerides) of total serum and of each lipoprotein fraction were determined at the same time using enzymatic methods. Collected fecal samples were weighed and kept at −20°C until analyzed. An aliquot of each fecal sample was hydrolyzed in order to separate the neutral sterols from bile acids, according to Miettinen et al. (20). Neutral sterols (cholesterol and its bacterial degradation products coprostanol and co-prostanone) were evaluated by gas liquid chromatography (GLC) after separation on thin layer chromatography. Total bile acids were measured after solvolysis by an enzymatic method (27), and bile acid patterns were determined by GLC (25). Fecal outputs of sterols have been corrected calculating the recovery of Cr_2O_3. The absorption of dietary cholesterol was measured in only six subjects using the radioisotope method (26), before and after 30 days of bran administration. Statistical comparison of the data from the two diet periods was done by the paired t-test.

RESULTS

Serum Lipids

After bran administration, the mean serum cholesterol levels fell from 199 to 160 mg/dl ($p < 0.02$) and the serum triglycerides from 150 to 126 mg/dl (NS) (Table 1). The lipid composition of lipoproteins is reported in Table 1. Significant changes are present only in the LDL fraction, where cholesterol decreased from 132.8 to 101.7 mg/dl. No significant changes were present in VLDL and HDL fractions.

Fecal Sterols

Neutral sterol loss increased from 876.6 to 1,092.0 mg/day, and the percentage of coprostanol plus coprostanone decreased from 72 to 54% (Table 2). Bile acid excretion increased significantly from 226.6 to 308.4 mg/day, whereas the percentage of deoxycholic acid decreased significantly.

During the 40 days, there were no changes in the subjects' weights. At the beginning of the study, defecation frequency was 7 to 9 in the first 10 days, and the average fecal weight was 96.2 ± 36.3 g/day; bowel frequency rose to 11 to 14 in the last 10-day period of bran administration, and the fecal weight increased to 216.8 ± 56.4 g/day.

The absorption of exogenous cholesterol decreased from 46.11 ± 3.29% to 40.96 ± 3.48% ($p < 0.01$) during the bran-rich diet. The values are within the normal range for our laboratory.

DISCUSSION

This study shows that a high dietary intake of bran increases daily fecal bile acid and neutral sterol output and decreases the total and LDL-cholesterol.

Serum Lipids

The effects of the addition of bran to the diet on serum lipids have been largely negative (30), but some authors found a decrease in serum cholesterol

TABLE 1. Changes of serum lipids and lipoproteins during bran administration[a]

Values	Plasma		VLDL		LDL		HDL
	C[b]	TG	C	TG	C	TG	(C)
Basal values	199.3 ± 18.6	150.7 ± 23.1	22.4 ± 4.1	78.2 ± 17.5	132.8 ± 18.9	35.1 ± 10.2	44.2 ± 5.2
After bran	160.1 ± 14.2[c]	126.7 ± 20.2[e]	16.0 ± 3.8[e]	58.8 ± 16.9[e]	101.7 ± 12.6[d]	36.2 ± 9.8[e]	46.6 ± 4.4[e]

[a] Results are given as the mean (mg/100 ml) ± SEM.
[b] C, cholesterol; TG, triglycerides.
[c] $p < 0.02$; [d] $p < 0.01$; [e] NS.

TABLE 2. Fecal outputs of neutral and acidic sterols during bran administration[a]

	Bile acids						Neutral sterols			
		Molar %						Molar %		
	mg/day	LCA[b]	DCA	CDCA	CA	Others	mg/day	C	CL	CN
Basal values	226.6 ± 41.8	52.7	36.4	3.1	1.9	5.5	876.6 ± 212.0	27.4	61.3	11.1
After bran	308.4 ± 32.6[d]	46.1	20.2[c]	8.6[c]	6.7[c]	18.0	1092.0 ± 128.4[e]	44.6[c]	46.8	8.4

[a] Mean values and SEM of eight subjects.
[b] C, cholesterol; CL, coprostanol; CN, coprostanone; LCA, lithocholic acid; DCA, deoxycholic acid; CDCA, chenodeoxycholic acid; CA, cholic acid.
[c] $p < 0.01$; [d] $p < 0.02$; [e] $p < 0.05$.

(4) and triglyceride (13) levels. The effect is more evident using other dietary fiber sources (7,16,17,21). In our study, by adding 5 g/day crude fiber to the diet, the total and LDL-cholesterol significantly decreased, probably because of the well-known increased fecal excretion of cholesterol and bile acids (3,23). Thus the reduction of serum cholesterol may depend on a mechanism similar to that described for bile acid sequestring resin as cholestyramine (10). Some studies demonstrated the binding capacity of dietary fibers, and even of bran, for cholesterol (31) and bile acids (8). In our subjects, the intestinal absorption of cholesterol was slightly reduced when bran was fed, whereas rats receiving bran showed a reduction of cholesterol absorption at a level of about 65% of controls (31). Whereas total and VLDL-triglycerides are frequently increased by cholestyramine administration (33), they are decreased by a bran-rich diet.

Fecal Sterol Loss

Normally, primary bile acids (cholic and chenodeoxycholic acids) are transformed by the intestinal flora in secondary bile acids (deoxycholic and lithocholic acids, respectively) (19). Hill and Aries (14) demonstrated that dietary fiber reduced bacterial conversion of primary bile acid. Others (6), however, found no changes of the intestinal flora during high fiber intake. It is known that a part of fecal bile acids is in a nondialyzable form because of their binding to fiber (11). The observed high fecal bile acid loss during bran feeding may be attributed to binding of bile acid to dietary fibers in such a way that both the intestinal absorption and the enzymatic activity of intestinal flora are avoided (2,23); in fact, the fecal bile acid pattern changes during a bran-rich diet because the secondary bile acids decrease in feces and in bile (23,32). Even in vegetarians, the deoxycholic acid pool size was smaller than in controls (23).

In man, intestinal bacteria transform cholesterol into poorly absorbed coprostanol and coprostanone (9). Bran administration reduces the percentage of these compounds in feces; but this change cannot determine the observed increased excretion of neutral sterols. In fact, germ-free rats, which do not have coprostanol in feces, excreted less fecal sterols than conventional rats (18). Reduction of cholesterol absorption could cause the high sterol excretion, even though the percentage of absorption decreased slightly in our subjects receiving bran.

CONCLUSION

The binding of sterols and bile acids to bran enhances excretion of cholesterol from the body and reduces serum cholesterol levels. Intestinal mucosa could play a key role in determining the changes of lipid metabolism during fiber intake. When intestinal mucosa are bypassed, both cholesterol and triglycerides in serum decrease greatly (5). In subjects ingesting fibers, there are some changes, such as reduction of postprandial hyperglycemia (11,15), increased daily fat excretion (1), and reduced postprandial chylomicronemia (1) which may depend on a reduced diffusion rate toward absorptive mucosal surface. Delayed intestinal absorption modifies energy intake (12) and may determine cholesterol metabolism changes during bran administration.

REFERENCES

1. Anderson, J. W., and Lin, W. J. (1979): *Am. J. Clin. Nutr.,* 32:346–363.
2. Birkner, H. J., and Kern, F., Jr. (1974): *Gastroenterology,* 67:237–244.
3. Cummings, J. H., Hill, M. J., Jenkins, D. H. A., Pearson, J. R., and Wiggins, H. S. (1976): *Am. J. Clin. Nutr.,* 29:1468–1473.
4. De Groot, A. P., Luyken, R., and Pikaar, N. A. (1963): *Lancet,* 2:303–304.
5. DenBesten, L., Reyna, R. H., Connor, W. E., and Stegink, L. D. (1973): *J. Clin. Invest.,* 52:1384–1398.
6. Drasar, B. S., Jenkins, D. J. A., and Cummings, J. H. (1976): *J. Med. Microbiol.,* 9:423–431.
7. Durringtòn, P. N., Manning, A. P., Bolton, C. H., Hartog, M. (1976): *Lancet,* 2:394–396.
8. Eastwood, M. A., and Hamilton, D. (1968): *Biochim. Biophys. Acta,* 152:165–173.
9. Eyssen, H., and Parmentier, G. (1974): *Am. J. Clin. Nutr.,* 27:1329–1340.
10. Grundy, S. M., Ahrens, E. H., and Salen, G. (1971): *J. Lab. Clin. Med.,* 78:94–121.
11. Gustafson, B. E., and Norman, A. (1968): *Scand. J. Gastroent.,* 3:625–631.
12. Heaton, K. W. (1973): *Lancet,* 2:1418–1421.
13. Heaton, K. W., and Pomare, E. W. (1974): *Lancet,* 1:49–50.
14. Hill, M. J., Aries, V. C. (1971): *J. Pathol.,* 104:129–139.
15. Jenkins, D. J. A., Hill, M. S., and Cummings, J. H. (1975): *Am. J. Clin. Nutr.,* 28:1408–1411.
16. Jenkins, D. J. A. (1978): In: *International Conference on Atherosclerosis,* edited by L. A. Carlson, R. Paoletti, C. R. Sirtori, and G. Weber, pp. 173–182, Raven Press, New York.
17. Jenkins, D. J. A., Leeds, A. R., Slavin, B., Mann, J., and Jepson, E. M. (1979): *Am. J. Clin. Nutr.,* 32:16–18.
18. Kellog, T. F., Knight, P. L., Wostmann, B. S. (1970): *J. Lipid Res.,* 11:362–366.
19. Midvedt, T. (1974): *Am. J. Clin. Nutr.,* 27:1341–1347.
20. Miettinen, T. A., Ahrens, E. H., and Grundy, S. M. (1965): *J. Lipid Res.,* 6:411–423.
21. Miettinen, T. A., and Tarpila, S. (1977): *Gut,* 19:137–145.
22. Persson, I., Raby, K., Founs-Bech, P., and Jensen, E. (1975): *Lancet,* 2:1209.
23. Pomare, E. W., and Heaton, K. W. (1973): *Br. Med. J.,* 4:262–264.
24. Raymond, T. L., Connor, W. E., Lin, D. S., Warner, S., Fry, M. M., and Connor, S. L. (1977): *J. Clin. Invest.,* 60:1429–1437.
25. Salvioli, G., Salati, R., Lugli, R., and Baldelli, M. V. (1974): *Il Fegato,* 20:77–88.
26. Samuel, P., Crouse, J. R., and Ahrens, E. H., Jr. (1979): *J. Lipid Res.,* 19:82–93.
27. Steensland, H. (1978): *Scand. J. Clin. Lab. Invest.,* 28:447–455.
28. Tarpila, S., Miettinen, T. A., and Metsäranta, L. (1978): *Gut,* 19:137–145.
29. Trowell, H. (1976): *Am. J. Clin. Nutr.,* 29:417–427.
30. Truswell, A. S., and Kay, R. M. (1976): *Lancet,* 1:367.
31. Vahouny, G. V., Roy, T., Gallo, L. L., Story, J. A., Kritchevsky, D., Cassidy, M., Grund, B. M., and Treadwell, C. R. (1978): *Am. J. Clin. Nutr.,* 21:208S–212S.
32. Watts, J. McK., Jablonski, P., and Touuli, J. (1978): *Surgery,* 135:321–324.
33. Witzum, J. L., Schoenfeld, G., and Weidman, S. W. (1976): *J. Lab. Clin. Med.,* 88:1008–1018.

Diet and Drugs in Atherosclerosis,
edited by G. Noseda, B. Lewis, and R. Paoletti.
Raven Press, New York © 1980.

Diet Analysis With an Automatic Computerized System

P. G. Da Col, G. Cappello, L. Cattin, M. Fonda, and P. Čok

Institute of Medical Clinic, University of Trieste, Trieste, Italy

The nutritional conditions of a population are assessed by measuring the amounts of calories and nutrients provided by the diet. Evidence provides a considerable degree of certainty that nutrition is closely related to the maintenance of a healthy state and to the prevention of many degenerative diseases, particularly atherosclerosis (7,10,16). It is hoped that information will now be forthcoming on the importance of the basic nutrients (amino acids, fatty acids, fiber), which can modify, positively or negatively, some metabolic pathways (3,8,9,11).

Clinicians and epidemiologists (14) have long had a special concern for the method of collecting data for dietary practice. Generally, the available tools for collecting data are diet history and special diet assistance. Diet history is inaccurate because memory often fails to indicate important details about the whole daily food intake. Another important source of error rises from the relatively vague amount of consumed food. Moreover, this method refers to "simple food," i.e., bread, milk, meat, and rice, and not to the cooking, preparation, and amount of ingredients. This is in contrast to the prevailing habit to eat elaborate, appetizing, and rich dishes. The problem in dietetic specialized assistance is the presence at home of a dietician over a long period of time. The next step in a nutritional assessment involves the dietetic analysis of the collected data. Generally, it is necessary to consult the food composition tables. Despite time and efforts employed, the results may be biased in regard to missing data or to contradictory information given in the tables. Finally, from the latter, the average nutritive value of a diet is calculated and expressed in the traditional way.

We present the preliminary results of a test carried out in order to verify the feasibility of a computerized dietetic analysis using an automatic computerized system for meal planning, which includes data records performed memorizing some food composition tables (1,2,4–6,12,13,15) and the data management system, and a new system for obtaining information about people's diet habits, that is, a personal diet journal. These memorized food composition tables, the "library," provide great advantages: (a) to fill a gap connected with the use of

TABLE 1. *Diet journal*

Date _____ Hour	Dishes	Sleep hours _____ Quantity	Homemade
7	Breakfast with biscuits	1 Portion	Yes
	Tea with sugar	1 Cup	Yes
13	Vegetable soup	1 Plate	Yes
	Grilled beef	1	Yes
	Carrots and salad	1 Plate	Yes
	Apple	1	
20	Rice with butter	1 Plate	Yes
	Fried eggs	2	Yes
	Cauliflower	1 Portion	Yes
	Strudel	1 Portion	Yes
	Orangeade Fanta	1	
	Coca Cola	1	
	Bar of chocolate	1	
	Bread	1	

a single table; thus average nutritive value for every item may be calculated; (b) a complete and homogeneous data set is available.

The nutrients taken into consideration are proteins, lipids, carbohydrates, fiber, mineral salts, vitamins, 12 amino acids, fatty acids, cholesterol, alcohol, and caloric equivalent. The control system of this library is able to define dishes, which, according to the nutrients of their ingredients, are codified in terms of "simple" foods, in order to analyze similarly the total food intake, illustrated by the journal. The so-called output of the program provides: (a) the definition of the dishes through a single component, and (b) daily nutritional balance, referring to the same parameters.

During an epidemiological study carried out on a sample of healthy, young women, we tried to apply a personal diet "journal," consisting of two parts. First, every subject is asked carefully to record, at least once a day, the whole daily food intake, expressed in terms of weights, units, or other domestic units of measure, e.g., one bowl of vegetable soup, one bottle of Coca Cola (Table 1). Second, the subject is asked to meticulously specify the recipes, listing the ingredients and indicating how many people the particular recipe serves (Table 2). In this second part, only weights or standardized domestic units of measure were used. Before beginning the study, each subject was trained to fill the journal and to use standardized domestic units of measure. We stressed taking notice of the entire daily food intake, including that consumed between meals. When food was not homemade, we referred to standardized recipes, according to the common literature and the information given by the same subjects. Finally, every schedule was reexamined with the subject to assess whether it was reliable. The interval to be recorded was 8 days, too short for concluding anything precise about real diet habits but enough to test our method.

TABLE 2. *Diet journal: Composition of dishes*

Breakfast with biscuits		Vegetable soup	
Portion 1, composition: Quantity of food		Portion 4, composition: Quantity of food	
Biscuits	50 g	Potatoes	320 g
Refined sugar	15 g	Carrots	120 g
Apricot jam	50 g	Courgettes	120 g
Tea	1 cup	Onions	40 g
		Cauliflower	120 g
		Celery	60 g
		Olive oil	60 g
		Butter	8 g
		Parmesan	60 g
		Soup cube	8 g
		Maize flour	60 g
		Water	2 liters

An example of the results of a diet analysis is shown in Table 3, which concerns a nutrient analysis of some dishes mentioned in the journal. Applying the same procedure to all dishes mentioned in the daily journal, a diet analysis of 1 day is performed and the caloric intake calculated (Table 4).

In conclusion, the analysis carried out by keeping records of food intake (diet journal) represents progress in comparison to diet history. It gives more information more precisely. The experiment proposed with a dietician in each home could be the best, but it is too expensive if adapted on a large scale. The computerized library gives more complete and homogeneous results.

Looking to the future, it would be helpful to plan a daily meal pattern with the average requirements to meet individual needs and especially the personal

TABLE 3. *Nutrient analysis: Vegetable soup*[a]

Proteins	18.3 g	Niacin	2.9 mg	Tryptophan	7.9[b]
Lipids	21.3 g	Ascorbic acid	49.9 mg	Valine	35.5[b]
Carbohydrate	32.3 g	Retinol	1,107 mg	Argynine	23.5[b]
Fiber	1.4 g	Isoleucine	32.4[b]	Histidine	14.9[b]
N_a	170.7 mg	Leucine	47.6[b]	Oleic acid	9.1
K	680.9 mg	Lysine	33.7[b]		
P	218.5 mg	Methionine	12.2[b]		
C_a	215.6 mg	Cysteine	5.5[b]		
F_e	1,509 μg	Phenylalanine	28.9[b]	Cholesterol	19.3 mg
Thiamine	224.5 μg	Tyrosine	19.5[b]	kcal	386
Riboflavin	452.6 μg	Threonine	20.4[b]		

[a] 1 portion.
[b] mg/g protein.

TABLE 4. Diet analysis, 8 days[a]

Protein	69.3 g	Niacin	13 mg	Tryptophan	723[b]
Lipid	106.9 g	Ascorbic acid	149 mg	Valine	3,507[b]
Carbohydrate	181.8 g	Retinol	3,330 mg	Arginine	3,111[b]
Fiber	3.5 g	Isoleucine	3,217[b]	Histidine	1,667[b]
Na	900 mg	Leucine	4,809[b]	Oleic acid	42 g
K	1,945 mg	Lysine	4,068[b]	Linoleic A.	19 g
P	900 mg	Methionine	1,452[b]	Cholesterol	439 mg
Ca	931 mg	Cysteine	755[b]	Sat. fat	45 g
Fe	16,680 µg	Phenylalanine	3,069[b]		
Thiamine	1,164 µg	Tyrosine	1,873[b]		
Riboflavin	2,948 µg	Threonine	2,398[b]	kcal	1,927

[a] Mean values for 1 day. Percentage of total kcal: protein, 262 (13.6%); lipid, 941 (48.8%); carbohydrate, 724 (37.6%).
[b] mg/total protein.

agreement of feasible and acceptable dishes, instead of the traditional single dietary components.

ACKNOWLEDGMENTS

The authors are indebted to Prof. Benedetto de Bernard and Mr. Oriano Radillo of the Institute of Biochemistry, University of Trieste, for their computer assistance.

REFERENCES

1. Altman, P. L., and Dittmer, D. S. (editors) (1968): *Metabolism.* Federation of American Societies for Experimental Biology, Bethesda, Maryland.
2. Carnovale, E., and Miuccio, F. C. (editors) (1976): *Tabelle di Composizione degli Alimenti.* Istituto Nazionale della Nutrizione, Rome.
3. Crawford, M. D., Gardner, M. J., and Morris, J. N. (1971): Changes in water hardness and local death rates. *Lancet,* II:327–329.
4. FAO Nutritional Studies (1970): *Amino Acid Content of Foods and Biological Data on Proteins.* Food and Agriculture Organization of the United Nations, Rome.
5. Feeley, R. M., Criner, P. E., and Watt, B. K. (1972): Cholesterol content of foods. *J. Am. Diet. Assoc.,* 61:134–149.
6. Fidanza, M. (1974): *Tabelle di Composizione degli Alimenti.* Institute of Food Science, University of Perugia, Perugia.
7. Glueck, C. J., Mattson, F., and Bierman, E. L. (1978): Diet and coronary heart disease. Another view. *N. Engl. J. Med.,* 298:1471–1474.
8. Heaton, K. W. (1973): Food fibre as an obstacle to energy intake. *Lancet,* II:1418–1421.
9. Jakubowsky, J. A., and Ardlie, N. G. (1978): Modification of human platelet function by a diet enriched in saturated or polyunsaturated fat. *Atherosclerosis,* 31:335–344.
10. Kannel, W. R., McGee, D., and Gordon, T. (1976): A general cardiovascular risk profile: The Framingham study. *Am. J. Cardiol.,* 38:46–51.
11. Mattson, F. H., Hollembach, E. J., and Kligman, A. M. (1975): Effect of hydrogenated fat on the plasma cholesterol and triglycerides levels of men. *Am. J. Clin. Nutr.,* 28:726–731.
12. Randoin, L., Le Gallic, P., Dupois, Y., Bernardin, A., Duchene, L., and Brun, P. (1961): *Tables de Composition des Aliments,* third edition, edited by J. Lanore. Institut Scientifique d'Hygiène Alimentaire, Centre National de la Recherche Scientifique, Paris.

13. Souci, S. W., Fachman, W., and Kraut, H. (1979): *Die Zusammensetzung der Lebensmittel. Naehrwerttabellen.* Wissenschaftliche Verlaggesellschaft, Stuttgart.
14. Walker, W. S. (1977): Changing United States life-style and declining vascular mortality: Cause or coincidence? *N. Engl. J. Med.,* 297:163–165.
15. Watt, B. K., and Merril, A. L. (1963): *Composition of Foods. Raw-Processed-Prepared.* Agriculture Handbook No. 8, Consumer and Food Economics Research Division, Agriculture Research Service, United States Department of Agriculture. Washington, D.C.
16. Wynder, L., and Reddy, B. S. (1975): Dietary fat and colon cancer. *J. Natl. Cancer Inst.,* 54:7–10.

Diet and Drugs in Atherosclerosis,
edited by G. Noseda, B. Lewis, and R. Paoletti.
Raven Press, New York © 1980.

Effect of Whey Feeding on Serum Lipids in Swine

H. B. Stähelin, A. Oberhänsli, M. Wanner, M. Jost, H. Schneeberger, and G. Ritzel

Geriatric Clinic Kantonsspital Basel, Swiss Federal Research Station for Animal Production Grangeneuve, Unit of Social and Preventive Medicine, University of Basel, Switzerland

In a survey of 4,500 volunteers in Basel in 1975 (11), we found high milk consumption to be correlated with low serum lipids. Mann (7) and Howard and Marks (5,8) reported a hypocholesterolemic effect of yogurt and milk in human volunteers. This hypocholesterolemic action was attributed to a number of different factors present in milk or milk products, such as calcium, orotic acid, beta-hydroxymethylglutarate, or lactose (10). These findings aroused much interest, since it was generally assumed that saturated fatty acids, as found in milk or butter, increase cholesterol.

To evaluate the effect of lactose, we studied the effect of whey in a preliminary study in human volunteers in whom we could observe a hypocholesterolemic trend under 100 g/day whey powder (14). Larger amounts of whey, however, are not easily tolerated by humans. The swine are routinely fed whey during rearing. The close physicochemical resemblance of porcine lipoproteins (2) to human lipoproteins renders swine an ideal test animal to study the effect of whey or other milk products on serum lipids. We thus investigated the effect of large quantities of whey in swine on their growth and serum lipids.

METHODS

Swine (20 to 25 kg) of both sexes were randomly allocated to two groups. The total group of animals consisted of six blocks of four litters each. Randomization was already achieved at the level of the litters in order to minimize genetic differences. The rearing was divided into five different food periods (Fig. 1). During period I, all animals received a control diet (Table 1). During period II, the animals of group A were fed a diet containing 50% dried whey (by weight) corresponding to 56 cal %. The available energy was equal in the control and experimental diets. One week was allowed for the change from control diet to whey. After 4 weeks, group B was switched to the whey feeding for 4 weeks (period III), and group A served as control. The same procedure was repeated for A and B, respectively, in period IV for 2 weeks. In the fifth period, all animals were on the control diet for 1 week. Growth was checked weekly,

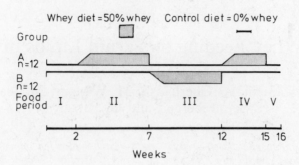

FIG. 1. Study design. Random allocation of 24 swine to two groups. Rearing period of swine (starting weight, 20 to 25 kg) divided into five feeding periods containing whey (50%) or control (0% whey) diets.

TABLE 1. *Feed composition*[a]

Feed	Diet (% weight)	
	Whey	Control
Whey powder	50	—
Barley	32.4	82.0
Corn	6.6	—
Soya (fat free)	6.4	6.4
Fish meal	3.0	3.0
Animal fat	—	4.5

[a] Minerals, amino acids, trace elements, and vitamins.

and venous blood was obtained by punctures of the jugular vein. Serum was separated and frozen. All samples were analyzed for cholesterol and triglycerides by standard enzymatic methods (15). HDL cholesterol was analyzed following the precipitation of VLDL and LDL by Mn^{2+} Cl_2 and heparin. Lipoprotein electrophoresis was performed using agarose gel and measuring the relative lipoprotein distribution by densitometry (15).

RESULTS

All 24 animals completed the rearing period. Growth was identical in both groups. Despite the large amount of whey fed, there were no serious gastrointestinal problems; however, an assimilation period of 1 week was necessary.

Whey feeding caused a significant drop in serum cholesterol in group A during period II ($p < 0.01$), averaging 20% and in group B by 20% during period III ($p < 0.02$). During the last two weeks of whey feeding (period IV), group

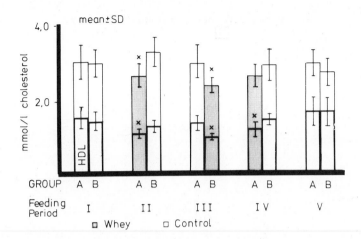

FIG. 2. Effect of whey on total cholesterol and HDL cholesterol in swine. Mean cholesterol and HDL cholesterol concentration in group A (*N* = 12) and group B (*N* = 12) is shown during the different feeding periods. For duration of feeding period, see Fig. 1; for *p* values (x), see Table 2.

A animals again showed a small drop in total cholesterol (Fig. 2). HDL cholesterol was significantly ($p < 0.01$) lowered by whey feeding in all feeding periods (Table 2; Fig. 2). The effect was more pronounced in periods III and IV than in period II. There was no difference between HDL cholesterol in groups A and B at the end of period II. Triglyceride concentration tended to be lower during whey feeding (Table 2); the difference is significant only in period IV. Group B animals had unusually high triglycerides, which regressed to normal values while they were still on the control diet.

Analysis of lipoprotein electrophoresis confirmed the results of the determination of the lipid fractions. The chylomicrons were more prevalent in animals fed the control diet, whereas in whey-fed animals, the beta-lipoproteins were slightly more prevalent. Differences were not statistically significant.

DISCUSSION

Animals fed the control diet showed regularly higher total cholesterol and HDL cholesterol than animals fed whey. The possibility of extraneous effects other than those produced by the diet is excluded, due to the careful randomization and crossover design of the experiment. Of some concern is the question of whether the small amount of fat (mainly animal fat) in the control diet could account for the observed differences. The slightly higher chylomicron concentration in control animals suggests an influence of fat ingested. The reduction in total cholesterol and HDL cholesterol by 20% is probably not attributable to the small difference of fat content in the food. However, it might be important

TABLE 2. Serum lipids in group A and group B[a] in different feeding periods

Food period	Total cholesterol (mmoles/liter)		HDL cholesterol (mmoles/liter)		Triglycerides (mmoles/liter)	
	A	B	A	B	A	B
I (Control)	3.00 ± 0.49	2.96 ± 0.38	1.54 ± 0.34	1.39 ± 0.24	0.54 ± 0.34	0.54 ± 0.29
II (A Whey)	2.62 ± 0.35[c]	3.27 ± 0.40	1.10 ± 0.11[c]	1.29 ± 0.16	0.33 ± 0.13	0.44 ± 0.26
III (B Whey)	2.96 ± 0.45	2.37 ± 0.21[b]	1.36 ± 0.22	0.97 ± 0.09[c]	0.46 ± 0.27	0.37 ± 0.17[a]
IV (A Whey)	2.61 ± 0.31	2.87 ± 0.42	1.2 ± 0.22[c]	1.46 ± 0.16	0.36 ± 0.14	0.61 ± 0.25[a]
V (Control)	2.94 ± 0.33	2.73 ± 0.38	1.68 ± 0.46	1.68 ± 0.40	0.44 ± 0.19	0.40 ± 0.21[a]

[a] N = 12 in each group.
[b] $p < 0.02$; [c] $p < 0.01$; [d] significant differences in group B between periods III and IV and IV and V but not III and V.

to investigate the effect of small amounts of saturated fat in HDL concentration, since it is known that large quantities of polyunsaturated fatty acids lower HDL cholesterol as well as total cholesterol (12). On the other hand, fat increased LDL as well as total cholesterol in swine (3) and probably stimulates hepatic lipid synthesis.

Nevertheless, the addition of whey appears to be of great influence in lowering total cholesterol and HDL cholesterol without ruling out the possible effect of food fat. Whey consists mainly of lactose (75%), protein (10%), and fat (1%), as well as a number of minerals. Calcium, which was also implicated (4), was of equal concentration in both diets. The amount of soya product fed was equal in both groups, excluding an effect of soya proteins on serum lipids (13). Milk and milk products contain a factor with a hypocholesterolemic action, possibly lactose, since the hypocholesterolemic effect is preserved in whey. There is some evidence that milk, orotic acid, and beta-hydroxymethylglutarate lower lipids by interfering with hepatic cholesterol synthesis (1,6,9). These observations were obtained in rats, in which HDL cholesterol represents the main fraction. In swine, whey apparently lowers not only the HDL cholesterol but also LDL cholesterol. It remains to be shown whether the observed effect on hepatic cholesterol synthesis is responsible for the lipid-lowering effect of the milk factor. Further work is needed to delineate the lipid-lowering mode of action of the implicated agents.

Our experiments emphasize the fact that the carbohydrate constituents in nutrition must receive more attention with respect to possible effects on lipid and lipoprotein metabolism. Long-term effects on serum lipids must be investigated under different experimental conditions; and studies are needed to determine whether the effects on lipid metabolism are relevant in atherogenesis.

SUMMARY

The hypocholesterolemic effect of milk was studied in swine by feeding large amounts of whey. Animals were randomly allocated to group A or B. After a 2-week control period, group A (N-12) was fed whey (50%) for 4 weeks. Group B (N-12), in a crossover study, received whey thereafter. All animals completed the study. Growth was identical in both groups over the total observation period. Whey diet reduced total cholesterol by 20% (2.62 ± 0.35 in whey-fed A versus 3.27 ± 0.40 mmoles/liter in B, $p < 0.01$; and 2.37 ± 0.21 in whey-fed B versus 2.96 ± 0.45 in control diet-fed A). HDL cholesterol was reduced by whey feeding in all food periods by 20.4%. Triglycerides were lowered to a smaller extent (not significant). It is suggested that the hypocholesterolemic milk factor is present in whey. This factor appears to reduce LDL as well as HDL cholesterol to a similar degree.

REFERENCES

1. Ahmed, A. A., McCarthy, R. D., and Porter, G. A. (1979): Effect of milk constituents on hepatic cholesterol genesis. *Atherosclerosis*, 32:347–357.

2. Chapman, M. J., and Goldstein, S. (1976): Comparison of the serum low density lipoprotein and of its apoprotein in the pig, rhesus monkey and baboon with that in man. *Atherosclerosis,* 25:267–291.
3. Chase, H. P., and Morris, T. (1976): Cholesterol metabolism following portacaval shunt in the pig. *Atherosclerosis,* 24:141–148.
4. Howard, A. N. (1977): The Masai, milk and the yogurt factor: an alternative explanation. *Atherosclerosis,* 27:383–385.
5. Howard, A. N., and Marks, J. (1978): Hypocholesterolemic effect on milk. *Lancet,* 2:255.
6. Kritchevsky, D., Tepper, S. A., Morrisey, R. B., Czarnecki, S. K., and Klurfeld, D. M. (1979): Influence of whole or skim milk on cholesterol metabolism in rats. *Am. J. Clin. Nutr.,* 32:597–600.
7. Mann, G. (1977): A factor in yogurt which lowers cholesterolemia in man. *Atherosclerosis,* 26:335–340.
8. Marks, J., and Howard, A. N. (1977): Hypocholesterolemic effect of milk. *Lancet,* 2:763.
9. Nair, C. R., and Mann, G. V. (1977): A factor in milk which influences cholesterolemia in rats. *Atherosclerosis,* 26:363–367.
10. Richardson, T. (1978): The hypocholesterolemic effect of milk—a review. *J. Food Protect.,* 41:226–235.
11. Ritzel, G. (1975): Evaluation von Ernährungserhebungen in Rahmen der Basler Studie III. In: *Zur Ernährungssituation der schweizerischen Bevölkerung,* edited by G. Brubacher and G. Ritzel, pp. 57–82. Huber, Bern.
12. Shepherd, J., Packard, C. J., Patsch, J. R., Gotto, A. M., Jr., and Taunton, O. D. (1978): Effects of dietary polyunsaturated and saturated fat on the properties of high density lipoproteins and the metabolism of apolipoprotein A-I. *J. Clin. Invest.,* 61:1582–1592.
13. Sirtori, C., Agradi, E., Conti, F., Matero, O., and Gatti, E. (1977): Soyabean-protein diet in the treatment of type II hyperlipoproteinemia. *Lancet,* 1:275–277.
14. Stähelin, H. B., and Ritzel, G. (1979): Effect of whey on plasma lipids. *Int. J. Vit. Nutr. Res.,* 49:229–230.
15. Stähelin, H. B., Seiler, W., and Pult, N. (1979): Erfahrungen mit dem Lipidsenker Procetofen (Lipanthyl®). *Schweiz. Rundschau Med. (Praxis),* 68:24–28.

Diet and Drugs in Atherosclerosis,
edited by G. Noseda, B. Lewis, and R. Paoletti.
Raven Press, New York © 1980.

Changes in Plasma Lipoprotein Concentration in Patients With Marked Hyperlipidemia on Lipid-Lowering Diet

M. Mancini, P. Rubba, A. Postiglione, C. Iovine, E. Farinaro, and F. Lamenza

Semeiotica Medica, Faculty of Medicine, University of Naples, Naples, Italy

Hyperlipidemia is a metabolic abnormality related to increased risk of atherosclerotic cardiovascular disease (4,5,10). Many studies, including ours, have shown that dietary treatment is effective in reducing plasma cholesterol and triglyceride concentrations in hyperlipidemic patients (6). In the present investigation, we sought to expand those previous observations and to evaluate the effect of a lipid-lowering diet on the individual lipoprotein fractions, separated by preparative ultracentrifugation. The patients under study were characterized by hyperlipidemia of a high degree, which is most frequently associated with clinical evidence of premature atherosclerosis.

PATIENTS AND METHODS

Twenty-eight patients with primary hyperlipidemia (HLP), seen in our lipid clinic, agreed to adhere to a lipid-lowering diet for at least 2 months. They had marked HLP, defined as plasma cholesterol and/or triglyceride concentrations above 320 and 460 mg/dl, respectively. These values correspond to the 99th percentile value of cholesterol and triglyceride distribution in a random sample of the Neapolitan population (3) after adjustment for sex and age (4).

Routine tests for exclusion of secondary forms of HLP were performed. No patient was on antidiabetic, hormonal, or antihypertensive therapy or on a weight-reducing diet.

Body mass index (BMI) was calculated by the equation body weight/height^2 (kg/m^2). Dietary history was taken by a dietician in order to evaluate adherence to the prescribed diet. Detailed dietary instruction were given to the patients.

Typing of HLP was performed according to WHO criteria (1,11). For this purpose, quantitative analysis of plasma lipoprotein fractions, separated by preparative ultracentrifugation (2), was performed. Plasma and lipoprotein cholesterol and triglycerides were determined by semiautomated methods (9).

47

DIETS

Two slightly different diets have been prescribed in our lipid clinic for the management of different types of HLP: (a) a diet which predominantly lowers plasma cholesterol (CL) (7) for patients with marked hypercholesterolemia (type. IIA and IIB), and (b) a diet which predominantly lowers plasma triglycerides (TL) (8) for patients with marked hypertriglyceridemia (types III, IV, and V). Both diets are characterized by a relatively high content of protein; saturated fat is very low (between 4 and 6% of total calories; and polyunsaturated fat represents 12 to 15%. Cholesterol intake is very low (300 mg/day). In the TL diet, the daily carbohydrate intake is reduced to 37 to 43% of total calories; at the same time, polyunsaturated fat is increased to 30 to 42%. In addition, in the TL diet, alcoholic beverages are completely excluded. Details of the two diets have been reported elsewhere (7,8).

RESULTS

Table 1 shows the decrease of plasma cholesterol and triglyceride concentrations in types IIA and IIB patients after 2 months of diet. An average cholesterol reduction of about 60 mg/dl can be observed without significant changes in plasma TG levels; BMI is only slightly reduced after the lipid-lowering diet.

Table 2 shows the changes taking place in plasma lipoprotein concentration

TABLE 1. *Changes of plasma cholesterol and triglyceride concentration (mg/dl) and BMI (kg/m²) in type II A and II B patients on CL diet for 2 months[b]*

Parameter	Cholesterol	Triglyceride	BMI
Basal	419 ± 53	188 ± 49	26 ± 2
On diet	360 ± 44[d]	130 ± 27	25 ± 1[c]

[a] Four males, seven females.
[b] X ± SEM.
[c] $p < 0.05$; [d] $p < 0.01$.

TABLE 2. *Changes of plasma lipoprotein concentration (mg/dl) in type II A and II B patients[a] on CL diet for 2 months[b]*

Parameter	VLDL		LDL cholesterol	HDL cholesterol
	Cholesterol	Triglyceride		
Basal	32 ± 10	133 ± 45	338 ± 61	52 ± 6
On diet	23 ± 7[c]	79 ± 23	270 ± 53[d]	54 ± 8

[a] Four males, seven females.
[b] X ± SEM.
[c] $p < 0.05$; [d] $p < 0.001$.

TABLE 3. *Changes of plasma cholesterol and triglyceride concentration (mg/dl) and BMI (kg/m²) in type IV and V patients[a] on TL diet for 2 months[b]*

Parameter	Cholesterol	Triglyceride	BMI
Basal	265 ± 27	1,148 ± 208	26 ± 1
On diet	212 ± 14[c]	506 ± 101[e]	25 ± 1[d]

[a] 16 males.
[b] X ± SEM.
[c] $p < 0.05$; [d] $p < 0.01$; [e] $p < 0.001$.

TABLE 4. *Changes of plasma lipoprotein concentration (mg/dl) in type IV and V patients[a] on TL diet for 2 months[b]*

Parameter	VLDL		LDL cholesterol	HDL cholesterol
	Cholesterol	Triglyceride		
Basal	174 ± 31	1,042 ± 210	57 ± 10	26 ± 3
On diet	88 ± 15[d]	435 ± 91[d]	87 ± 13[c]	36 ± 4[d]

[a] 16 males.
[b] X ± SEM.
[c] $p < 0.05$; [d] $p < 0.01$.

for the same patients. LDL and VLDL cholesterol are significantly reduced; HDL cholesterol is unmodified.

Tables 3 and 4 describe the results obtained in types IV and V patients. Total plasma cholesterol and triglyceride and BMI are significantly reduced; VLDL cholesterol and triglyceride are more than halved. On the other hand, LDL and HDL cholesterol are significantly increased after 2 months of diet.

A type III patient (Fig. 1), typically showing a high VLDL cholesterol/total triglyceride ratio (> 0.30), agreed to adhere to three different dietary regimens, for 1 month each: (a) an ordinary TL diet, 1,200 cal, low in fat and carbohydrate; (b) a diet relatively enriched in carbohydrate, 2,000 cal, and (c) a diet low in carbohydrate and enriched in saturated fat content, 1,600 cal. After 1 month on an ordinary TL diet, marked reduction of VLDL cholesterol and triglyceride is observed; however, the VLDL cholesterol/total triglyceride ratio is still abnormal (0.39). Normalization of the ratio is achieved by a carbohydrate-poor diet, not by a fat-restricted regimen.

DISCUSSION

This study demonstrates that patients with marked hyperlipoproteinemia benefit greatly from a lipid-lowering diet. The lipid-lowering effect has been achieved

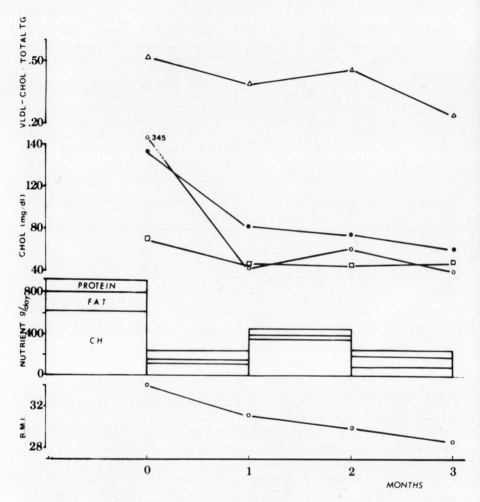

FIG. 1. Effect of different diets on VLDL *(open circles)*, LDL *(solid circles)*, and HDL *(squares)* cholesterol concentration in a 30-year-old type III patient.

in these outpatients by prescribing a diet in some respect similar to that usually consumed in Mediterranean countries. In this area, dietary intake of saturated fatty acid is much lower than that in Northern Europe and the United States. The fall in plasma cholesterol observed in type II patients after diet is mainly due to a decrease in LDL concentration but also reflects some reduction in VLDL. In types IV and V, VLDL cholesterol and triglyceride are decreased; HDL cholesterol is increased. All these diet-induced changes can be regarded as useful. LDL cholesterol is still low in types IV and V patients, despite a small rise observed after diet.

The finding of normalization of VLDL cholesterol/total plasma triglyceride ratio in a type III patient is interesting. We take this result as a good evidence of the usefulness of carbohydrate restriction in the management of type III hyperlipoproteinemia.

SUMMARY

Twenty-eight patients (21 males, 7 females) with plasma cholesterol and/or triglyceride over the 99th percentile value for healthy adults in Naples (320 mg/dl and 426 mg/dl, respectively) received dietary treatment.

With a diet low in saturated fat and cholesterol (high P/S) LDL and VLDL cholesterol were significantly reduced ($p < 0.01$ and 0.05) after 2 months in eleven type IIA and IIB patients, without concomitant changes in HDL concentration. In five type V patients and 11 type IV patients, besides limitation of saturated fatty acid and cholesterol, moderate carbohydrate restriction and alcohol exclusion were prescribed. This reduced VLDL cholesterol and triglyceride ($p < 0.01$); HDL and LDL cholesterol were slightly increased ($p < 0.01$ and 0.05).

A patient with type III hyperlipoproteinemia and VLDL abnormally rich in cholesterol was better managed with carbohydrate- rather than fat-restricted diet.

REFERENCES

1. Beaumont, J. L., Carlson, L. A., Cooper, G. R., Fejfar, Z., Fredrickson, D. S., and Strasser, T. (1970): Classification of hyperlipidemias and hyperlipoteinemias. *WHO Bull.*, 43:891–908.
2. Carlson, K. (1973): Lipoprotein fractionation. *J. Clin. Pathol. [Suppl.]*, 5:32–37.
3. Farinaro, E., Oriente, P., Paggi, E., Panico, S., and Mancini, M. (1978): L'indagine di Pozzuoli "Olivetti." In: *Rapporto conoscitivo sullo stato delle indagini epidemiologiche in Italia nel campo dell'arteriosclerosi.*" Consiglio Nazionale delle Ricerche: Collana di Medicina Preventiva, Vol. II, pp. 177–201.
4. Goldstein, J. L., Hazzard, W. R., Schrott, H. G., Bierman, E. L., and Motulsky, A. G. (1973): Hyperlipidemia in coronary heart disease. *J. Clin. Invest.*, 52:1533–1543.
5. Keys, A. (1970): Coronary heart disease in seven countries. *Circulation, [Suppl. I]*, 41:1–111.
6. Mancini, M., Farinaro, E., Moro, C. O., Di Marino, L., Rubba, P., Postiglione, A., and Oriente, P. (1975): In: *"Lipid, lipoproteins, drugs,"* edited by D. Kritchevsky, R. Paoletti, and W. L. Holmas, pp. 201–219. Plenum, New York.
7. Moro, C. O., Mancini, M., Cuzzupoli, M., Di Marino, L., and Caputo, V. (1968): La dieta nell'arteriosclerosi umana. *Quad. Nutr.*, 28:31–43.
8. Moro, C. O., Mancini, M., and Di Marino, L. (1970): Dieta per la correzione dell'ipertrigliceridemia endogena. *Quad. Nutr.*, 30:93–105.
9. Oriente, P., Di Marino, L., Patti, L., Mastranzo, P., and Iovine, C. (1979): Determinazione enzimatica simultanea del colesterolo e dei trigliceridi del siero e delle frazioni lipoproteiche isolate mediante ultracentrifugazione preparativa e tre differenti metodi di precipitazione. In: *Atti del Convegno Nazionale del Progetto Finalizzato Medicina Preventiva I*, pp. 185–193. Consiglio Nazionale delle Ricerche, Rome.
10. Rhoads, G. G., Gulbrandsen, C. L., and Kagan, A. (1976): Serum lipoproteins and coronary heart disease: A prospective case-control study. *N. Engl. J. Med.*, 294:293–298.
11. Rubba, P., Farinaro, E., Postiglione, A., Strazzullo, P., Oriente, P., and Mancini, M. (1978): Multiple lipoprotein abnormalities in primary hyperlipidemia in Naples. In: *International Conference on Atherosclerosis*, edited by L. A. Carlson, R. Paoletti, C. R. Sirtori, and G. Weber, pp. 117–122. Raven Press, New York.

Diet and Drugs in Atherosclerosis,
edited by G. Noseda, B. Lewis, and R. Paoletti.
Raven Press, New York © 1980.

The Influence of Various Diets on Type V Hyperlipoproteinemia in Children

*G. M. Kostner, H. Rosegger, S. Otto, and W. D. Müller

*Institute of Medical Biochemistry, University of Graz, and Universitätskinderklinik,
A-8010 Graz, Austria*

Type V hyperlipoproteinemia (HLP) is characterized by fasting chylomicrone-mia in addition to elevated very low density lipoprotein (VLDL) values. Whether or not this form of HLP leads to early development of atherosclerosis is still a matter of discussion. Recent reports indicate that at least certain affected individuals are not at higher risk when compared with normolipemics (5). Secondary type V HLP is rather frequently recognized in association with chronic pancreatitis, hypothyroidism, diabetes mellitus, nephrosis, dysglobulinemia, and glycogen storage disease. Under these conditions, the serum lipoprotein abnormalities return to normal if the underlying disorder is successfully treated (4). On the other hand, the metabolic disorder on a molecular level of the primary form of type V HLP remains obscure. Primary and secondary forms are sometimes hard to distinguish (3). Type V HLP usually occurs in adults only, and case reports in subjects less than 20 years of age are rare. Clinical features and treatment are best summarized by Fredrickson et al. (4). In addition, it is known from various reports that type V HLP is hardly accessible to drug treatment, and strictly observed dietary advice should be of value. This report deals with two primary type V HLP children under the age of 5 years who have been treated successfully, to a certain extent, with a special diet.

PATIENTS

Case I

Patient G.S., male, was born at the local university hospital for obstetrics and gynecology. During a routine checkup at the age of 3 days, a milky serum was found by the clinician in charge. The patient was then transferred to the children's hospital and checked thouroughly for possible abnormalities or diseases. Except for the high serum lipid values (Table 1), there were no indications for the presence of disorders of the liver, pancreas, thyroid gland, or kidneys, or for various forms of inherited metabolic diseases. During these examinations, ·the ophthalmologist noticed a transient fundus lipemicus. Eruptive xanthoma

TABLE 1. *Serum lipid and lipoprotein values of patient G.S. on various diets*

Age	Diet[b]	EQ^a (kcal/kg)	Serum lipids (mg/dl)			Lipoprotein electrophoresis	Remarks
			TG	Chol	PL		
5 days	A	36	2,250	300	470	chylom. pre-β ↑	
10 days	B	50	274	115	212	pre-β ↑	Fundus lipemicus
14 days	C	101	4,780	550	ND	chylom. pre-β ↑	
19 days	C	101	7,480	830	660	chylom. pre-β ↑	Eruptive xanthoma
35 days	D	123	720	150	280	chylom. pre-β ↑	
4.5 months	D'	135	1,650	330	300	chylom. pre-β ↑	
8 months	E	100	705	145	193	chylom. pre-β ↑	
10 months	F	91	2,150	220	305	chylom. pre-β ↑	
11 months	G	91	7,000	580	ND	chylom. pre-β ↑	Eruptive xanthoma
12 months	F	93	3,300	360	420	chylom. pre-β ↑	

a Energy quotient: caloric intake in kilocalories per kilogram body weight.

b The diet was given from the day of life shown in the previous line until the day indicated in this line. Diet A, 4 days ad libitum breastfeeding, then 24 hr fasting. Diet B, parenteral nutrition: infusion of glucose, amino acids, plus minerals. Diet C, delipidated human milk plus carbohydrates. Diet D, Tricery[®], which is a formula diet from Sopharga, France, containing 30 g/liter (44 cal %) lipids, mostly medium chain triglycerides, 35 g/liter (23 cal %) protein, and 50 g/liter lactose (33 cal % carbohydrates). Diet D', equal to D plus one meal of mixed vegetables. Diet E, carbohydrate rich mixed diet composed of skimmed milk, vegetables, starch, and fruits: 13 cal % lipids, four-fifths of which are MCT, 13 cal % protein, and 74 cal % carbohydrate. Diet F, richer in lipid compared to E: 31 cal % lipids, one-fifth of which are MCT, 13 cal % protein, and 56 cal % carbohydrate. Diet G, protein-rich diet: 30 cal % lipids, four-tenths of which are polyunsaturated fat, one-tenth saturated, and four-tenths MCT; 22 cal % protein, and 48 cal % carbohydrate.

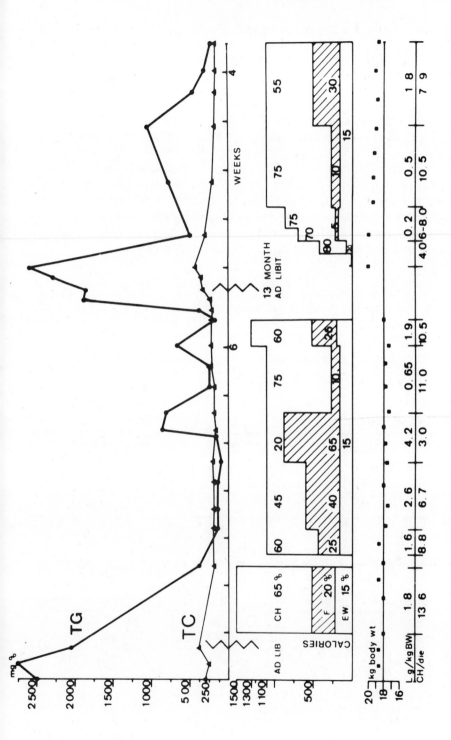

FIG. 1. Serum triglyceride (TG) and total cholesterol (TC) values of patient K.B. after various diets. L (F), lipids; CH, carbohydrates; EW, proteins.

were also observed on several occasions on elbows, face, and forearms. The grandmother and uncle of the patient also showed a typical type IIb/V HLP, whereas the mother seemed to be affected by type IV HLP.

Case II

Patient K.B., female, was brought to the children's hospital at the age of 5 years with observed signs of acute pancreatitis. Besides the usual childhood infections, she grew normally in full health. Clinical tests excluded a secondary form of type V HLP. A report of all clinical data has been published earlier (6). The only striking abnormality was fasting chylomicronemia with elevated VLDL (see Fig. 1), a reduced postheparin lipolytic activity (PHLA) to approximately 30% of normal, and the presence of eruptive xanthomas on the elbows. The patient was put on a formula diet of various composition in two consecutive periods, and changes of serum lipoproteins were observed.

RESULTS

Patient G.S. was hospitalized for the first 3 weeks of his life and then controlled as an outpatient. The serum lipid and lipoprotein values in relation to various

TABLE 2. *Lipid and lipoproteins of some relatives of patient G.S.*

| Subject | Relation | Age (years) | Serum lipids (mg/dl) | | | Lipoproteins and Fredrickson type |
			TG	Chol	PL	
A. S.	Mother	26	345	245	300	pre-β ↑↑, IV
A. S.	Father	34	196	174	232	pre-β ↑, ?
F. Z.	Uncle	28	4,180	572	683	chylom. pre-β ↑↑, V
A. R.	Grandmother	55	460	305	398	β and pre-β ↑↑, IIb

TABLE 3. *Postheparin lipolytic activity of patient G.S.*

| Subject | Minutes after heparin administration | Lipolytic activity (μmoles/ml/hr) | | |
		Total	Extrahepatic	Hepatic[a]
Propositus	0	0.61	ND	ND
Propositus	10	19.4	ND	ND
Propositus	20	18.3	7.3	11.0
Normal males[b]	10	18.6 ± 5.3	5.5 ± 1.7	13.1 ± 5.0
Eight type V patients (males)[b]	10	22.7 ± 5.3	5.2 ± 1.1	17.5 ± 5.0

[a] Hepatic lipase was measured after inactivation of lipoprotein lipase with protamine sulfate.
[b] Values taken from ref. 5.

dietary changes are shown in Table 1. Table 2 shows the lipid values of some relatives underlining the presence of a primary form of type V. In Table 3, the PHLA values are listed, which were measured at the age of 6 weeks. No abnormality was seen.

Additional Investigation of the Lipoproteins

Investigation of the serum lipoproteins at several time intervals showed a distinct type V pattern with grossly elevated VLDL of S_f 20 to 400 and $S_f >$ 400. The LDL were reduced to approximately one-third. At the age of 31 weeks, we measured lipoprotein lipids and found the following values: Total cholesterol (TC), 330 mg/dl; HDL-C, 24 mg/dl; LDL-C, 53 mg/dl. Since there is a report in the literature of a type I/V patient with apoCII deficiency (2), we also measured various apolipoproteins immunochemically. All apolipoproteins, including AI, AII, B, CI, CII, CIII, D, E, and F, were qualitatively demonstrable. VLDL were also isolated and investigated by TMU-polyacrylamide gel electrophoresis. Densitometric scan revealed a normal distribution of apoE: CI: CII: CIII.

Comments

The laboratory data of patient G. S., which will be published in detail elsewhere, (6a) clearly revealed the presence of a primary type V HLP with normal PHLA. To our knowledge, this is the first report of this disorder in newborns. In this study, PHLA was measured with intralipid as substrate. It must be stated, however, that other investigators observed some forms of type V HLP where normal PHLA values were found if intralipid was used, whereas very low levels were found with chylomicrons of the same patient or of normal individuals (7). This observation led the authors to the conclusion that a structurally altered lipoprotein lipase might have been present in those patients. Excluding this as a possible cause of the hypertriglyceridemia in our patient, there are no indications of the presence of the underlying defect. As can be seen from Table 1, dietary treatment of the propositus had only moderate influence on the serum lipoprotein concentrations. It seemed that both lipid- and carbohydrate-rich diets induced a massive hypertriglyceridemia. Only during partial parenteral feeding did the serum lipid values tend to return to normal. The patient is still under observation.

Patient K. B. was studied several years ago during hospitalization for 6 and 5 weeks, respectively. She was massively hypertriglyceridemic with elevated chylomicrons and VLDL. LDL and HDL were reduced by approximately 50%. PHLA measured after administration of 10 U heparin/kg body weight was reduced to 30% of normal. The changes of serum lipids occurring during dietary treatment are shown in Fig. 1. In the first period of investigation, the patient started with serum triglyceride values of 2,700 mg/dl and TC of 325 mg/dl. On a 1,500 kcal/day, 65% carbohydrate, 20% lipid, and 15% protein diet,

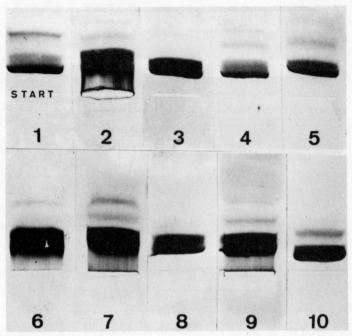

FIG. 2. Lipoprotein electrophoresis in 0.5% agarose gels of the serum of patient K.B. on various diets. Sera were drawn after an overnight fast. **1:** Normal control. **2:** K.B. on the first day of her visit. **3–10:** K.B. on various diets. **3:** Day 10 on 1,500 kcal with 20% lipids. **4:** Day 4 on 1,100 kcal with 25% lipids. **5:** Day 10 on 1,100 kcal with 40% lipids. **6** and **7:** Days 6 and 7 on 1,100 kcal with 65% lipids. **8:** Day 4 on 1,100 kcal with 75% carbohydrate. **9:** Day 10 on 1,100 kcal with 75% carbohydrate. **10:** Day 3 on 1,300 kcal with 55% carbohydrate. For explanation, see scheme in Fig. 1.

serum triglyceride was drastically reduced, but fasting chylomicronemia did not disappear. Lowering the caloric intake to 1,100 kcal/day with various carbohydrate/lipid ratios led to an almost complete normalization of the lipoprotein pattern (Fig. 2). Only if the lipid content of the diet was raised to 65% did fasting chylomicronemia and elevated VLDL reappear. Reduction of the lipid intake to 10 cal % with 75% carbohydrate first gave a normalization of the serum lipoprotein pattern; but on the third day on this diet, a massive hypertriglyceridemia developed. Finally, it was found that a 1,300 kcal/day diet with 60 cal % carbohydrate, 25 cal % lipid, and 15 cal % protein gave a normalization and stabilization of the serum lipoprotein profile. At the second investigation period 12 months later, the patient returned to the hospital with lipid values identical to those of the first observation. Reduction of the caloric intake first to 500 kcal/day and then to 1,000 kcal/day with a low fat content led to rapid normalization of the serum triglyceride. Raising caloric intake to 1,100 kcal/day with a carbohydrate content of 75% was accompanied by a gradual increase of serum triglyceride and the appearance of fasting chylomicronemia. A drastic reduction of serum triglyceride, on the other hand, was observed with a 1,100 kcal/day diet of 55% carbohydrate, 30% lipid, and 15% protein.

Serum lipoproteins investigated by agarose gel electrophoresis on several occasions (Fig. 2) gave further insight in the changes occurring in serum lipoproteins. A characteristic change of LDL was also noticed in the analytical ultracentrifuge by switching from high lipid to high carbohydrate diets.

CONCLUSION

We have shown that type V HLP can be demonstrated in early life and even a few days after birth. The two investigated cases differed with respect to the PHLA, which apparently was completely normal in patient G.S. but reduced to 30% in patient K.B. A thorough investigation of serum lipids, lipoproteins, and all known clinical parameters gave no indication of the basic metabolic defect of this HLP. There seems to be little doubt about the fact that triglyceride clearance in these patients is markedly diminished, leading to an accumulation of exogenous (chylomicrons) and endogenous (VLDL) triglyceride-rich particles. This has been demonstrated earlier in three type V patients (1). The metabolic block in primary type V patients does not concern the lipoprotein lipase or the hepatic lipase. Several other possibilities may also be discussed, e.g., lack or impaired function of other lipases or an impaired uptake of chylomicron remnants.

With respect to the treatment of these patients, it must be emphasized that with the exception of a hypocaloric diet, there exist only a few possibilities to normalize serum triglyceride values. As the present study has shown, an optimal diet for type V children is a moderate, balanced diet, with approximately 55 cal % carbohydrate, 30 cal % lipid, and 15% proteins.

The substitution of long chain triglycerides for medium chain triglycerides seems to have no effect, nor is the substitution for polyunsaturated fats of considerable value.

Further investigations are in progress, aimed at disclosing the underlying metabolic defect and evaluating diets which can be used in long-term treatment.

ACKNOWLEDGMENTS

Parts of this study have been supported by the Fonds zur Förderung der wissenschaftlichen Forschung (Proj. No. 3734). The technical assistance of H. Grillhofer is appreciated.

REFERENCES

1. Ballantyne, F. C., Ballantyne, D., Olsson, A. G., Rössner, S., and Carlson, L. A. (1977): Metabolism of VLDL of S_f 100–400 in Type V hyperlipoproteinemia. *Acta Med. Scand.*, 202:153–161.

2. Breckenridge, W. C., Little, J. A., Steiner, G., Chow, A., and Poapst, M. (1978): Hypertriglyceridemia associated with deficiency of apolipoprotein CII. *N. Engl. J. Med.,* 298:1265–1273.
3. Fallat, R. W., and Glueck, C. J. (1976): Familial and acquired hyperlipoproteinemia. *Atherosclerosis,* 23:41–62.
4. Fredrickson, D. S., and Levy, R. I. (1972): Familial hyperlipoproteinemia. In: *The Metabolic Basis of Inherited Diseases,* third edition, pp. 545–614. McGraw Hill, New York.
5. Greenberg, B. H., Blackwelder, W. C., and Levy, R. I. (1977): Primary Type V hyperlipoproteinemia: A descriptive study in 32 families. *Ann. Intern. Med.,* 87:526–534.
6. Müller, W. D., and Kostner, G. M. (1974): Einfluss von Fett bzw. Kohlenhydratreicher Nahrung auf das Serumlipoproteinmuster bei primärer Hypertriglyceridämie im Kindesalter. *Wien. Klin. Wochenschr.,* 86:757–762.
6a. Otto, S. et al. (1980): *(in preparation).*
7. Schreibman, P. H., Arons, D. L., Saudeck, C. D., and Arky, R. A. (1973): Abnormal lipoprotein lipase in familial exogenous hypertriglyceridemia. *J. Clin. Invest.,* 52:2075–2082.

Diet and Drugs in Atherosclerosis,
edited by G. Noseda, B. Lewis, and R. Paoletti.
Raven Press, New York © 1980.

Effects of Soybean Protein Diet on Serum Lipids, Plasma Glucagon, and Insulin

Giorgio Noseda and Claudia Fragiacomo

Ospedale Beata Vergine, 6850 Mendrisio, Switzerland

Some studies have suggested that a soybean protein diet has a hypocholesterolemic effect in animals (2) and man (9). This research has been carried out in hospitalized patients whose dietary prescriptions were followed in detail. Our research is part of a multicentric trial conceived to verify the hypocholesterolemic effect of the soybean protein diet in outpatients. Fifteen patients with type II hyperlipidemia were chosen. Most had already been treated with a hypolipidemic diet and/or hypolipidemic drugs without success.

Another aim of our study was to investigate the hypothetical role of glucagon and insulin on the lipid-lowering effect of a soybean protein diet by determining these two hormones at regular intervals during and after the diet.

MATERIAL AND METHODS

Patients and Diet

Fifteen patients (7 with type IIa and 8 with type IIb hyperlipidemia as characterized by lipoprotein electrophoresis) were treated with the soybean protein diet according to the following protocol. First, there were 4 weeks of washout, during which the patients followed a hypolipidemic diet with a low amount of cholesterol and a P/S ratio of ≥ 1.8. The composition of the hypolipidemic diet was proteins, 20%; lipid, 25%; carbohydrate, 55%; and cholesterol, 80 to 90 mg/1,000 kcal. This was followed by 8 weeks of a soybean protein diet replacing most animal proteins and with a P/S ratio ≥ 2.2. The composition of the soybean protein (Cholsoy, Ghimas, Bologna, Italy) was protein, 52%; water, 6%; lipid, 1%; fiber, 3.5%; minerals (ash), 6%; carbohydrate, 31.5%; and kcal 280/100 g. This product was employed in the preparation of various foods. The composition of the soybean protein diet was protein, 21%; lipid, 22%; carbohydrate, 55%; and cholesterol, 0 to 10 mg/1,000 kcal. This was followed by 6 weeks of a hypolipidemic diet, as during the washout period. For the formulation of the diets, we considered the following parameters: age, sex, weight, height, and physical activity.

Plasma Lipid Analysis

Blood samples were drawn after a 12 hr overnight fast. Cholesterol and tri-glycerides were analyzed by automated techniques (1,7). Electrophoresis of plasma lipoproteins was carried out on agarose gel, as described by Noble (6). Fasting VLDL (density < 1.006 g/ml) were isolated by ultracentrifugation, according to the method of Havel et al. (5). HDL cholesterol levels were determined after precipitation of LDL with heparin-$MnCl_2$, and LDL cholesterol was calculated by the difference.

Plasma Glucagon and Insulin

The two hormones were determined by radioimmunoassay (Hypolab, Coinsins, Switzerland).

RESULTS

The modifications of plasma lipids before, during, and after treatment with a soybean protein diet are summarized in Table 1. During our study, we noted a nonsignificant decrease of total cholesterol in the first period of the hypolipidemic diet (from 331 to 314 mg/dl). For the following 8 weeks, a marked lowering of total cholesterol levels (from 314 to 267 mg/dl) was noted. Levels did not increase at the end of the soybean protein period. LDL cholesterol levels did not change during washout (from 254 to 241 mg/dl) but decreased significantly during the soybean protein diet (from 241 to 194 mg/dl). HDL cholesterol levels increased slightly but not significantly from 38 to 40 mg/dl during treatment with soybean proteins.

Plasma triglycerides were not markedly modified. They decreased at the beginning of treatment but increased afterwards. After 8 weeks, the difference was not statistically significant. The changes of plasma glucagon, insulin, and glucagon insulin ratio before, during, and after treatment with soybean protein diet are summarized in Table 2. During 8 weeks of soybean protein treatment, a significant increase in plasma glucagon from 218 to 247 pg/ml was measured. After cessation of the soybean protein diet, the plasma glucagon levels returned to the same values as at the beginning. Plasma insulin decreased during 8 weeks of the soybean protein diet only slightly and not significantly from 19.9 to 16.4 pg/ml and increased in the following 6 weeks to 18.7 pg/ml.

As a consequence of the variations of the plasma glucagon and insulin levels, the plasma glucagon insulin ratio rose significantly during the soybean protein diet from 11.5 to 15.7 and decreased afterwards to 11.8.

DISCUSSION

Our study shows that the soybean protein diet is effective not only in hospitalized patients but also in outpatients, whose dietary prescriptions cannot be con-

TABLE 1. Plasma lipids[a] before, during, and after treatment with soybean proteins

Plasma lipid (mg/dl)	Before (weeks)		During (weeks)					After (weeks)	
	4	2	0	1	2	4	8	3	6
Total cholesterol	331 ± 28	318 ± 26	314 ± 24	292 ± 38	285 ± 35	279 ± 33	267 ± 30[b]	275 ± 37	272 ± 39
Triglycerides	200 ± 78	172 ± 67	175 ± 78	171 ± 70	152 ± 58	163 ± 67	164 ± 71	161 ± 77	171 ± 76
LDL-cholesterol	253 ± 31		241 ± 26			207 ± 36	194 ± 32[b]		197 ± 38
HDL-cholesterol	37 ± 8		38 ± 7			39 ± 8	40 ± 8		40 ± 8

[a] $\overline{X}$ ± 1 SD.
[b] $p < 0.001$.

TABLE 2. *Plasma glucagon, insulin, and glucagon: Insulin ratio[a] before, during, and after treatment with soybean proteins*

Hormone (pg/ml)	Before	During (weeks) 4	During (weeks) 8	After (6 weeks)
Glucagon	218 ± 114	252 ± 98	247 ± 95[b]	215 ± 101
Insulin	19.9 ± 5.3	19.2 ± 4.7	16.4 ± 4.9	18.7 ± 6.5
Glucagon insulin ratio	11.5 ± 6.3	13.9 ± 7.1	15.7 ± 6.8[c]	11.8 ± 5.2

[a] $\overline{X} \pm SD$.
[b] $p < 0.05$; [c] $p < 0.01$.

troled in detail. Total and LDL cholesterol decreased significantly. HDL cholesterol increased slightly and not significantly. The HDL-cholesterol increase may be significant in a long-term study. The triglycerides decreased only slightly and not significantly.

The soybean protein diet induces some hormonal changes, significantly increasing plasma glucagon, inversely but not significantly decreasing plasma insulin, and consequently significantly increasing the plasma glucagon insulin ratio. These hormonal modifications can explain the hypolipidemic effects of the soybean protein diet. Glucagon and insulin have been reported in animal (8) and human (3) experiments to have opposite effects on the mechanisms regulating plasma lipid concentrations. Glucagon in excess of insulin, as in our cases, may lower serum lipids. The mechanism by which soybean proteins increase glucagon secretion is probably due to alpha-cell stimulation by amino acids liberated during protein digestion. It is well known that glucagon secretion is stimulated by certain amino acids, among which arginine is an outstanding example (3).

Another possibility is that protein intake influences alpha-cell function by stimulating release of gastrointestinal hormones, e.g., cholezystokinin-pancreozymin (4). This hypothesis needs further experimental confirmation.

REFERENCES

1. Block, W. D., Janett, J., and Levine, J. B. (1965): Use of a single color reagent to improve the automated determination of serum cholesterol. In: *Technicon Symposia on Automation in Analytical Chemistry.* Mediad, New York.
2. Carrol, K. K., and Hamilton, R. M. G. (1975): Effect of dietary protein and carbohydrate on plasma cholesterol levels in relation to atherosclerosis. *J. Food Sci.,* 40:18–23.
3. Eaton, R. P., and Schade, D. S. (1974): Effect of clofibrate on arginine-stimulated glucagon and insulin secretion in man. *Metabolism,* 23:445–454.
4. Eisenstein, A. B., Strack, I., Gallo-Torres, H., Georgiadis, A., and Miller, O. N. (1979): Increased glucagon secretion in protein-fed rats: lack of relationship to plasma amino acids. *Am. J. Physiol.,* 236(1):E20-E27.
5. Havel, R. J., Eden, H. A., and Bragdon, J. H. (1955): The distribution and chemical composition of ultracentrifugally separated lipoproteins in human serum. *J. Clin. Invest.,* 34:1345–1353.

6. Noble, R. P. (1968): Electrophoretical separation of plasma lipoproteins on agarose gel. *J. Lipid Res.,* 9:693–700.
7. Noble, R. P., and Campbell, F. M. (1970): Improved accuracy in automated fluorimetric determination of plasma triglycerides. *Clin. Chem.,* 16:166.
8. Paloyan, E., and Harper, P. V. (1961): Glucagon as a regulating factor of plasma lipids. *Metabolism,* 10:315–323.
9. Sirtori, C. R., Agradi, E., Conti, F., Mantero, O., and Gatti, E. (1977): Soybean protein diet in the treatment of type II hyperlipoproteinemia. *Lancet,* 5:275–277.

Diet and Drugs in Atherosclerosis,
edited by G. Noseda, B. Lewis, and R. Paoletti.
Raven Press, New York © 1980.

Lipoproteins and Apolipoproteins A_1 and B in Obese Subjects in Basal State and Following a Hypocaloric Diet

P. Avogaro, G. Bittolo Bon, G. Cazzolato, and G. B. Quinci

Regional General Hospital, Unit for Atherosclerosis, National Council for Researches, 30100 Venice, Italy

There is a weak correlation between obesity and lipid and/or lipoprotein plasma levels (1,2,5,6,10). Triglycerides (TG) and very low density lipoproteins (VLDL) are usually higher in obese than in normal subjects (1,2,5,6,10).

BODY WEIGHT AND HIGH DENSITY LIPOPROTEINS

Recently, it has been shown that obesity is associated with reduced levels of high density lipoprotein cholesterol (HDL-C) (7,8,11). Epidemiological data from the Framingham Study (7) and the Trømso Study (9), however, did not reveal any close relationship between HDL-C and relative body weight.

Recently, we stressed an inverse correlation between body weight index (BWI) and plasma levels of HDL-C and apo-A_I (7). We studied 120 subjects (60 males and 60 females) with a BWI between 0.8 and 1.2. Lower levels of HDL and apo-A_I were found in men than in women; the difference was not significant. A high negative correlation was found between BWI, HDL-C, and apo-A_I in both males and females, whereas no correlation was found between BWI and apo-B.

When values of HDL-C and apo-A_I were considered according to quartiles of BWI in both sexes, significant variations were found between the mean values of the lowest and the highest quartile. These data are even more significant as they were obtained from "normal" people with a BWI kept within normal limits by exclusion of both obese and very lean subjects. Recently, emphasis has been placed on the role of HDL-C and apo-A_I as a biochemical marker of human atherosclerosis (3,8). As the difference in concentration of HDL-C between normal and atherosclerotic patients is a few milligrams, the relevant influence of body weight on these parameters must be emphasized.

LIPOPROTEINS AND APOLIPOPROTEINS A_I AND B IN OBESE

Research was undertaken to ascertain the plasma levels of the major plasma lipoprotein classes and of the two major apolipoproteins, apo-B and apo-A_I,

TABLE 1. Concentrations of plasma lipids, lipoproteins, apo-B and apo-A$_I$ in 30 obese subjects and 30 controls

Subjects	BWI (%)	Total plasma (mg%)				VLDL (mg%)			LDL (mg%)		HDL-C (mg%)
		C	TG	apo-B	apo-A$_I$	C	TG	apo-B	C	apo-B	
Controls											
m̄	102	258	160	119	144	31	89	16	165	103	62
SE	2	9	13	5	4	5	7	1	7	4	2
Obese											
m̄	153[a]	257	162	129	112[a]	30	87	17	180	112	46[a]
SE	4	9	13	5	3	5	7	1	6	4	2

[a] $p < 0.01$ versus controls.

TABLE 2. *Ratios of plasma lipids and apolipoproteins in 30 obese subjects and 30 controls*

Subjects	$\dfrac{C}{HDL\text{-}C}$	$\dfrac{LDL\text{-}C}{HDL\text{-}C}$	$\dfrac{apo\text{-}B}{apo\text{-}A_I}$	$\dfrac{LDL\text{-}C}{LDL\text{-}B}$	$\dfrac{HDL\text{-}C}{apo\text{-}A_I}$
Controls					
$\bar{m}$	4.14	2.64	0.83	1.59	0.43
SE	0.27	0.19	0.06	0.13	0.03
Obese					
$\bar{m}$	5.56[a]	3.91[a]	1.15[a]	1.61	0.41
SE	0.29	0.26	0.16	0.13	0.02

[a] $p < 0.01$ versus controls.

in obese people. Thirty obese subjects were included in the study (BWI, between 1.30 and 1.75; mean, 1.53). Their plasma lipid levels matched with those recorded in a control series (BWI, 0.82 to 1.11; mean, 1.02). For controls, subjects were selected having plasma levels of cholesterol and TG close to the baseline lipid levels of the obese. Before inclusion in the study, both obese subjects and controls followed a typical Italian diet (50% carbohydrate, 35% fat, 15% protein; cholesterol, 400 to 600 mg; P/S, 0.8 : 1). In the comparison between obese subjects and controls, the only significant variations were that obese subjects had lower values of HDL-C and apo-A_I and higher ratio values of total cholesterol (TC)/ HDL-C, LDL-C/HDL-C, and apo-B/apo-A_I (Tables 1 and 2).

LIPOPROTEINS AND APOLIPOPROTEINS A_I AND B IN OBESE FED A HYPOCALORIC DIET

After the first analysis for a period of 40 to 60 days, the obese subjects were fed a hypocaloric, hypocholesterolemic diet (1,000 kcal; 45% carbohydrate, 35% fat, 20% protein; cholesterol, 300 mg/day; P/S, 1). A new analysis was performed at a time when a major loss of weight was not obtainable and the body weight had been stable for days.

Following dietary treatment, the BWI decreased significantly in all subjects (between 5 and 18%) (Fig. 1). A significant decrease of TC, VLDL-C, LDL-C, total TG, VLDL-TG, VLDL-apo-B, and of ratios C/HDL-C, LDL-C/ HDL-C, apo-B/apo-A_I, and LDL-C/LDL-apo-B was recorded following dietary treatment, while the HDL-C/apo-A_I ratio remained unchanged, and a significant increase of both HDL-C and apo-A_I was observed (Fig. 1, Table 3). It is relevant that even if VLDL-TG in obese subjects following a diet are lower than in controls, values of apo-A_I and HDL-C are still significantly lower than in controls. Another reason may be the origin of the decreased levels of apo-A_I and HDL-C in obese, which are unrelated to the levels of VLDL-TG.

The relationship between the degree of the weight loss and the variations of

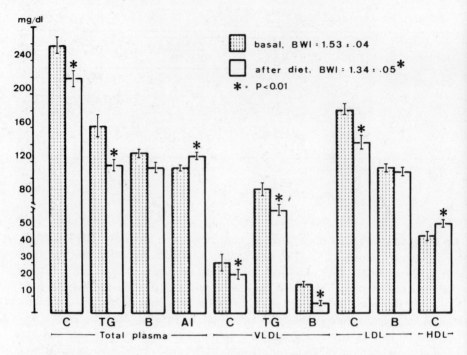

FIG. 1. Behavior of lipids and apo-A_I and apo-B in total plasma and in the major lipoprotein classes following a hypocaloric diet (1,000 kcal) in obese subjects.

the various examined parameters was ascertained (Table 4). A significant relationship between the degree of the various weight decreases and the increase of plasma levels of apo-A_I and HDL-C has been stressed. No other correlations have been observed.

This finding may mean that only apo-A_I and HDL-C values are directly correlated to body weight (and to adipose tissue size), while variations of

TABLE 3. *Behavior of various ratios in obese subjects following a hypocaloric diet[a]*

State	$\dfrac{C}{HDL\text{-}C}$	$\dfrac{LDL\text{-}C}{HDL\text{-}C}$	$\dfrac{apo\text{-}B}{apo\text{-}A_I}$	$\dfrac{LDL\text{-}C}{LDL\text{-}B}$	$\dfrac{HDL\text{-}C}{apo\text{-}A_I}$
Basal					
m̄	5.56	3.91	1.15	1.61	0.41
SE	0.29	0.26	0.16	0.13	0.02
After diet					
m̄	4.03[b]	2.62[b]	0.89[b]	1.34[b]	0.42
SE	0.28	0.18	0.05	0.12	0.02

[a] 1,000 kcal.
[b] $p < 0.01$ versus basal.

TABLE 4. *Correlations between the decrease of BWI and variations of the various parameters*

ΔTC	R = −0.09
ΔTG	R = 0.26
ΔB	R = 0.10
ΔA-I	R = 0.37[a]
ΔVLDL-C	R = 0.08
ΔVLDL-TG	R = 0.20
ΔVLDL-B	R = 0.13
ΔLDL-C	R = −0.04
ΔLDL-B	R = 0.02
ΔHDL-C	R = 0.49[b]

[a] $p < 0.05$.
[b] $p < 0.01$.

LDL-C and/or apo-B are more dependent on variations of food quantity and/or quality.

SUMMARY

The chemical composition of major plasma lipoprotein classes and plasma levels of apolipoproteins A$_I$ and B have been studied in 30 obese subjects. When matched with controls, obese subjects showed lower values of HDL-C and apo-A$_I$ and higher values of ratios TC/HDL-C, LDL-C/HDL-C, and apo-B/apo-A$_I$. The same subjects were fed a hypocaloric diet (1,000 kcal) for 45 to 60 days. Following dietary treatment, a significant decrease of TC, VLDL-C, LDL-C, total-TG, VLDL-TG, VLDL-apo-B, and ratios C/HDL-C, LDL-C/HDL-C, apo-B/apo-A$_I$, and LDL-C/LDL-apo-B was recorded.

REFERENCES

1. Albrink, M. J., and Meigs, J. W. (1964): Interrelationship between skinfold thickness, serum lipids and blood sugar in normal men. *Am. J. Clin. Nutr.,* 15:255.
2. Albrink, M. J., Meigs, J. W., and Granoff, M. A. (1962): Weight gain and serum triglycerides in normal men. *N. Engl. J. Med.,* 266:484.
3. Avogaro, P., Bittolo Bon, G., Cazzolato, G., and Quinci, G. B. (1979): Are apoliproproteins better discriminators than lipids for atherosclerosis? *Lancet,* I:901–903.
4. Avogaro, P., Cazzolato, G., Bittolo Bon, G., Quinci, G. B., and Chinello, M. (1978): HDL-cholesterol, apolipoproteins A$_I$ and B, age and index body weight. *Atherosclerosis,* 31:85–91.
5. Avogaro, P., Crepaldi, G., Enzi, G., and Tiengo, A. (1967): Association of hyperlipaemia, diabetes mellitus and mild obesity. *Acta Diabetol. Lat.,* 4:572–590.
6. Gofman, J. W., and Jones, M. B. (1952): Obesity, fat metabolism and cardiovascular disease. *Circulation,* 5:514–518.
7. Gordon, T., Castelli, W. P., Hjortland, M. C., Kannel, W. B., and Damber, T. R. (1977): High density lipoprotein and a protective factor against coronary heart disease. *Am. J. Med.,* 62:707–714.
8. Miller, C. J., and Miller, N. E. (1975): Plasma high density lipoprotein concentration and development of ischaemic heart disease. *Lancet,* I:16–19.
9. Miller, N. E., Forde, O. H., Thelle, D. S., and Mjos, O. D. (1977): The Trømso Heart Study.

High density lipoprotein and coronary heart disease: a prospective case-control study. *Lancet,* I:965–968.
10. Walker, W. J., Weiner, N., and Milch, L. J. (1957): Differential effect of dietary fat and weight reduction on serum levels of beta-lipoprotein. *Circulation,* 15:31–37.
11. Wilson, D. E., and Lees, R. S. (1972): Metabolic relationship among the plasma lipoproteins. Reciprocal changes in the very-low and low-density lipoproteins in man. *J. Clin. Invest.,* 51:1051–1057.

Diet and Drugs in Atherosclerosis,
edited by G. Noseda, B. Lewis, and R. Paoletti.
Raven Press, New York © 1980.

HDL-Cholesterol Levels and Coronary Alterations: A Clinical and Angiographic Study

Oreste Mantero, Giuseppe Catenazzo, Gianluca Fiorini, and
*Bruno Brusoni

*Vergani Medical Division and Center E. Grossi Paoletti; and * De Gasperis Division,
Ospedale Ca' Granda, 20100 Milan, Italy*

It can be seen from the literature that plasmatic concentrations of cholesterol bound up with high density lipoproteins (C-HDL) are inversely correlated to coronary disease in man (3,5,6). Although the actual mechanism of action of the antiatherogenic role of HDL is not clear (4), the epidemiologic and clinical contributions made to the literature demonstrate that a low level of C-HDL becomes a risk factor independent of the value of total cholesterolemia itself (5).

Recent clinical studies (2,8) suggest that the predictive value of atherogenic risk of HDL is linked, above all, to the apoprotein fractions (apo-A and apo-B). In fact, a significant lowering of plasma levels of apo-A exists in myocardial infarction and in peripheric arteriopathy (8). Others (1) find an even more specific reduction in the apo-A_I fraction in coronary disease. Even in transient ischemic attacks (TIA) a significant lowering of C-HDL levels has been found (7).

MATERIALS AND METHODS

The authors selected 24 male patients, ages 22 to 70, with clinical symptoms of coronary heart failure yet without the main coronary risk factors, i.e., arterial hypertension, cigarette smoking, diabetes mellitus, total cholesterol (TC) levels between 137 and 257 mg% (with the exception of one patient with a TC level of 317 mg%), triglyceride (TG) levels between 62 and 200 mg% (with the exception of one patient with a level of 263 mg%), and no family history of ischemic heart disease (Tables 1 and 2). TC was calculated with the enzymatic method (Boehringer CHOD-PAP). TG was calculated using the Wahlefeld enzymatic method.

Blood samples were centrifuged and preserved at −22°C. Values were determined, in block, later. Blood plasma concentrations of C-HDL were evaluated using the precipitation method, with destran-sulfate and magnesium chloride. Coronary angiograms were carried out following the Judkins and Sones tech-

TABLE 1. *Clinical data in 24 males*

Patient	Age (years)	TC (mg/dl)	TG (mg/dl)	C-HDL (mg/dl)	Coronary angiogram	Friesinger's score
T.E.	54	222	200	25	IVA + C	10
R.R.	53	219	227	32	3 vessels	13
M.G.B.	38	227	127	26	3 vessels	12
A.D.	52	228	170	35	3 vessels	8
M.S.	48	241	133	24	3 vessels	11
P.E.	40	179	145	30	3 vessels	10
T.L.	49	224	177	34	LM	8
Z.G.	67	188	195	35	IVA + R	7
S.G.	54	247	143	35	3 vessels	14
P.V.	70	219	267	40	3 vessels	12
C.T.	52	183	103	34	IVA	4
R.G.	22	224	100	27	IVA	4
T.L.	38	210	204	38	IVA + C	10
V.L.	58	257	263	32	3 vessels	13
S.A.	59	246	62	28	3 vessels	12
L.M.	39	137	110	29	IVA + R	7
L.C.	44	252	166	29	IVA	4
B.L.	57	206	196	30	IVA	4
A.E.	47	235	164	31	IVA + R	7
C.A.	48	238	128	41	3 vessels	11
L.G.	48	241	120	36	IVA + R	7
O.R.	53	217	108	52	3 vessels	10
S.I.	46	211	98	33	IVA + R	8
S.D.	57	317	146	37	IVA + R	8

TABLE 2. *Mean values of TC, TG, and C-HDL*

Group	Age (years)	TC (mg/dl)	TG (mg/dl)	C-HDL (mg/dl)
Controls (males)	41.2	167 ± 5	109 ± 5	45 ± 10
Patients with positive coronary angiogram	49.7	223	156	33

nique, and angiographic findings were interpreted according to the Friesinger method of scoring from 0 to 5.

DISCUSSION

With respect to the lipemic composition, it should be emphasized that none of our patients (with the exception of M.S., age 48) was treated with hypolipemic drugs, since TC and TG levels were different from those normally considered to require drug therapy. The mean TC value in our cases was 223 mg% versus 167 ± 5 mg% in the control group. TG was 165 mg% versus 109 ± 5; C-HDL was 33 mg% versus 45 ± 10 in the control group. Angiograms were positive in all these patients, and coronary lesions varied in both extension and severity (Friesinger score, 4 to 14).

In this group of patients, the interventricular artery appeared to be the most frequently affected by the atherosclerotic process, both as a single vessel and in association with the other vessels. C-HDL levels in our patients increased, albeit moderately, with age (Table 3). However, this is not contradictory to known facts inasmuch as we are dealing with an abnormal group and, therefore, the lower C-HDL level in the younger members determined an earlier clinical manifestation of the atherosclerotic disease.

We studied the correlation between the extension and severity of coronary lesions and the average age of patients (Table 4). It was clearly seen that coronary atherosclerosis increased with age, first affecting the interventricular artery, followed by the circumflex branch, and then the right coronary artery. As is known, age actually seems to condition the extension of lesions, thus becoming a serious

TABLE 3. *Mean C-HDL levels in 22 patients with positive coronary angiogram*

Age (years)	C-HDL (mg/dl)
<41	30.75
41–50	32.57
51–60	34.00

TABLE 4. *Relationship between severity and extension of coronary lesions and average ages*[a]

Lesion		Average age (years)
Single vessel (IVA or LM)		44
Double	(IVA + C)	46
	(IVA + R)	50
Triple	(IVA + C + R)	52

[a] $N = 22$.

independent risk factor on its own. If we go on to analyze relationships between this correlation and respective C-HDL levels, however, we will see how lower levels condition the precocious appearance of atherosclerotic lesions, especially in the interventricular artery. As age increases, and consequently the extension of coronary lesions, a slight increase in C-HDL mean values is also seen. This slight increase in C-HDL cannot be considered a protective factor capable of staving off the appearance of clinical symptoms. Therefore, if low C-HDL levels are capable of influencing the precocity and severity of the coronary lesion, the extension, as far as we know, appears to be linked to age and still-unidentifiable factors.

SUMMARY

Twenty-four male patients, ages 22 to 70, with the clinical symptoms of coronary heart disease but without recognizable major risk factors were studied.

Plasma concentrations of C-HDL were evaluated by means of the precipitation technique with $MgCl_2$ + dextran-sulfate. Coronary angiograms were carried out using the Judkins and Sones techniques, and findings were interpreted according to the Friesinger method.

The mean C-HDL levels of studied patients were significantly lower than those of the control group (33 ± 9 versus 45 ± 10 mg%). The earliest lesions were detected in the interventricular artery, the extension of coronary lesions increasing with age. The low concentrations of C-HDL found in patients in the younger age groups is positively correlated to obstructive coronary heart disease. Plasma C-HDL levels increase, yet not significantly, with age.

REFERENCES

1. Avogaro, P., Cazzolato, G., Bittolo Bon, G., Quinci, G. B., and Chinello, M. (1978): HDL-cholesterol, apolipoproteins A_1 and B. Age and index body weight. *Atherosclerosis,* 31:85–91.
2. Avogaro, P., Cazzolato, G., Bittolo Bon, G., and Quinci, G. B. (1979): Are apolipoproteins better discriminators than lipids for atherosclerosis? *Lancet;* I:901–903.
3. Castelli, W. P., Doyle, J. T., Gordon, T., Hames, C. G., Hjortland, M. C., Hulley, S. B.,

Kagan, A., and Zukel, W. J. (1977): HDL-cholesterol and other lipids in coronary heart disease. The cooperative lipoprotein phenotyping study. *Circulation,* 5:767–772.

4. Haiat, R., Bugugnani, M. J., and Fouyè, H. (1979): Le HDL-cholesterol: un nouvel indice d'appreciation du risque cardio-vasculaire? *Coeur Med. Int.,* 2:213–217.

5. Hulley, S. B., Cohen, R., and Widdowson, G. (1977): Plasma HDL-cholesterol level. Influence of risk factor intervention. *JAMA,* 238:2269.

6. Miller, G. J., and Miller, N. E. (1975): Plasma HDL concentration and development of ischemic heart disease. *Lancet,* 1:16.

7. Sirtori, C. R., Gianfranceschi, G., Gritti, I., Nappi, G., Brambilla, G., and Paoletti, P. (1979): Decreased HDL cholesterol levels in male patients with transient ischemic attacks. *Atherosclerosis,* 32:205–211.

8. Vergani, C., Trovato, G., and Dioguardi, N. (1978): Serum total lipids, lipoproteins, cholesterol, apoproteins A and B in cardiovascular disease. *Clin. Chim. Acta,* 87:127.

Diet and Drugs in Atherosclerosis,
edited by G. Noseda, B. Lewis, and R. Paoletti.
Raven Press, New York © 1980.

The Brisighella Study: A 6-Year Follow-Up

G. C. Descovich, *G. Mannino, U. Montaguti, and S. Lenzi

*Istituto di Clinica Medica II dell'Università di Bologna, Bologna; and *Cattedra di Analisi Numerica dell'Università di Modena, Modena, Italy*

A reduction in the risk of myocardial infarction and other atherosclerotic diseases, obtained with the control of some risk factors, was the aim of the Brisighella study started in the Bologna Lipid Clinic in 1972.

The study had three distinct phases. During the first period, some population characteristics were recorded, related to the main coronary heart disease (CHD) risk factors. The nutritional behavior and environmental situation were also investigated. These prevalence results were adopted to classify subjects into risk classes.

During the second period, the general mortality and morbidity were recorded to evaluate incidence rates of CHD and other atherosclerotic vascular diseases. The main aim was to obtain risk coefficients for every factor under survey, specific to the Brisighella population.

The third phase consisted of preventive intervention directed at a substantial modification of those factors shown by the findings of the second period as being primarily connected to atherosclerotic cardiovascular diseases.

This chapter concerns the cross-sectional and 6-year follow-up results.

MATERIALS AND METHODS

The population sample consisted of 2,939 subjects over age 14 (1,491 males and 1,448 females). Recruitment response was very high (93%).

From the risk factors considered in this study, only results on plasma total cholesterol, blood pressure, and cigarette smoking habits are reported. Total plasma cholesterol was carried out by semiautomatic methods advised by the Italian Lipid Clinic Group.

Quality control was performed together with the Prague WHO Reference Laboratory and three Italian reference centers (Padua, Rome, and Naples).

Blood pressure was taken in accordance with WHO-advised methods. Smoking habits and myocardial infarction, angina pectoris, and claudicatio intermittens histories were obtained using the London School of Hygiene Questionnaires. A 12-lead electrocardiogram was made and classified according to Minnesota Code.

Death causes are classified according to the eighth revision of the WHO International Classification of Diseases and Death Causes.

Subjects who died from myocardial infarction and its late complications and sudden death subjects were considered CHD deaths when other causes could be reasonably excluded. In sudden death, the WHO Infarction Register Criteria (death within 24 hr from the onset of symptoms) were used. Statistical evaluation was performed with univariate and multivariate analysis.

RESULTS

Average plasma cholesterol levels (Fig. 1) increased with age in both sexes. While previous values for females are lower, after the fourth decade, an even more pronounced increase takes place in males. The same trend occurs in plasma triglyceride levels and diastolic and systolic blood pressure.

A hyperlipoproteinemic pattern is evident in 36.6% of males and 34.6% of

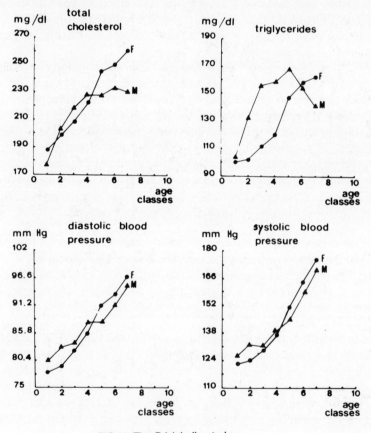

FIG. 1. The Brisighella study.

females. In both sexes, type IIa is more frequent. Type IV pattern is relatively uncommon in females, while in males its frequency is nearer to that of type IIa. More than 50% of males smoked, 36% being heavy smokers. The female group was predominantly composed of nonsmokers, and only 10% were heavy smokers.

After obtaining the prevalence rates, the next step was to divide the population according to the situation with respect to freely determined cutoff points: 240 mg/dl for total cholesterol, 160 mm/Hg for systolic blood pressure, 95 mm/Hg for diastolic blood pressure, and 10 or more cigarettes per day for heavy smokers. Thus females without risk factors are more frequently found than males (28.90 versus 32.04%), while subjects with three risk factors are about five times more often male than female (Table 1).

During the 6-year follow-up period in Brisighella, 52 males and 16 females died. Here only males are considered because of the low statistical significance of the general and CHD female mortality rate.

Comparing the mortality in Italy with that of Brisighella (Table 2), the general and specific death rates are always lower in Brisighella, except for trauma, injuries, and accidents (Table 2). In Brisighella, the most frequent cause of death is cardiovascular disease, and the ratio between cardiovascular diseases and all neoplastic diseases is about 2:1, as in Italy.

In the CHD group, the mean values of total cholesterol and systolic and diastolic blood pressure are higher than in the whole population and in the group of other death causes (Table 3). Such a pronounced difference cannot be demonstrated for blood pressure, even if values shown by the CHD group are always the highest. This aspect is particularly evident in diastolic blood pressure (Table 3).

With respect to the lipoprotein pattern in the CHD group, normals are only 12.5 against 63.3% of subjects who died from other causes, and 64.4% of the total population. The most frequent hyperlipoproteinemic pattern in the CHD group is type IIa, while type IIb and IV frequencies are similar, being slightly less than one-half of type IIa.

TABLE 1. *Brisighella Study: subjects with or without 1, 2, 3 main risk factors*

| | Males | | Females | |
	n	%	n	%
No R.F.	424	28.43	464	32.04
TC	161	10.79	178	12.29
BP	203	13.61	341	23.54
HS	272	18.24	75	5.17
TC + BP	143	9.59	315	21.75
TC + HS	118	7.91	25	1.72
BP + HS	93	6.23	28	1.93
TC + BP + HS	77	5.16	22	1.51

TC = hypercholesterolemia, BP = hypertension, HS = heavy smokers.

TABLE 2

BRISIGHELLA STUDY:

DEATH RATES (x 10.000, x year)

♂	Brisighella (1972-77)	Italy (1969-73)
infectious	———	2.1
neoplasms	15.6	21.9
mental	———	1.3
circulatory	33.5	44.3
respiratory	———	10.5
digestive	2.2	7.7
trauma	8.9	7.6
other causes	———	11.1
TOTAL	60.3	106.8

Using the same cutoff points, the number of subjects who were hypercholesterolemic, hypertensive, and heavy smokers in CHD and other death groups as compared with the total population (Table 3) was verified. Hypercholesterolemic subjects are predominant in the CHD group, but in the group of other causes, the frequency of hypertension is similar to that in the CHD group. This result cannot be explained, but it might be due to the apparent similarity in the mean death age. Heavy smoker frequency in the CHD group is higher than in the group of other causes of death, but it does not reach the level of the total population.

Since the total population contains young people in whom heavy smoking habits are more common, this result may once again be explained in terms of mean death age.

Isolating subjects in 0, 1, 2, and 3 risk factor groups determined as above, and comparing the CHD group to the other causes of death group and to the total population, no subject who died from CHD was shown to be free from risk factors. Furthermore, more than 87% had at least two risk factors.

Although definitive conclusions cannot be drawn because of the low number of deaths, it may be emphasized that CHD seems to be more frequent in subjects with higher levels of plasma cholesterol and systolic and diastolic blood pressure, and appears to occur more frequently in subjects with two or three risk factors.

TABLE 3. *Brisighella study: Risk factors and causes of death*

Risk factor	Total population	CHD	Other causes
Total cholesterol (mg ± SD; mx̄/dl)	222 ± 43	276 ± 45	213 ± 41
Blood pressure (x̄ ± SD, mm Hg)			
Systolic	143 ± 22	169 ± 29	157 ± 32
Diastolic	87 ± 12	96 ± 11	94 ± 18
Nonsmokers (%)	31.05	37.5	16.6
Exsmokers (%)	17.03	16.6	43.3
Smokers (≤10 cig./day) (%)	13.81	12.5	16.6
Smokers (>10 cig./day) (%)	36.28	33.3	23.3
Hypercholesterolemia (no.; all; %)	499/1,491 33.46	21/24 87.50	8/30 26.66
Hypertension (no./all; %)	516/1,491 34.60	21/24 87.50	26/30 86.66
Smokers (10 cig./day) (no.; %)	560/1,491 37.55	8/24 33.33	7/30 23.33
Risk factor (%)			
0	28.90	—	10.0
1	42.64	12.50	56.66
2	23.73	66.66	20.0
3	5.16	20.83	13.33

An attempt to calculate multiple logistic function applying the classic method to age, total cholesterol, systolic and diastolic blood pressure, and smoking habits indicates that systolic blood pressure and total cholesterol are the most important risk factors.

Smoking habits and diastolic blood pressure give results that cannot be explained at present. The suggestion, which might be clarified by the 8-year follow-up findings, is that this is a population sample with a mortality trend different from those shown by populations previously investigated.

The efficacy of the third phase, concerning preventive intervention, is linked to the solution of this problem.

Diet and Drugs in Atherosclerosis,
edited by G. Noseda, B. Lewis, and R. Paoletti.
Raven Press, New York © 1980.

HDL$_2$ and HDL$_3$ Variations During the Postprandial Phase in Humans

R. Fellin, G. Baggio, M. R. Baiocchi, S. Martini, G. Baldo, E. Manzato, and G. Crepaldi

Department of Internal Medicine, Division of Gerontology and Metabolic Diseases, University of Padua, 35100 Padua, Italy

Substantial evidence indicating that different plasma lipoprotein fractions are interrelated in both their protein and lipid portion has accumulated over the past years (6). Many of the processes involved are mediated through the activity of various lipolytic enzymes, some of which are affected by apolipoproteins acting either as cofactors or inhibitors (9). More recently, correlations between the metabolism of chylomicrons and very low density lipoproteins (VLDL) and high density lipoproteins (HDL) have been investigated (3,11). Eisenberg et al. (2) demonstrated *in vitro* that formation of HDL-like particles takes place during the lipoprotein lipase-mediated conversion of triglyceride-rich lipoprotein to intermediate density lipoprotein (IDL). In addition, Patsch et al. (7) showed that HDL$_3$ added to the system during this process is converted to HDL$_2$. In the present study, the relationship between triglyceride-rich lipoprotein and HDL$_2$ and HDL$_3$ during alimentary lipemia in humans was evaluated. During this phase, there is a physiological increase in chylomicrons and VLDL, as well as an activation of lipoprotein lipase activity.

MATERIAL AND METHODS

Subjects

Six male and six female healthy volunteers were studied in the outpatient clinic. The average age in each group was 27.8 and 25.8 years, respectively. All subjects had normal body weight and normal blood lipid levels (Table 1).

Experimental Plan

Following an overnight fast, a blood sample was collected at 11 a.m. At 12:30 p.m., a meal containing 1,500 calories and consisting of 40% fat, 40% carbohydrate, and 20% protein was administered. Cholesterol content was about 500 mg, and alcohol, in the form of wine, about 7.5 g. The polyunsaturated/

TABLE 1. *Cholesterol, triglyceride, and phospholipid basal levels[a] in whole serum, VLDL, LDL, HDL, HDL₂ and HDL₃ fractions in 12 healthy volunteers[b]*

Fraction	Cholesterol (mg/dl)		Triglyceride (mg/dl)		Phospholipid (mg/dl)	
	Males	Females	Males	Females	Males	Females
Whole serum	187.2 ± 15.4	183.7 ± 11.1	78.9 ± 12.9	72.0 ± 8.0	183.0 ± 11.8	209.3 ± 10.1
VLDL	9.5 ± 3.2	6.3 ± 1.4	28.2 ± 6.3	17.7 ± 5.3	—	—
LDL	127.7 ± 15.5	115.2 ± 11.9	34.2 ± 5.9	32.7 ± 3.5	75.2 ± 14.0	97.8 ± 10.3
HDL	50.2 ± 3.9	62.2 ± 6.0	16.8 ± 2.0	21.5 ± 1.0	99.5 ± 8.9	105.8 ± 9.5
HDL₂	7.5 ± 0.9	11.4 ± 1.5^{c}	—	—	13.0 ± 2.2	15.5 ± 2.8^{c}
HDL₃	31.4 ± 2.8	34.6 ± 2.6	—	—	45.9 ± 3.8	49.2 ± 4.6

[a] Mean ± SE.
[b] Six males and six females.
[c] $p < 0.05$.

saturated fatty acid ratio was $2:6$. This meal reflects the alimentary habits of Northern Italy. At 4:30 and 9:00 p.m., blood samples were taken. During the study, the volunteers were required to avoid all stressing psychological and physical activity; they were forbidden to smoke or take drugs (contraceptives included).

Lipoprotein Isolation

Blood specimens were collected in 0.01% EDTA. Plasma was separated immediately in a low speed centrifuge and stored at 4°C. VLDL were isolated by ultracentrifugation for 22 hr at $120,000 \times g$ at 10°C, using a Beckman L5-65B ultracentrifuge and the Ti50 rotor at 1.006 g/ml hydrated density. Floating VLDL were removed by tube slicing technique. Another plasma aliquot was precipitated with 5% (v/v) sodium-heparin (Liquemin 5000, Hoffmann-LaRoche AG, Grenzach) and 5% 1 M $MnCl_2$, kept at 4°C for 16 hr, and then centrifuged for 30 min at 4,000 rpm at room temperature. The filtrate containing HDL was ultracentrifuged for 40 hr at $145,000 \times g$ at 10°C and 1.22 g/ml density. The top fraction was ultracentrifuged again under the same conditions at 1.21 g/ml density, and the succeeding top fraction containing plasma protein-free HDL was ultracentrifuged for 30 hr at $145,000 \times g$ at 10°C and 1.11 g/ml density. Thus HDL₂ were obtained in the supernatant and HDL₃ in the infranatant (4).

Chemical Analysis

Whole plasma and all the fractions were assayed for free and esterified cholesterol [Roschlau's enzymatic method (8)], triglycerides [Wahlefeld's (12) enzymatic method], phospholipids [Zilversmit's (14) colorimetric test], and proteins [according to Lowry et al. (5)].

RESULTS

Basal lipid levels in plasma and in the lipoprotein fractions (Table 1) were similar in males and females. HDL levels were higher in females, but the difference was not statistically significant. In agreement with Shepherd et al. (10), however, we observed significantly higher HDL₂ levels in females compared to males.

Where the behavior of HDL₂ and HDL₃ is studied in the two sexes in the postprandial phase, a mirror-like tendency at 4.5 hr postprandial is observed, especially in the females; a significant increase in HDL₂ corresponds to a decrease in HDL₃ (Fig. 1). At 9 hr postprandial, the HDL₂ level is still significantly higher than basal value. The phenomenon is less marked in the males, in whom HDL₂ increase is slight and gradual up to the 9th hr (Fig. 2), while HDL₃ decrease is similar to that seen in females, but less pronounced. Therefore,

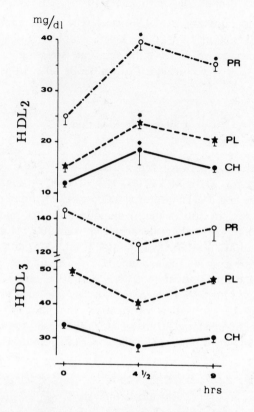

FIG. 1. Protein (PR), phospholipid (PL), and cholesterol (CH) variations (mean ± SE) in HDL_2 and HDL_3 at 4.5 and 9 hr postprandial in six females. $^*p < 0.05$.

the HDL_2/HDL_3 ratio is the parameter that undergoes greatest modification during the postprandial phase (Fig. 3). This ratio increases significantly in the females compared to both basal levels and levels in males and shows maximum increase at 4.5 hr postprandial (lower part of Fig. 3). On the other hand (upper part of Fig. 3), despite similar basal levels, triglycerides increase significantly in both sexes in the postprandial phase but more markedly in the males. This increase is determined by an accumulation of VLDL (chylomicrons and VLDL) that reaches statistically significant levels only in the male at 4.5 hr compared to 0 hr.

DISCUSSION

The results of this study show that in the postprandial phase, the HDL_2 and HDL_3 subfractions present significant variations, but HDL_2, which are

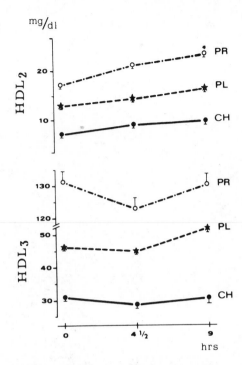

FIG. 2. Protein (PR), phospholipid (PL), and cholesterol (CH) variations (mean ± SE) in HDL_2 and HDL_3 at 4.5 and 9 hr postprandial in six males. *$p < 0.05$.

about one-quarter of the HDL_3, show greater fluctuation. During the postprandial phase, moreover, the HDL_2 increase in the female, compared to the male, is more evident, as already demonstrated in fasting plasma (10). Therefore, the postprandial phase may represent a physiological moment during which the female regulates HDL_2 at higher levels, compared to the male. The reasons for this behavior are not known. However, since HDL_2 formation is related to chylomicron metabolism (2,3), it may be hypothesized that the higher increase in HDL_2 in the fertile female is due to a more pronounced capacity to remove triglyceride-rich particles. It is possible that the transformation of HDL_3 into HDL_2 contributes to the increase in the latter. *In vitro* studies favor this possibility (7).

It has been recently suggested that the putative protection against atherosclerosis in premenopausal women may be related to their higher HDL_2 subfraction (1). It is of interest to evaluate the HDL_2/HDL_3 ratio in relation to the formation and catabolism of chylomicrons in the postprandial phase in order to detect possible alterations in subjects with signs of premature atherosclerosis. This hypothesis is now gaining experimental evidence in animals as well as humans (13).

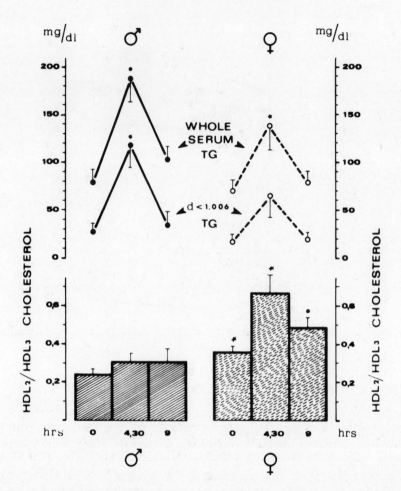

FIG. 3. Variations of whole serum and VLDL (density class < 1.006 g/ml), triglycerides *(upper section)*, and HDL₂/HDL₃ cholesterol ratio *(lower section)* at 4.5 and 9 hr postprandial in six males and six females. *$p < 0.01$.

ACKNOWLEDGMENTS

We thank Eugenia Fellin for skillful preparation of the meals, and Patricia Segato for help in translating this manuscript.

REFERENCES

1. Cheung, M. C., and Albers, J. J. (1977): Distribution of cholesterol and apolipoproteins A-I and A-II in human high density lipoprotein subfractions separated by CsCl equilibrium gradient centrifugation: Evidence for HDL subpopulations with differing A-I/A-II. *J. Clin. Invest.,* 60(3):473–485.

2. Eisenberg, S., Patsch, J. R., Olivecrona, T., and Gotto, A. M., Jr. (1978): Effects of lipolysis on human high density lipoproteins (HDL). *Circulation,* 58:15.
3. Havel, R. J., Kane, J. P., and Kashyap, M. L. (1973): Interchange of apolipoproteins between chylomicrons and high density lipoproteins during alimentary lipaemia in man. *J. Clin. Invest.,* 52:32–38.
4. Kostner, G. M., and Holasek, A. (1977): The separation of human serum high density lipoproteins by hydroxyapatite column chromatography. *Biochim. Biophys. Acta,* 488:417–431.
5. Lowry, O. H., Rosebrough, N. J., Farr, A. L., and Randall, R. J. (1951): Protein measurement with the Folin phenol reagent. *J. Biol. Chem.,* 193:265–275.
6. Nikkilä, E. (1953): Studies on the lipid-protein relationships in normal and pathologic sera and the effect of heparin on serum lipoproteins. *Scand. J. Clin. Lab. Invest. [Suppl.],* 5:158–171.
7. Patsch, J. R., Gotto, A. M., Jr., Olivecrona, T., and Eisenberg, S. (1978): Formation of high density lipoprotein₂-like particles during lipolysis of very low density lipoproteins *in vitro. Proc. Natl. Acad. Sci. USA,* 75:4519–4523.
8. Roschlau, P. (1974): Enzymatische Bestimmung des Gesamt-Cholesterins in Serum. *Chem. Klin. Biochim.,* 12:226–231.
9. Schaefer, E. J., Eisenberg, S., and Levy, R. I. (1978): Lipoprotein apoprotein metabolism. *J. Lipid Res.,* 19:667–687.
10. Shepherd, J., Packard, C. J., Patsch, J. R., Gotto, A. M., Jr., and Taunton, O. D. (1978): Metabolism of apolipoproteins A-I and A-II and its influence on the high density lipoprotein subfraction distribution in males and females. *Eur. J. Clin. Invest.,* 8:115–120.
11. Tall, A. R., and Small, D. M. (1978): Plasma high density lipoproteins. *N. Engl. J. Med.,* 299:1232–1236.
12. Wahlefeld, A. M. (1974): Triglycerides determination after enzymatic hydrolysis. In: *Methoden der enzymatische Analyse,* edited by H. U. Bergmeyer, vol. 2, p. 1878. Verlag Chemie, Weinheim.
13. Zilversmit, D. B. (1979): Atherogenesis: a postprandial phenomenon. *Circulation,* 60(3):473–485.
14. Zilversmit, D. B., and Davis, A. K. (1950): Microdetermination of plasma phospholipids by trichloroacetic. *J. Lab. Clin. Med.,* 35:155–163.

Diet and Drugs in Atherosclerosis,
edited by G. Noseda, B. Lewis, and R. Paoletti.
Raven Press, New York © 1980.

Vascular Prostacyclin Synthesis, Platelet Sensitivity, Plasma Factors, and Platelet Function in Patients With Peripheral Occlusive Arteriopathy With and Without Diabetes Mellitus

Helmut Sinzinger, Josef Kaliman, Kurt Klein, and Karl Silberbauer

Atherosclerosis Research Group, Department of Medical Physiology, Atherosclerosis and Thrombosis Research Commission of the Austrian Academy of Sciences, Department of Cardiology and Second Department of Internal Medicine, University of Vienna, Austria

Prostacyclin (PGI_2), originally discovered by Moncada and co-workers (8), has been shown to be a powerful inhibitor of platelet aggregation. Earlier studies of our group (13,14) demonstrated that in juvenile onset diabetes, the vascular PGI_2 synthesis in forearm venous biopsy specimen was statistically significantly decreased. Similar data were reported for experimental diabetes (3,11). These data demonstrated that in humans, a diminished vascular PGI_2 formation accompanied by an altered platelet function might be responsible by a disturbed thromboregulation (16) for initiation and progression of atherosclerotic vascular disease.

The aim of our study was to prove the functional PGI_2 and platelet behavior in patients with advanced atherosclerosis, i.e., in patients with significant, angiographically documented, peripheral occlusive arteriopathy (POA).

MATERIAL AND METHODS

We studied 80 male patients with occlusive arteriopathy for the following functional tests. In 10 patients with and in 10 without diabetes mellitus, as well as in 10 age-matched controls, the PGI_2, activity of the forearm vein was estimated using our modification (15) of Moncada's bioassay. The activity was expressed in picograms PGI_2 per milligram per minute.

The sensitivity of the platelets of the same patients to exogenous, synthetic PGI_2 in different doses (0.6, 1.2, and 2.4 ng), and the amount of PGI_2 necessary to suppress the ADP-induced platelet aggregation response to the half, were examined (ID_{50}). The synthetic prostacyclin standard was kindly provided by Dr. John E. Pike, The Upjohn Company, Kalamazoo, Michigan. The stimulating effect of patients' plasma on PGI_2 synthesis of vascular rings *in vitro* was tested as described earlier (7). The following platelet function tests were performed:

platelet count, ADP (1 μM/liter)-induced aggregation, collagen-induced aggregation, and the test for circulating microaggregates (17).

RESULTS

The synthesis of PGI_2 in forearm veins of patients with POA is with 1.59 ± 0.73 pg PGI_2/mg/min statistically significantly ($p < 0.0001$) diminished in comparison to the age-matched controls (8.81 ± 2.6 pg PGI_2). In patients with POA and diabetes mellitus, no further change in PGI_2 formation could be found (1.60 ± 0.70 pg PGI_2).

Platelet sensitivity to synthetic PGI_2 *in vitro,* which might be a parameter for the platelet membrane receptor of PGI_2 (10), is not significantly different between POA and controls. However, a statistically significant decrease in sensitivity ($p < 0.05$) in the patients with maturity onset diabetes was observed. This difference was the same for the ID_{50}, as well as for the three doses of PGI_2 used to inhibit ADP-induced platelet aggregation (6).

The plasma is able to stimulate PGI_2 synthesis *in vitro* in comparison to incubation of the vascular rings in buffer. No difference in the effect of the plasma in the three patient groups was found. The Wu index in controls was 0.96 ± 0.03, in patients with POA 0.86 ± 0.10, and in patients with POA and diabetes mellitus 0.85 ± 0.07. The difference was statistically significant between both controls and both patient groups ($p < 0.01$).

The platelet count was not significantly different between the groups. The ADP- and collagen-induced platelet aggregation exhibited hyperreactive platelets. However, the differences between the groups were not statistically significant. The values for the specific platelet proteins β-thromboglobulin and the platelet factor 4 were significantly different between controls and patients (12).

DISCUSSION

Our data demonstrate a statistically significantly diminished PGI_2 synthesis in patients with POA with and without diabetes mellitus (5). No difference could be detected for platelet sensitivity to PGI_2 in POA (6), as it was reported recently for atherosclerotic rabbit platelets (1). However, the sensitivity of platelets of diabetics with POA was significantly altered (6), which confirms data from diabetics (2). This is important, as this sensitivity might correlate to the PGI_2 receptors on the platelet membrane and be, at least in diabetics, in part responsible for the disturbed thromboregulation (16) in this disease. No additional influence by plasma factors was found using normal vascular rings, as reported for uremics (7,9). However, we did not work with diabetic vascular rings, which might detect a different behavior (4). The general finding of a somewhat activated platelet function behavior in combination with diminished vascular PGI_2 formation and platelet sensitivity might be important factors for perpetuation and progression of the atherosclerotic process.

REFERENCES

1. Dembinska-Kiec, A., Rücker, W., and Schönhofer, S. (1979): Prostacyclin-dependent differences in TxA_2 formation by platelets from normal and atherosclerotic rabbits. *Atherosclerosis,* 33:217.
2. Garcia-Conde, J., Amado, J. A., Merino, J., and Benet, I. (1979): Prostaglandin and platelet function in diabetes. *Thromb. Haemost.,* 42:798.
3. Harrison, H. E., Reece, A. H., and Johnson, M. J. (1978): Decreased vascular prostacyclin synthesis in experimental diabetes. *Life Sci.,* 23:351.
4. Johnson, M. J., and Harrison, H. E. (1979): *Personal communication.*
5. Kaliman, J., Schweiger, E., Klein, K., Sinzinger, H., and Silberbauer, K. (1980): Thrombiozyten-funktion und Prostaglandin I_2-Synthese in der Gefässwand bei diabetischen und nicht diabetischen Patienten mit peripherer Verschlusskrankheit. *Verh. Dtsch. Ges. Angiol. (in press).*
6. Klein, K., Kaliman, J., Sinzinger, H., and Silberbauer, K. (1980): Plättchensensitivität für Prostacyclin bei diabetischen und nicht-diabetischen Patienten mit atherosklerotischen Gefässveränderungen—ein Mass für die Prostacyclinrezeptoren der Plättchenmembran? *VASA (in press).*
7. Leithner, Ch., Winter, Ch., Silberbauer, K., Wagner, O., Pinggera, W. F., and Sinzinger, H. (1978): Enhanced prostacyclin availability of blood vessels in uraemic humans and rats. In: *Dialysis, Transplantation Nephrology,* edited by H. Robinson, vol. 15, p. 418. *Proc. Eur. Dialysis Transplant. Assoc.*
8. Moncada, S., Gryglewski, R., Bunting, S., and Vane, J. R. (1976): An enzyme isolated from arteries transforms prostaglandin endoperoxides to an unstable substance that inhibits platelet aggregation. *Nature,* 263:663.
9. Remuzzi, G., Bertani, T., Livio, M., and Cavenaghi, A. E., Mysliwiec, M., Marchesi, D., Donati, M. B., DeGaetano, G., and Mecca, G. (1978): Vascular factors in the pathogenesis of uraemic bleeding. In: *Dialysis Transplantation Nephrology,* edited by H. Robinson, vol. 15, p. 449. *Proc. Eur. Dialysis Transplant. Assoc.*
10. Siegl, A. M., Smith, J. B., Silver, M. J., Nicolaou, K. C., and Ahern, D. (1979): Selective binding site for (^3H) prostacyclin on platelets. *J. Clin. Invest.,* 63:215.
11. Silberbauer, K., Schernthaner, G., Sinzinger, H., Clopath, P., Piza-Katzer, H., and Winter, M. (1979): Diminished prostacyclin generation in human and experimentally induced (streptozotocin, alloxan) diabetes mellitus. *Thromb. Haemost.,* 42:334.
12. Silberbauer, K., Schernthaner, G., Sinzinger, H., and Kaliman, J. (1979): *Unpublished data.*
13. Silberbauer, K., Schernthaner, G., Sinzinger, H., Piza-Katzer, H., and Winter, M. (1979): Decreased vascular prostacyclin in juvenile onset diabetes. *N. Engl. J. Med.,* 300:366.
14. Silberbauer, K., Schernthaner, G., Sinzinger, H., Piza-Katzer, H., and Winter, M. (1979): Elevated plasma β-thromboglobulin and decreased vascular prostacyclin in diabetes mellitus. *Eur. J. Clin. Invest.,* 31:9.
15. Silberbauer, K., Sinzinger, H., and Winter, M. (1978): Prostacyclin production by vascular smooth muscle cells. *Lancet,* i:1356.
16. Sinzinger, H., Silberbauer, K., and Winter, M. (1979): Vaskulärer Faktor als Thromboregulations-mechanismus. In: *Therapiekontrolle in der Angiologie,* edited by R. Hild and G. Spaan, p. 405. Verlag Witzstrock, Baden-Baden.
17. Wu, K. K., and Hook, J. C. (1974): A new method for the quantitative detection of platelet aggregates in patients with arterial insufficiency. *Lancet,* i:24.

Diet and Drugs in Atherosclerosis,
edited by G. Noseda, B. Lewis, and R. Paoletti.
Raven Press, New York © 1980.

Procetofen in Four Types of Hyperlipoproteinemia: Effect on Apo-A and Apo-B Lipoproteins

H. Micheli, D. Pometta, and *A. Gustafson

Division de Diabétologie, Département de Médecine, Hôpital Cantonal, Geneva, Switzerland

Increasing evidence has been obtained in recent years that a substantial decrease of total serum cholesterol reduces significantly the development of atherosclerotic disease in hypercholesterolemic patients. However, the hypolipemic drugs commonly used in addition to diet to obtain this goal are still few, and there is a need for alternative medications when one drug is not well tolerated or not active enough. Therefore, we studied a relatively recent drug, procetofen (Lipanthyl®), which was introduced in Switzerland a year ago (8,11), although it has been used in France for more than 5 years (5,9).

PATIENTS AND METHODS

There were 31 patients in the study. All had a diet appropriate to their type of hyperlipoproteinemia for more than 3 months. Any other hypolipemic drugs were stopped 2 months before the control period. Fasting blood samples were taken at 1-month intervals, twice during the pretest period, and on three occasions during the treatment period. The dose of procetofen was 300 mg/day in all but one patient, in whom it was 200 mg. Patients were seen at each visit by one of us (HM) for checking drug adherence, body weight, and possible side effects. Three other patients were rejected from the study. In two, the reason was a gain or a loss of more than 1.5 kg during the study. The third patient disappeared before the last two controls.

The number of patients with each type of hyperlipoproteinemia is given in Table 1. Six of the 31 patients were females (five type IIa and one type III). Secondary hyperlipoproteinemias were excluded. Seven of the type IIa had a family history of other cases with hypercholesterolemia, and three had tendinous xanthomas. Type IIb and type III hyperlipoproteinemia were diagnosed after two preparative ultracentrifugations at density 1.006 and 1.063. One type II had no floating beta-band on electrophoresis of the $d = 1.006$ supernatant.

---

* *Present address:* University Hospital, Lund, Sweden.

TABLE 1. *Effect of 3 months treatment with procetofen (300 mg) in 31 patients with four types of hyperlipoproteinemia*[a]

Type	Cholesterol (mmoles/liter ± SD)			Triglycerides (mmoles/liter ± SD)		
	Control	Treatment	Mean of individual (% change)	Control	Treatment	Mean of individual (% change)
IIa N=15, t-test	10.49 ± 1.92	8.30 ± 2.25 ($p < 0.001$)	−22%	1.36 ± 0.61	0.92 ± 0.37 ($p < 0.01$)	−32%
IIb (N=10, t-test)	8.70 ± 1.01	7.04 ± 0.85 ($p < 0.01$)	−19%	3.87 ± 2.82	2.38 ± 1.48 ($p < 0.05$)	−38%
III (N=2)	12.20	5.99	−51%	5.67	2.29	−60%
IV (N=4, t-test)	6.35 ± 0.52	6.02 ± 1.25 (NS)	−5%	6.46 ± 2.29	3.08 ± 1.38 NS[a]	−52%

[a]Calculations are based on two individual pretreatment samples (control) and three samples obtained during treatment in each patient. Paired t-test of the difference was $p < 0.05$ at month 1 and 2 even if degree of freedom was 3 only.

Very low density lipoproteins (VLDL) in this patient, however, were excessively rich in cholesterol; low density lipoproteins (LDL) were excessively rich in triglycerides. The patient was considered as having intermediary lipoproteins. Cholesterol was measured by a modification of the Abel-Kendall method using hydrolyzation, extraction with nonane (nonane fraction, Fluka), evaporation, and Liebermann-Burchard reagent (7). For triglycerides, a manual method was used (10).

In a subsample of 11 patients from the type IIa group, we also measured apolipoprotein A (apo-A) and apolipoprotein-B (apo-B) by electroimmunoassay, according to Laurell (3,4). Anti-alpha-lipoprotein serum was purchased from Behring. Anti-apo B was prepared in our laboratory by injecting rabbits with lipoproteins isolated by ultracentrifugation between density 1.030 and 1.050 g/ml. An internal reference serum was used as standard. In each patient, the five serum samples were tested the same day on the same EIA plate while the serum was kept frozen at $-20°C$ up to 6 months (6). Alpha-lipoprotein cholesterol was also measured in these 11 patients after precipitation of apo-B-containing lipoproteins (VLDL and LDL) by heparin-manganese chloride (2).

RESULTS

Results of the effect of procetofen treatment on serum cholesterol and triglycerides are summarized in Table 1. The mean concentrations and percentage changes are calculated in each type from individual mean values obtained from the two blood controls before treatment and of the three samples obtained during treatment.

In the 11 patients in whom it was measured, apo-A increased by 19% after 1 month and up to 28% after 3 months of procetofen medication (Table 2).

TABLE 2. *Percent changes of apo-A, apo-B, alpha-lipoprotein-cholesterol, and serum cholesterol during 3 months treatment with procetofen in 11 patients with type IIa hyperlipoproteinemia*[a]

Parameter	Month		
	1	2	3
Apo-A	+19	+24	+28
(*t*-test)	<0.001	<0.001	<0.001
Alpha-cholesterol	+14	+14	+5
(*t*-test)	<0.05	<0.05	NS
Apo-B	−14	−13	−15
(*t*-test)	<0.001	<0.01	<0.001
Serum cholesterol	−18	−21	−25
(*t*-test)	<0.01	<0.001	<0.001

[a] Apo-A and Apo-B in arbitrary units against a reference serum (see Methods). Statistical differences are calculated by paired *t*-test.

Apo-B decreased by 13 to 15% during the same period. Alpha-lipoprotein cholesterol showed a slightly significant increase at the first two controls, whereas
the small increase seen at the third month was not significant.

SIDE EFFECTS

No side effects were observed, except in one subject who suffered a rash at
the end of 3 months' treatment. The rash disappeared 4 days after withdrawal
of the drug but reappeared within 2 days when the drug was resumed. Two
female patients complained transitorily of fatigue, which was explained in one
case by other reasons. The patient who received only 200 mg/day had this
dose because serum creatinine was 25 mg/liter before the study. The creatinine
concentration increased during the treatment period to 35 mg/liter but was
stable later while procetofen medication was maintained at a lower dosage of
100 mg/day. No increase of serum transaminases were found in those patients
($N = 18$) in whom these enzymes were evaluated after 2 or 3 months of procetofen
treatment.

COMMENTS

Most patients in this study had received other hypolipemic drugs before procetofen, and a number of them had poorly responded to or tolerated these
other drugs. Therefore, this may be a selection of patients difficult to treat.
On the other hand, patients with type IIa had a high mean cholesterol concentration (10.5 mmoles/liter or about 400 mg/100 ml). Such hyperlipoproteinemias
are known to be little influenced by diet alone and difficult to treat efficiently
with hypolipemic drugs. Thus decreases of cholesterol concentrations by 22%
in type IIa and by 19% in type IIb during 3 months' treatment with procetofen
are notable. These figures are similar to but somewhat lower than in most
previous studies with this medication, which are between 24 and 30% (5,9,11);
but they are higher than in one recent study, where starting values of serum
cholesterol were lower (315 mg/100 ml) (8) than in our patients. In the study
where cholesterol decreased by 30% in type IIa and by 27% in type IIb (11),
cholesterol concentrations were rather close to ours in both types. Thus, hyperlipoproteinemias with serum cholesterol as high as seen in familial heterozygote
type IIa are favorably influenced in many cases. In our material, while combining
results of patients with type IIa and IIb ($N = 25$), there were eight patients
in whom the cholesterol value decreased by 29% or more. In other words, 13
of the 25 patients had their cholesterol levels reduced to below 300 mg/100
ml during procetofen treatment, and 11 of these had this value below 280 mg/
100 ml.

Changes in diet are unlikely to have played a role in the improvement of
cholesterol and triglycerides, as body weight was changed by no more than
1.5 kg during the study. During treatment, triglycerides diminished in type

IIa, but cholesterol was not significantly lowered in type IV. While alpha-lipoprotein cholesterol only slightly increased under procetofen, apo-A impressively increased up to 28% at the end of 3 months. This shows a quantitative difference in the action of procetofen on two components of alpha-lipoproteins. The action on apo-A is of major interest, as apo-AI seems to play a role in the esterification of cholesterol (1). However, we do not know from our antiserum whether apo-AI or apo-AII was elevated by procetofen.

The lowering of apo-B was 14%, which was less than the 21% decrease of serum cholesterol in these 11 patients. Interestingly, the effect on apo-B was obtained after 1 month, whereas the lowering of cholesterol was progressive in a few patients, giving as a mean a decrease of 18% at the first month up to 25% at the third month.

SUMMARY

Procetofen (300 mg/day) was given for 3 months to 31 patients with four types of hyperlipoproteinemia. Serum cholesterol decreased by 22% in type IIa ($N = 15$), by 19% in type IIb ($N = 10$), by 51% in the two type III, and by 5% in type IV. Serum triglyceride was lowered, respectively, by 32, 38, 60, and 52% in these four types.

Apo-A in 11 patients with type IIa was increased up to 28%, while alpha-lipoprotein cholesterol was only slightly elevated (mean, 11%). Apo-B in these patients decreased by 14% under procetofen treatment.

Procetofen was well tolerated, except in one patient who developed a rash at the end of 3 months.

REFERENCES

1. Albers, J. J., Lin, J., and Roberts, G. P. (1979): Effects of human plasma apolipoproteins on the activity of purified lecithin:cholesterol acyltransferase. *Artery,* 5:61–75.
2. Burstein, M., Scholnick, H. R., and Morfin, R. (1970): Rapid method for isolation of lipoproteins from human serum by precipitation with polyanions. *J. Lipid Res.,* 11:583–593.
3. Curry, M. D., Alaupovic, P., and Suenram, A. (1976): Determination of apolipoprotein A and its constitutive AI and AII polyseptides by separate electroimmunoassays. *Clin. Chem.,* 22:315–322
4. Curry, M. D., Gustafson, A., Alaupovic, P., and Mc Conathy, W. J. (1978): Electroimmunoassays, radioimmunoassays and radial immunodiffusion assay evaluated for quantification of human apolipoprotein B. *Clin. Chem.,* 24:280–286.
5. Drouin, P., Mejean, L., Sauvanet, J. P., Pointel, J. P., and Debry, G. (1976): Etude de l'action hypolipémiante du procétofène chez des malades porteurs d'une HLP de type IIa ou IIb. *Gaz. Med. France,* 83:3848–3860.
6. Micheli, H., Pometta, D., and Gustafson, A. (1979): Treatment of hyperlipoproteinemia (HLP) type IIa with a new phenoxy-acetic acid derivative procetofen. *Clin. Pharmacol. Biopharm.,* 17:12.
7. Micheli, H., Pometta, D., Jornot, C., and Scherrer, J. R. (1979): High-density lipoprotein cholesterol in male relatives of patients with coronary heart disease. *Atherosclerosis,* 32:269–276.
8. Mordasini, R., Grandjean, E. M., Nobile, P. C., Paumgartner, G., and Riva, G. (1979): Proceto-

fen—Eine Alternative in der Behandlung der Hypercholesterolämie? *Schweiz. Med. Wochenschr.,* 109:1140–1143.

9. Rouffy, J. (1975): A propos du traitement de 100 observations d'hyperlipoprotéinémies essentielles athérogènes. *Sem. Hop. Paris Ther.,* 51:467.

10. Soloni, F. G. (1971): Simplified manual micromethod for determination of serum triglycerides. *Clin. Chem.,* 17:529–534.

11. Staehelin, H. B., Seiler, W., and Pult, N. (1979): Erfahrungen mit dem Lipidsenker Procetofen (Lipanthyl). *Praxis,* 68:24–28.

Diet and Drugs in Atherosclerosis,
edited by G. Noseda, B. Lewis, and R. Paoletti.
Raven Press, New York © 1980.

Drug-Induced Hypolipidemic Effects in Rats: Real Decrease or Altered Tissue Distribution?

C. R. Sirtori, *G. d'Atri, *P. Gomarasca, *E. Galimberti, **D. M. Klurfeld, and **D. Kritchevsky

Center E. Grossi Paoletti and Chemotherapy Chair, University of Milan, 20129 Milan, Italy; *LPB Cinisello Balsamo, Milan, Italy; and **The Wistar Institute, Philadelphia, Pennsylvania 19104

The mechanism of the hypolipidemic activity of drugs chemically related and unrelated to clofibrate (CPIB) is still incompletely understood. Several biochemical changes, among which a reduced liver cholesterol and triglyceride biosynthesis (1) and an enhanced lipoprotein catabolism via lipoprotein lipase (9) have been suggested.

In rodents, all these drugs cause liver enlargement, probably secondary to mitochondrial and peroxisomal proliferation (3). Peroxisome proliferation is associated with an increase of lipid-oxidating enzymes (6) and of the carnitine acyltransferase activity (10). The relevance of these observations, in the clinical realm of application of these drugs, is not clear.

Recent experimental data have also suggested that, in rats, a significant tissue cholesterol accumulation may be the consequence of drug treatments for hyperlipidemia (13). Cholesterol retention and not changes in tissue cholesterol biosynthesis would thus be the suggested mechanism of the hypocholesterolemic effect. These conclusions, based on the analysis of plasma time activity curves of labeled cholesterol, are open to criticism since total radioactivity and not cholesterol specific activity was measured. However, in view of the current interest in the long-term effects of hypolipidemic agents (2), a detailed study was carried out on CPIB and chemically unrelated drugs, with the objective of determining tissue cholesterol distribution in two strains of rats on normal and high fat diets.

CPIB and the chemically unrelated pirinixil (BR-931) (11) were examined in the Sprague-Dawley and Wistar rats. The first strain is a well-known responder to hypolipidemic treatments, whereas the latter usually shows a poor plasma response to these agents (4). In some experiments, Wy 14,643 (13) and tiadenol (7), the former chemically related to pirinixil and the latter unrelated to other hypolipidemic agents, were also tested.

MATERIALS AND METHODS

Animals and Treatments

Male Sprague-Dawley rats (230 to 240 g) and Wistar rats (170 g for the pirinixil experiment, 350 g for the tiadenol study) were used in the experiments. Sprague-Dawley rats received two different dietary treatments; a standard Charles River diet and a cholesterol-cholic acid-supplemented diet (8). Wistar rats received a semipurified, low lipid diet (5).

Drug treatment was carried out by daily administration of the drugs by gastric tube in the Sprague-Dawley rats; the Wistar rats received drugs as a fixed percentage in the diet.

Experimental Protocol

Groups of five Sprague-Dawley rats were treated for 7- and 15-day periods with the standard diet and the concomitant administration of CPIB (200 mg/kg), Wy 14,643 (20 mg/kg), and pirinixil (20 mg/kg) and killed thereafter. Another group of five Sprague-Dawley rats was treated with the cholesterol-cholic acid diet and similar doses of the three drugs; they were killed after 15 days.

All the experiments in the Wistar rats were carried out for 21 days by administration of the semipurified diet or of the diet mixed with appropriate drug concentrations. Animals were killed at the end of treatment.

Biochemical Analyses

Cholesterol and triglyceride levels were determined in the plasma of both rat strains. In addition, liver cholesterol levels were estimated in the Wistar rats, whereas liver, spleen, kidney, heart, lung, duodenum, ileum, colon, and aortic cholesterol levels were assayed in the Sprague-Dawleys. Fragments of the selected tissues were homogenized and saponified in alcoholic KOH. Lipids were extracted by chloroform/methanol (2:1) and cholesterol assayed as in plasma. Serum volume was estimated as 3% of body weight.

RESULTS

Sprague-Dawley Rats

On a standard diet, the three tested drugs (Wy 14,643, pirinixil, and CPIB) all significantly reduced plasma cholesterol levels after 7 and 15 days of treatment (Table 1). All three drugs also significantly increased liver weight, most markedly Wy 14,643, followed by CPIB and pirinixil. However, total liver cholesterol levels were only moderately increased by the three agents. The only statistically significant liver cholesterol increase was found with Wy 14,643 after 15 days

TABLE 1. Normal diet: 7-day and 15-day treatments

Tissues	Days	Control	Wy 14,643 (20 mg/kg)	Pirinixil (20 mg/kg)	CPIB (200 mg/kg)
Plasma-cholesterol (mg/100 ml)	7	82.5 ± 1.69	58.9 ± 6.07[a]	63.9 ± 5.72[a]	56.2 ± 7.22[a]
	15	64.2 ± 5.61	43.9 ± 4.10[a]	52.7 ± 2.83[a]	42.5 ± 5.37[a]
Liver					
Relative weight (100 g/bw)	7	4.260 ± 0.215	6.558 ± 0.195[b]	5.543 ± 0.213[a]	5.442 ± 0.083[b]
	15	4.664 ± 0.147	6.610 ± 0.236[b]	6.082 ± 0.249[b]	5.963 ± 0.330[a]
Total cholesterol (mg)	7	32.83 ± 1.43	38.62 ± 1.37[a]	38.05 ± 0.740[a]	35.35 ± 1.11
	15	37.08 ± 1.75	46.48 ± 2.58[a]	41.36 ± 3.12	42.58 ± 3.03
Spleen: total cholesterol (mg)	7	2.53 ± 0.03	1.96 ± 0.09[b]	1.99 ± 0.09[b]	2.02 ± 0.25
	15	2.68 ± 0.13	3.02 ± 0.14	3.12 ± 0.03[a]	3.24 ± 0.26
Kidney: total cholesterol (mg)	7	3.90 ± 0.21	3.93 ± 0.19	3.97 ± 0.14	3.22 ± 0.07[a]
	15	3.61 ± 0.33	3.18 ± 0.18	3.56 ± 0.18	3.55 ± 0.25
Heart: total cholesterol (mg)	7	1.25 ± 0.09	1.37 ± 0.04	1.39 ± 0.08	1.41 ± 0.06
	15	1.75 ± 0.02	1.67 ± 0.10	1.72 ± 0.11	1.69 ± 0.04
Lung: total cholesterol (mg)	7	5.30 ± 0.30	6.01 ± 0.49	6.91 ± 0.33[a]	6.43 ± 0.77[a]
	15	6.36 ± 0.43	7.31 ± 0.46	8.55 ± 0.14[b]	8.26 ± 0.57[a]
Duodenum: cholesterol (mg/g tissue)	7	2.51 ± 0.07	2.35 ± 0.02	2.42 ± 0.17	2.10 ± 0.03[b]
	15	2.16 ± 0.12	3.96 ± 0.39[a]	3.46 ± 0.57	2.74 ± 0.51
Jejunum: cholesterol (mg/g tissue)	7	2.41 ± 0.16	2.37 ± 0.21	2.42 ± 0.13	2.40 ± 0.14
Ileum: cholesterol (mg/g tissue)	15	3.01 ± 0.15	3.16 ± 0.08	2.91 ± 0.06	1.94 ± 0.63
Colon: cholesterol (mg/g tissue)	7	1.81 ± 0.38	1.98 ± 0.43	1.12 ± 0.35	2.33 ± 0.31
	15	1.25 ± 0.18	1.15 ± 0.36	1.34 ± 0.38	3.33 ± 0.38[b]
Aorta: cholesterol (mg/g tissue)[c]	7	2.22	2.28	2.14	1.90
	15	2.60	2.99	2.12	2.85

x̄ ± SEM. Rats were intubated daily.
[a] $p < 0.05$ versus control.
[b] $p < 0.01$ versus control.
[c] Pools of five arteries.

TABLE 2. *Nath diet: 15-day treatment*

Tissue	Control	Nath diet	Wy 14,643 (20 mg/kg)	Pirinixil (20 mg/kg)	Clofibrate (200 mg/kg)
Plasma-cholesterol (mg/100 ml)	71.5 ± 6.83	1776 ± 365.6	533 ± 90.2[b]	763 ± 69.6[b]	662 ± 99.1[b]
Liver					
Relative weight (100 g/bw)	4.540 ± 0.15	5.380 ± 0.06	7.865 ± 0.32[a]	6.820 ± 0.22[b]	6.957 ± 0.15[b]
Total cholesterol (mg)	29.58 ± 4.03	630.50 ± 174.1	708.96 ± 196.2	418.97 ± 87.7[b]	640.65 ± 181.8
Spleen: total cholesterol (mg)	2.42 ± 0.18	4.97 ± 0.99	2.83 ± 0.23[b]	3.05 ± 0.45[a]	2.48 ± 0.34[b]
Kidney: total cholesterol (mg)	2.36 ± 0.06	3.03 ± 0.29	2.22 ± 0.15[b]	2.48 ± 0.33[a]	2.48 ± 0.22[a]
Heart: total cholesterol (mg)	1.41 ± 0.03	2.52 ± 0.21	1.45 ± 0.06[a]	1.41 ± 0.10[a]	1.40 ± 0.12[a]
Lung: total cholesterol (mg)	6.75 ± 0.38	7.92 ± 0.51	7.09 ± 0.36	7.11 ± 0.35	6.95 ± 0.27[a]
Duodenum: cholesterol (mg/g tissue)	2.96 ± 0.13	6.98 ± 0.66	4.25 ± 0.32[b]	7.55 ± 2.16	5.82 ± 0.72[a]
Jejunum: cholesterol (mg/g tissue)	2.26 ± 0.18	5.82 ± 0.92	3.71 ± 0.53[b]	5.70 ± 1.23	5.05 ± 0.53
Ileum:					
Colon: cholesterol (mg/g tissue)	2.88 ± 0.13	5.86 ± 0.77	3.77 ± 0.29[a]	4.64 ± 0.36[a]	4.31 ± 0.20[a]
Aorta: cholesterol (mg/g tissue)[c]	2.26	3.24	2.38	2.59	3.85

$\bar{x}$ ± SEM. Rats were intubated daily.

[a] $p \pm 0.05$ versus Nath diet.
[b] $p < 0.01$ versus Nath diet.
[c] Pools of five arteries.

of treatment. No changes were found in the spleen and kidney weight and cholesterol content at the two intervals of treatment. Only in the lungs was a significant cholesterol increase detected with the pirinixil and CPIB treatments; the increase was statistically significant with CPIB only at the 7-day interval, and with pirinixil after both 7 and 15 days of treatment. Wy 14,643 and pirinixil did not modify the intestinal cholesterol concentration, whereas CPIB markedly increased the cholesterol concentration of the colonic wall after 7 and 15 days.

On a high fat regimen, all three drugs exerted a marked reduction of plasma cholesterol levels (Table 2). This was most significant with Wy 14,643, less so with CPIB and pirinixil. Liver weight and cholesterol content were also markedly raised by the diet. The three drugs again all increased the relative liver weight, Wy 14,643 being the most active, followed by CPIB and pirinixil. However, total liver cholesterol content was only increased about 10% by Wy 14,643; it was not changed by CPIB, and it was significantly reduced by pirinixil. Total cholesterol content was also reduced in the spleen, kidney, and heart by all three drugs. Analyses of the cholesterol concentrations in the intestinal wall gave variable findings. Wy 14,643 significantly reduced duodenal and colonic cholesterol concentrations. CPIB and pirinixil caused negligible changes in the duodenal and ileal cholesterol concentrations, but both these drugs decreased the cholesterol concentration in the colonic wall approximately 20%.

Wistar Rats

Tiadenol (0.10% in the diet) and pirinixil (0.05%) were tested in two separate experiments on a 21-day schedule. Both compounds failed to reduce plasma cholesterol and triglyceride levels (Table 3); indeed, pirinixil significantly increased plasma cholesterol. Both increased liver weight; however, pirinixil decreased liver cholesterol concentrations and total liver cholesterol 50 to 25%,

TABLE 3. *Plasma and liver lipid charges in Wistar rats following pirinixil and tiadenol treatments*

	Cholesterol ($\bar{x} \pm$ SEM)	
Treatment	Control	Drug
Pirinixil 0.05%[a]		
Plasma (mg/dl)	68 ± 7	93 ± 7^c
Liver (total mg)	47 ± 2	37 ± 3^b
Plasma + Liver (mg)	53.5	43.7
Tiadenol 0.10%[a]		
Plasma (mg/dl)	144 ± 6	162 ± 14
Liver (total mg)	21 ± 1	33 ± 1^b
Plasma + Liver (mg)	35.3	49.9

[a] Drug concentration in the ad lib diet.
[b] $p < 0.05$.
[c] $p < 0.01$.

respectively, whereas tiadenol only moderately reduced liver cholesterol concentrations and increased, by approximately 20%, the total liver content. The liver + plasma cholesterol pools were reduced 18% by pirinixil and increased about 28% by tiadenol.

DISCUSSION

The results presented here do not support the hypothesis that cholesterol retention in the body may explain the plasma cholesterol reduction observed in rats after hypolipidemic treatments. Indeed, even in the case of the Wistar rats, who do not respond with a plasma lipid lowering effect to these agents, pirinixil, like its analog Wy 14,643 and CPIB *(unpublished data),* induced a significant liver cholesterol depletion. The only contrasting findings were obtained with tiadenol, tested only in the Wistar rats. Tiadenol increased total liver cholesterol while not changing plasma cholesterol levels. Similar findings were obtained with this agent in younger rats.

A more detailed analysis was carried out with CPIB, Wy 14,643, and pirinixil in the Sprague-Dawley rats on both standard and high fat regimens. On a standard diet, after 7 and 15 days of treatment, all three drugs significantly reduced plasma cholesterol levels and increased liver weight. However, none of the three, with the possible exception of Wy 14,643 after 15 days, significantly increased total liver cholesterol. An inconstant cholesterol increase was detected in the lungs with all three agents. The marked cholesterol increase in the colonic wall induced by CPIB was an unexpected finding. The relevance of this observation, in view of the reported high incidence of colon tumors in CPIB-treated individuals (2), should be further evaluated.

During the high lipid regimen in the Sprague-Dawley rats, all three tested drugs showed a remarkable plasma cholesterol lowering effect, as already noted by Tomarelli et al. (13). However, even in these conditions, none of the three drugs enhanced cholesterol retention in the liver. Indeed, pirinixil significantly reduced liver cholesterol levels. Cholesterol retention in the colon was not confirmed on this dietary regimen, all three agents generally decreasing the cholesterol content of the spleen, kidney, and major portions of the gastrointestinal system.

In conclusion, this detailed analysis of cholesterol distribution in two different rat strains treated with chemically related and unrelated hypolipidemic agents supports the hypothesis that tissue cholesterol depletion, rather than cumulation, similar to that noted in humans (12), is a likely mechanism for plasma cholesterol reduction.

REFERENCES

1. Adams, L. L., Webb, W. W., and Fallon, H. J. (1971): Inhibition of hepatic triglyceride formation by clofibrate. *J. Clin. Invest.,* 50:2339–2347.

2. Committee of Principal Investigators (1978): A cooperative trial in the primary prevention of ischemic heart disease using clofibrate. *Br. Heart J.,* 40:1069–1118.
3. Hess, R., Staubli, W., and Riess, W. (1965): Nature of the hepatomegalic effect produced by ethylchlorophenoxyisobutyrate in the rat. *Nature,* 208:856–858.
4. Kritchevsky, D., Klurfeld, D. M., Tepper, S. A., Mueller, M. A., Puglisi, L., and Sirtori, C. R. (1980): Increased plasma cholesterol and decreased body lipid levels in Wistar rats following pirinixil (BR 931) treatment. *Pharmacol. Res. Commun.,* 11:475–485.
5. Kritchevsky, D., Whitehouse, M. W., and Staple, E. (1960): Oxidation of cholesterol-26-C^{14} by rat liver mitochondria: Effect of nicotinic acid. *J. Lipid Res.,* 1:154–158.
6. Lazarow, P. B. (1978): Rat liver peroxisomes catalyze the β oxidation of fatty acids. *J. Biol. Chem.,* 253:1522–1528.
7. Martin, E., and Feldmann, G. (1974): Etude hystologique et ultrastructurale du foie chez le rat aprés administration subaigue d'un nouvel agent hypolipidémiant, le bis-(hydroxyethyl-thio) 1.10 decane. *Pathol. Biol.,* XXII–II:179–188.
8. Nath, N., Wiener R., Harper, A. E., and Elvehjem, C. A. (1959): Diet and cholesterolemia. Part 1 (Development of a diet for the study of nutritional factors affecting cholesterolemia in rats.) *J. Nutr.,* 67:289–301.
9. Nikkila, E. A., Huttunen, J. K., and Ehnholm, C. (1977): Effect of clofibrate on postheparin plasma triglyceride lipase activities in patients with hypertriglyceridemia. *Metabolism,* 26:179–186.
10. Reddy, J. K., Moody, D. E., Azarnoff, D. L., and Rao, M. S. (1977): Hepatic catalase is not essential for the hypolipidemic action of peroxisome proliferators. *Proc. Soc. Exp. Biol. Med.,* 154:483–487.
11. Sirtori, C. R., Gomarasca, P., d'Atri, G., Cerutti, S., Tronconi, G., and Scolastico, C. (1978): Pharmacological profile of BR-931, a new hypolipidemic agent that increases high-density lipoproteins. *Atherosclerosis,* 30:45–56.
12. Sodhi, M. S., Kudchodkar, B. J., and Horlick, L. (1973): Hypocholesterolemic agents and mobilization of tissue cholesterol in man. *Atherosclerosis,* 17:1–19.
13. Tomarelli, R. M., Bauman, L. M., and Savini, S. (1978): Effect of Wy-14,643 on cholesterol metabolism in normal and hypercholesterolemic rats. *Atherosclerosis,* 30:301–311.

Diet and Drugs in Atherosclerosis,
edited by G. Noseda, B. Lewis, and R. Paoletti.
Raven Press, New York © 1980.

Effect of Antilipidemic Agents on the Proliferative Activity and Glycosaminoglycan Synthesis of Cultured Aortic Endothelial Cells

Magdolna Bihari-Varga, Eva Csonka, and H. Jellinek

Second Department of Pathology, Semmelweis Medical University, Budapest, 1091 Hungary

In our experiments, the *in vitro* effect of two antilipidemic agents, pyrido-1,2 pyrimidine [Chinoin-123 (CH-123)] and clofibrate (Miscelron®), on the proliferation and on the glycosaminoglycan (GAG) synthesis of pig aortic endothelial cells has been examined.

MATERIAL AND METHODS

Culture Methods

Endothelial cell monolayers (BAEC) were prepared from the carotid arteries of Minnesota minipigs as described earlier (3). Based on the results of our previous investigations (1), the most favorable conditions to study the effect of drugs on endothelial cells was chosen. CH-123 and clofibrate were added in increasing concentrations (10^{-8} to 10^{-3}) to the medium of parallel series of cultures of the sixth passage. The alterations caused were checked on the ninth day in culture. The medium was not changed during the course of the experiment.

Cell Count

Cell number was estimated by triplicate counting in Bürker's chamber.

GAG Analysis

GAG contained in the cells and in the growth medium were analyzed separately. Proteolytic digestion of the cell samples or medium was performed with papain (Merck, Darmstadt) (0.1 M EDTA; 0.01 M cysteine. HCl; pH, 5.8). Total GAG content was measured by hexuronic acid determination, according to Bitter and Muir (2).

Characterization of GAG was based on enzymatic (7), electrophoretic (6), and degradation (5) methods. The relative amount of the different GAG was

111

estimated by densitometric scanning of cellulose acetate electrophoretograms (0.3 M calcium acetate; pH, 4.1; 5 V/cm; 4 hr) stained with Alcian blue. Protein determination was carried out as described by Lowry et al. (4).

RESULTS AND DISCUSSION

CH-123 was found to be effective in concentrations between 0.1 and 100 μmoles. In this range, CH-123 increased cell proliferation and inhibited GAG synthesis, as reflected by the decreased GAG content of the cells and of the medium. The most expressed change took place when 10 μmoles CH-123 was present in the medium (Fig. 1a). The GAG pattern of the cells was also influenced

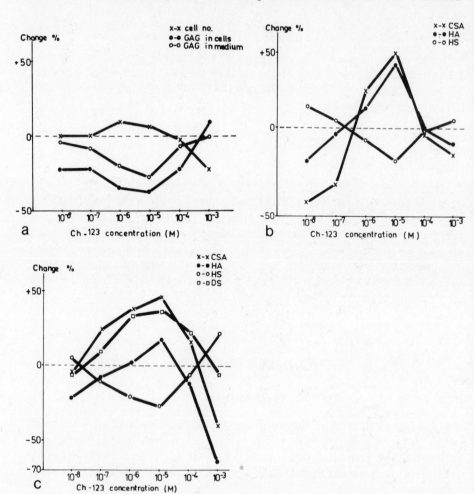

FIG. 1. Changes in the count of endothelial cells and in the GAG content of the cells and of the media **(a)**, in the GAG composition of endothelial cells **(b)**, and in the GAG composition of endothelial culture medium as a function of CH-123 concentration **(c)**.

by the addition of CH-123; the relative amount of chondroitin sulfate (CSA) and of hyaluronic acid (HA) increased, showing peak values at 10 μmoles CH-123 concentration, while the concentration of heparan sulfate (HS) varied inversely (Fig. 1b). Alterations in the rate of excretion showed similar tendencies: CSA, HA, and dermatan sulfate (DS) varied according to a maximum curve and HS to a minimum curve (Fig. 1c).

The addition of clofibrate to the culture medium resulted in somewhat different alterations. The proliferation rate was not altered by the presence of clofibrate within the concentration range investigated by us. GAG synthesis and excretion was stimulated by lower concentrations of the drug and inhibited by higher concentrations (Fig. 2a). From among the individual GAG, in contrast to CH-123

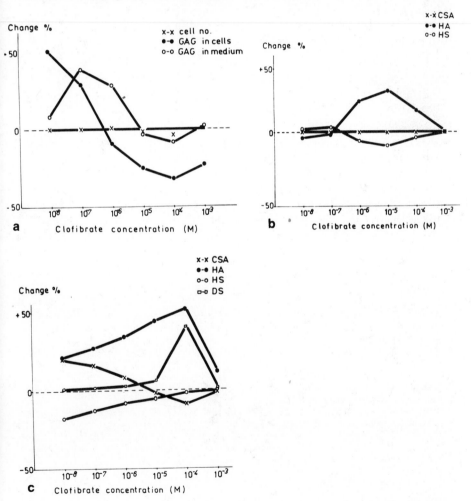

FIG. 2. Changes in the count of endothelial cells and in the GAG content of the cells and of the media **(a)**, in the GAG composition of endothelial cells **(b)**, and in the GAG composition of endothelial culture medium as a function of clofibrate concentration **(c)**.

clofibrate did not influence CSA synthesis within the cells. The increase in HA concentration and the decrease in HS content could be demonstrated (Fig. 2b). Changes in the GAG pattern of the culture medium differed also from those caused by CH-123. The addition of clofibrate resulted in a minimum curve in CSA content, when it was plotted as a function of the concentration of the drug. HS concentrations also were decreased; the effect was most expressed at 0.01 μmoles. Alterations in HA and DS content showed similar tendencies to those measured in the presence of CH-123 (Fig. 2c).

From the results presented above, it might be concluded that both investigated drugs caused alterations in the GAG synthesis and excretion of cultured pig endothelial cells. The changes in the GAG content and pattern of the cells and of the culture media, as well as the most effective drug concentration, was characteristic of the drug. CH-123, in addition, had an influence on cell proliferation.

SUMMARY

The effect of CH-123 and clofibrate on endothelial cells was examined by adding them in increasing concentrations (10^{-3} to 10^{-8} M) to the medium of monolayer cultures prepared from pig carotid arteries. The extent to which cellular GAG content and distribution were influenced was studied. CH-123 showed a slight enhancement of cell proliferation, accompanied by a dose-dependent decrease in GAG synthesis and secretion. From among the individual GAG components, the amount of chondroitin-4-sulfate and of HA was elevated in both the cells and the culture medium.

The addition of clofibrate did not influence cell proliferation and increased GAG synthesis.

REFERENCES

1. Bihari-Varga, M., Csonka, E., Gruber, E., and Jellinek, H. (1980): Age-related changes in the glycosaminoglycans and collagen of cultured pig endothelial cells. *Artery (in press)*.
2. Bitter, T., and Muir, H. (1962): A modified uronic acid carbazole reaction. *Anal. Biochem.,* 4:330.
3. Csonka, E., Kerényi, T., Koch, A. S., and Jellinek, H. (1975): In vitro cultivation and identification of aortic endothelium from miniature pig. *Arterial Wall*, 3:31.
4. Lowry, O. H., Rosenbrough, V. J., Farr, L. A., and Randall, R. J. (1951): Protein measurement with the Folin phenol reagent. *J. Biol. Chem.,* 193:265.
5. Malmström, A., Carlstedt, I., Aberg, L., and Fransson, L. A. (1975): The copolymeric structure of dermatan sulfate. *Biochem. J.,* 151:477.
6. Merrilees, M. J., Merrilees, M. A., Birnbaum, P. S., Scott, P. J., and Flint, M. H. (1977): The effect of centrifugal force on glycosaminoglycan production by aortic smooth muscle cells in culture. *Atherosclerosis,* 27:259.
7. Murata, K., Ogura, T., and Oknyama, T. (1974): The acidic glycosaminoglycans in leukocytes, an application of enzymatic methods. *Connect. Tissue Res.,* 2:101.

Diet and Drugs in Atherosclerosis,
edited by G. Noseda, B. Lewis, and R. Paoletti.
Raven Press, New York © 1980.

Effects of Biguanides on Lipid Metabolism

Sergio Muntoni

Center for Metabolic Diseases and Atherosclerosis, Regional General Hospital,
09100 Cagliari, Italy

Biguanides affect both carbohydrate and lipid metabolism. Their most typical effects include lowering hyperglycemia in the maturity-onset obese-diabetic syndrome and hypertriglyceridemia in type IV hyperlipoproteinemia, two frequently associated conditions (2). However, a deeper insight into the mechanism of their metabolic effects showed that biguanides must be considered as drugs acting primarily on lipid metabolism (15).

We first analyzed the action of biguanides at the subcellular level and then considered the resulting effects at the integrated metabolic level.

MECHANISM OF ACTION OF BIGUANIDES

Owing to their molecular structure, biguanides interact with biological membranes, particularly those of mitochondria (23), wherein they accumulate against the concentration gradient (7).

Whether the resulting effects are toxic or therapeutic depends on drug concentrations. High concentrations inhibit the oxidative phosphorylation and hence ATP generation (20), the main consequences at the integrated metabolic level being anaerobic glycolysis and lactic acidosis. Low concentrations (10^{-5} to 10^{-4} M), corresponding to those occurring in various tissues after therapeutic doses (12,14,27), were shown by us (17) to (a) depress selectively the oxidation rate of fatty acids (FA), while leaving unaffected the oxidative capacity of mitochondria, and (b) restore the glucose oxidation depressed by palmitic acid, indicating that such an increase in glucose oxidation was due to the depression of FA oxidation produced by biguanides.

The above data suggest that (a) the FA oxidase system is more sensitive, or its site more accessible, to biguanides than other enzymatic systems of the mitochondrial machinery (such differences are reflected by the "therapeutic index" of biguanides), and (b) the effects of biguanides on carbohydrate and lipid metabolism are tightly coupled (the primary effect being the depression of FA oxidation), which produces a shift in the glucose-FA cycle (21) toward a metabolic setting more favorable to glucose utilization (15).

115

EFFECTS ON LIPID METABOLISM

The effects of biguanides on lipid metabolism, at both the cellular and integrated levels, appear to be rather more complex than would be expected from the sole depression of the FA oxidation rate. In fact biguanides, at concentrations (or doses) within the therapeutic range (a) depress lipogenesis in adipose tissue (19) and liver (1); (b) depress basal and hormone-stimulated lipolysis in adipocytes (4); (c) depress FA oxidation in muscle (17); (d) lower plasma FFA turnover rate (16,24,28,29), as a consequence of the effects in (b) and (c); and (e) lower circulating triglyceride levels in endogenous hypertriglyceridemia (6,9,11,13, 26,28).

In addition, in cholesterol-fed rabbits, metformin exerts an antiatherosclerotic effect independent of any changes in plasma lipid levels (1,32). This action is ascribed to changes in the structure and composition of atherogenic very low density lipoproteins (VLDL) toward less atherogenic features (18,22,25).

The hypotriglyceridemic action of biguanides takes place specifically in endogenous hypertriglyceridemia (6,9,11,13,26,28), predominantly through reduction of triglyceride synthesis and VLDL production (28). Such an effect has been recently confirmed in livers from hyperlipemic rats treated with metformin (30).

The mechanism of the hypotriglyceridemic action of biguanides, although incompletely understood, is likely to result from reduction of both hyperinsulinemia (11,28,31) and plasma FFA turnover (16,28,29). It is worthy to note that both hyperinsulinemia (10) and increased turnover of plasma FFA (3) are typical features of obesity, and that biguanides are effective on the metabolic derangements of the obese-diabetic syndrome (15). Therefore, the antidiabetic and hypotriglyceridemic effects of biguanides are likely to stem from an underlying common mechanism. Such a mechanism can be outlined as follows (see also Fig. 1): The simultaneous depression of lipolysis in adipose tissue (4) and of

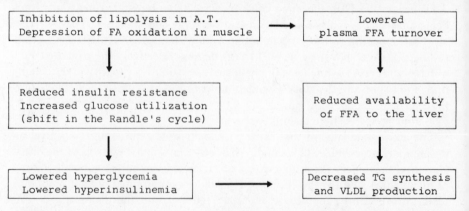

FIG. 1. Outline of the mechanisms of the antidiabetic and hypotriglyceridemic activities of biguanides.

FA oxidation in muscle (15) results in a decrease in plasma FFA turnover (16,29) and an increase in peripheral glucose utilization, and hence a reduction of hyperinsulinemia (10,11), as a consequence of reduced insulin resistance. The combination of decreased FFA supply to the liver and of lowered hyperinsulinemia results in decreased triglyceride synthesis and VLDL production. A more detailed outline of the hypotriglyceridemic effect of biguanides with respect to the feeding condition has been proposed elsewhere (15,16).

In addition to the above actions which are exerted by all the antidiabetic biguanides, metformin has been shown to modify composition (25), turnover (22), and aortic uptake (22) of VLDL. The protection of the arterial walls by metformin (1,32) seems to be related to structural alterations of VLDL. These changes are likely to be produced at some steps of the intestinal lipoprotein biosynthesis, owing to the fact that metformin accumulates in the intestinal mucosa (32). The modifications observed in the VLDL structure of hypercholesterolemic rabbits (22) and of type III patients treated with metformin (18), resulting in less atherogenic features, may explain the antiatherosclerotic activity, independent of the reduction of plasma lipid levels, exerted by metformin in both experimental animals (1,32) and humans (5,8).

CONCLUSIONS

Besides possessing antidiabetic activity, biguanides are effective lipid-lowering agents in type IV hyperlipoproteinemia. In addition, metformin exerts an antiatherosclerotic action independent of its effect on plasma lipid levels through modifications of composition, turnover, and arterial uptake of VLDL.

REFERENCES

1. Agid, R., Marquié, G., and Lafontan, M. (1975): Effets comparatifs des sulfamides hypoglycémiants et des biguanides antidiabétiques sur les lésions vasculaires et les troubles lipidiques entraînés par des régimes athérogènes chez le lapin. In: *Journées annuelles de Diabétologie de l'Hôtel-Dieu,* edited by M. Rathery, pp. 259–278. Flammarion, Paris.
2. Bagdade, J. D., Bierman, E. L., and Porte, D., Jr. (1971): Influence of obesity on the relationship between insulin and triglyceride levels in endogenous hypertriglyceridemia. *Diabetes,* 20:664–672.
3. Birkenhäger, J. C., and Tjabbes, T. (1969): Turnover rate of plasma FFA and rate of esterification of plasma FFA to plasma triglycerides in obese humans before and after weight reduction. *Metabolism,* 18:18–32.
4. Brown, J. D., Stone, D. B., and Steele, A. A. (1969): Mechanism of action of antilipolytic agents: Comparison of the effects of insulin, tolbutamide and phenformin on lipolysis induced by dibutyryl cyclic AMP plus teophyllin. *Metabolism,* 18:926–929.
5. Conti, F., Sirtori, M., Gianfranceschi, G., Tremoli, E., and Sirtori, C. R. (1976): Impiego della metformina nel trattamento delle arteriopatie arteriosclerotiche degli arti inferiori. *Giorn. Arterioscl.,* 1:53–57.
6. Crepaldi, G. (1974): Treatment of hyperlipoproteinemia with metformin. In: *Atherosclerosis III,* edited by F. G. Schettler and A. Weizel, p. 801. Springer-Verlag, Berlin.
7. Davidoff, F. (1971): Effects of guanidine derivatives on mitochondrial function. III. The mechanism of phenethylbiguanide accumulation and its relationship to in vitro respiratory inhibition. *J. Biol. Chem.,* 246:4017–4027.

8. Descovich, G. C., Montaguti, U., Ceredi, C., Cocuźza, E., and Sirtori, C. R. (1978): Long-term treatment with metformin in a large cohort of hyperlipidemic patients. *Artery,* 4:348–359.

9. Fedele, D., Tiengo, A., Nosadini, R., Marchiori, E., Briani, G., Garotti, M. C., and Muggeo, M. (1976): Hypolipidemic effects of metformin in hyperprebetalipoproteinemia. *Diabete Metab.,* 2:127–134.

10. Grodsky, G. M., Karam, J. H., Pavlatos, F. C., and Forsham, P. H. (1963): Reduction by phenformin of excessive insulin levels after glucose loading in obese and diabetic subjects. *Metabolism,* 12:278–286.

11. Gustafson, A., Bjöntorp, P., and Fahlen, M. (1971): Metformin administration in hyperlipidemic states. *Acta Med. Scand.,* 190:491–494.

12. Hall, H., Ramachander, G., and Glassman, J. M. (1968): Tissue distribution and excretion of phenformin in normal and diabetic animals. *Ann. NY Acad. Sci.,* 148:601–611.

13. Lang, P. D., Vollmar, J., Klemens, U. H., Löwis of Menar, P., Gries F. A., Koschinsky, T., Huth, K., Pilz, E., Schlierf, G., Kremer, G. J., Lenhart, P., Schwandt, P., Hammel, H., and Studlar, M. (1973): Die Lipidskende wirkung von Phenformin bei primärer Hyperlipoproteinämie Typ IV. *Dtsch. Med. Wochenschr.,* 98:2280–2286.

14. Lintz, W., Berger, W., Aenishaenslin, W., Kutova, V., Baerlocher, Ch., Kapp, J. P., and Beckmann, R. (1974): Butylbiguanide concentration in plasma, liver, and intestine after intravenous and oral administration to man. *Eur. J. Clin. Pharmacol.,* 7:433–448.

15. Muntoni, S. (1974): Inhibition of fatty acid oxidation by biguanides: Implications for metabolic physiopathology. *Adv. Lipid Res.,* 12:311–377.

16. Muntoni, S., Tagliamonte, P., and Pintus, F. (1978): Metformin and plasma FFA turnover in man. In: *International Conference on Atherosclerosis,* edited by L. A. Carlson, R. Paoletti, C. R. Sirtori, and G. Weber, pp. 333–338. Raven Press, New York.

17. Muntoni, S., Tagliamonte, P., Sirigu, F., and Corsini, G. U. (1973): Demonstration of the mechanism of action of biguanides. *Acta Diabetol. Lat.,* 10:1300–1307.

18. Paoletti, R., Ghiselli, G. C., Fumagalli, R., and Sirtori, C. R. (1976): New advances in antiatherosclerotic drugs. In: *International Conference on Atherosclerosis,* edited by L. A. Carlson, R. Paoletti, C. R. Sirtori, and G. Weber, pp. 29–34. Raven Press, New York.

19. Pereira, J. N., Jangaard, N. O., and Pinson, E. R. (1967): Some metabolic effects of phenformin in rat adipose tissue. *Diabetes,* 16:869–874.

20. Pressman, B. C. (1963): The effects of guanidine and alkylguanidines on the energy transfer reactions of mitochondria. *J. Biol. Chem.,* 238:401–409.

21. Randle, P. J., Garland, P. B., Newsholme, E. A., and Hales, C. N. (1963): The glucose fatty acid cycle: its role in insulin sensitivity and the metabolic disturbances of diabetes mellitus. *Lancet,* 1:785–789.

22. Rodriguez, J., Catapano, A., Ghiselli, G. C., and Sirtori, C. R. (1976): Turnover and aortic uptake of very low density lipoproteins (VLDL) from hypercholesterolemic rabbits as a model for testing antiatherosclerotic compounds. In: *Atherosclerosis Drug Discovery,* edited by C. E. Day, pp. 169–189. Plenum, New York.

23. Schäfer, G. (1976): Some new aspects on the interaction of hypoglycemia-producing biguanides with biological membranes. *Biochem. Pharmacol.,* 25:2015–2024.

24. Schönborn, J., Heim, K., Rabst, U., and Kasper, H. (1975): Effect of metformin on turnover and oxidation of free fatty acids in maturity onset diabetes. *VI International Congress of Pharmacology,* Helsinki. Abstr. 1246.

25. Sirtori, C. R., Catapano, A., Ghiselli, G. C., Innocenti, A. L., and Rodriguez, J. (1977): Metformin: An antiatherosclerotic agent modifying very low density lipoproteins in rabbits. *Atherosclerosis,* 26:79–89.

26. Sirtori, C. R., Tremoli, E., Sirtori, M., Conti, F., and Paoletti, R. (1977): Treatment of hypertriglyceridemia with metformin. *Atherosclerosis,* 26:583–592.

27. Stauffacher, W., and Berger, W. (1973): Recent notions concerning the mode of action of biguanides. In: *Proceedings of the Geneva XII International Therapeutic Union Congress,* edited by B. Glasson and A. Benakis, pp. 129–140. Medecine et Hygiene, Geneve.

28. Stout, R. W., Brunzell, J. D., Porte, D., Jr., and Bierman, E. L. (1974): Effect of phenformin on lipid transport in hypertriglyceridemia. *Metabolism,* 23:815–828.

29. Tagliamonte, P., Sirigu, F., Corsini, G. U., and Muntoni, S. (1973): Influence of phenformin on plasma FFA turnover in man. *Riv. Farmacol. Ter.,* 4:151–157.

30. Tiengo, A., Fedele, D., Nosadini, R., and Crepaldi, G. (1978): Hypotriglyceridemic effect of metformin in human and rat hyperlipidemia. In: *International Conference on Atherosclerosis,* edited by L. A. Carlson, R. Paoletti, C. R. Sirtori, and G. Weber, pp. 327–331. Raven Press, New York.

31. Tzagournis, M., Seidensticker, J. F., and Hamwi, G. I. (1968): Metabolic abnormalities in premature coronary disease: effect of therapy. *Ann. NY Acad. Sci.,* 148:945–957.

32. Weber, G., Catapano, A., Ghiselli, G. C., and Sirtori, C. R. (1978): Experimental studies on the antiatherosclerotic effect of metformin. In: *International Conference on Atherosclerosis,* edited by L. A. Carlson, R. Paoletti, C. R. Sirtori, and G. Weber, pp. 319–325. Raven Press, New York.

Diet and Drugs in Atherosclerosis,
edited by G. Noseda, B. Lewis, and R. Paoletti.
Raven Press, New York © 1980.

Dipyridamole as an Antithrombotic Agent: An Intricate Mechanism of Action

G. Di Minno, S. Villa, V. Bertelé, and G. de Gaetano

Istituto di Ricerche Farmacologiche Mario Negri, 20157 Milan, Italy

The mechanism of action of dipyridamole as an antithrombotic agent has been controversial (1,3,6). In a recent report, Moncada and Korbut (6), working on rabbit blood *in vitro,* concluded that the antithrombotic activity depended on its inhibition of phosphodiesterase activity in circulating blood. This would potentiate the stimulatory effect of prostacyclin (PGI_2) on increasing platelet levels of cAMP, thus decreasing platelet aggregability. In another report, Best and colleagues (1), working on *in vitro* human platelets, suggested that the mechanism of action of this drug is related to the inhibition of platelet thromboxane (TX) A_2 activity, the most potent stimulus of platelet aggregation.

The aim of our study was to evaluate the mechanism of action of dipyridamole on some *in vitro, in vivo,* and *ex vivo* parameters of platelet function. The first approach was to study its effect on *in vitro* human platelet aggregation induced by arachidonic acid (AA). The second approach was to study the inhibition of platelet aggregation induced by adenosine and PGI_2 before and after dipyridamole ingestion in healthy human subjects. The third approach, done in rats, was aimed at evaluating the possible interaction between dipridamole and PGI_2 on bleeding time.

Preincubation of human platelets at 37°C for 10 min with 50 μM dipyridamole, the concentration used by others, resulted in a complete inhibition of platelet aggregation induced by threshold concentrations of arachidonic acid (AA). On the other hand, 5 μM dipyridamole (a concentration within the range of plasma levels observed after administration) was uneffective but strongly potentiated the inhibitory activity of exogenous PGI_2. Therefore, although dipyridamole could inhibit AA metabolism in platelets, this effect was only observed at concentrations of the drug much higher than that which can be reached in plasma during treatment. At therapeutic concentrations, *in vitro* potentiation of PGI_2 inhibitory activity may be the most important mechanism of action of this drug (3).

To further assess the clinical significance of this pharmacological interaction, we studied the inhibition of platelet aggregation induced by exogenous PGI_2 and by adenosine in 10 volunteers both before and 90 to 180 min after the ingestion of a single dose of 100 mg dipyridamole. The purpose of this experiment

TABLE 1. *PGI₂ and adenosine inhibition of human platelet aggregation before and 90 to 180 min after ingestion of dipyridamole (100 mg)*[a]

Agent	Threshold aggregating concentration	Threshold inhibiting concentration	
		PGI₂ (nM)	Adenosine (μM)
ADP (μM)			
Before dipyridamole	4.5 ± 0.9	5.9 ± 1.6	22.0 ± 6.8
90 min after dipyridamole	4.0 ± 0.7	6.2 ± 1.6	16.3 ± 9.5
180 min after dipyridamole	6.6 ± 1.3	5.5 ± 1.2	11.2 ± 7.2
AA (mM)			
Before dipyridamole	0.7 ± 0.04	3.1 ± 1.6	2.1 ± 0.7
90 min after dipyridamole	0.8 ± 0.04	2.9 ± 1.6	2.5 ± 1.1
180 min after dipyridamole	0.9 ± 0.08	2.5 ± 0.9	4.4 ± 1.8

[a] Mean ± SE of five subjects.

was to see whether following dipyridamole ingestion, a lower concentration of exogenous PGI_2 would be required to inhibit *in vitro* platelet aggregation. The threshold aggregating concentration (4) for ADP and AA (that is, the minimal concentration inducing maximal aggregation) was unchanged before and 90 to 180 min after drug administration.

On the other hand, the concentration of PGI_2 required to inhibit platelet aggregation following dipyridamole ingestion was not lower, as could be expected, but similar or even higher than that required before dipyridamole. In contrast, adenosine-induced inhibition of ADP-induced platelet aggregation was strongly potentiated (Table 1). When subjects ingested a single dose of 150 mg dipyridamole, similar results were found for both PGI_2 and adenosine (Table 2).

TABLE 2. *PGI₂ and adenosine inhibition of human platelet aggregation before and 90 to 180 min after ingestion of dipyridamole (150 mg)*[a]

Agent	Threshold aggregating concentration	Threshold inhibiting concentration	
		PGI₂ (nM)	Adenosine (μM)
ADP (μM/liter)			
Before dipyridamole	6.1 ± 0.5	15.6 ± 6.3	22.0 ± 9.2
90 min after dipyridamole	6.3 ± 0.9	9.7 ± 2.9	15.2 ± 7.3
180 min after dipyridamole	7.3 ± 0.8	11.2 ± 2.5	13.5 ± 10.2
AA (mM)			
Before dipyridamole	0.7 ± 0.02	3.4 ± 1.5	2.5 ± 1.9
90 min after dipyridamole	0.8 ± 0.04	3.7 ± 1.6	7.6 ± 6.4
180 min after dipyridamole	0.8 ± 0.01	3.4 ± 0.7	7.1 ± 6.5

[a] Mean ± SE of five subjects.

TABLE 3. *Effect of aspirin, PGI₂, and dipyridamole on tail bleeding time in rats*[a]

Group	Interval (min)	Bleeding time (min)
Control	—	102 ± 10
Aspirin (200 mg/kg i.p.)	—	149 ± 18
Dipyridamole (30 mg/kg i.p.)	—	118 ± 8
PGI₂ (3.8 µg/kg i.v.)	5	314 ± 40
PGI₂ (3.8 µg/kg i.v.) + dipyridamole (30 mg/kg i.p.)	5	517 ± 50
Aspirin + dipyridamole	30	>600

[a] Saline, 37°C.

In some cases, we found that the threshold inhibitory concentration of PGI_2 was greater after dipyridamole ingestion. Similar results were found when two other antiaggregatory PGs (4,5,7,8), namely, PGD_2 and PGE_1, were tested in similar conditions. These *ex vivo* results do not support the hypothesis that dipyridamole acts *in vivo* potentiating the inhibitory effect of circulating PGI_2.

The last part of our study was performed in an animal model of platelet function. We studied bleeding time on rat tails by a standardized template technique (2). Neither aspirin (5 to 200 mg/kg i.p.) nor dipyridamole (30 mg/kg) significantly modified bleeding time. The latter strongly potentiated the prolonging effect of exogenous PGI_2 on bleeding time, but inhibition of the formation of endogenous PGI_2 by aspirin resulted in a marked lengthening of bleeding time. Thus in our model, dipyridamole appeared to potentiate aspirin in the absence of endogenous PGI_2 (Table 3).

CONCLUSION

These data do not support the hypothesis that dipyridamole acts as an antithrombotic agent only by interacting with platelet and vascular prostaglandins. Indeed, the potentiation of adenosine-induced inhibition of human platelet aggregation suggests that this physiological antiaggregating agent could have an important role in explaining some properties of dipyridamole.

REFERENCES

1. Best, L. C., Martin, T. J., McGuire, M. B., Preston, F. E., Russel, R. G. G., and Segal, D. S. (1978): Dipyridamole and platelet function. *Lancet,* 1:846.
2. Dejana, E., Callioni, A., Quintana, A., and de Gaetano, G. (1979): Bleeding time in laboratory animals II. *Thromb. Res.,* 15:191.
3. Di Minno, G., de Gaetano, G., and Garattini, S. (1978): Dipyridamole and platelet function. *Lancet,* 1:1258.
4. Di Minno, G., Silver, M. J., and de Gaetano, G. (1979): Prostaglandins as inhibitors of human platelet aggregation. *Br. J. Haematol.,* 63:637.
5. Mills, D. C. B., Macfarlane, D. E., and Nicolau, K. C. (1977): Interaction of prostacyclin (PGI₂) with the prostaglandin receptors on human platelets that regulate adenylate cyclase activity. *Blood [Suppl. I],* 50:247.

6. Moncanda, S., and Korbut, R. (1978): Dipyridamole and other phosphodiesterase inhibitors act as anti-thrombotic agents by potentiating endogenous prostacyclin. *Lancet,* 1:1286.
7. Siegl, A. M., Smith, S. B., Silver, M. J., Nicolau, K. C., and Ahern, D. (1979): Selective binding site for (^{3}H) prostacyclin on platelets. *J. Clin. Invest.,* 63:215.
8. Whittle, B. J. R., Moncada, S., and Vane, J. R. (1978): Comparison of the effects of prostacyclin (PGI$_2$), prostaglandin E$_1$ and prostaglandin D$_2$ in platelet aggregation in different species. *Prostaglandins,* 16:387.

Diet and Drugs in Atherosclerosis,
edited by G. Noseda, B. Lewis, and R. Paoletti.
Raven Press, New York © 1980.

Effect of Inhibition of Lysosomal Activity in Mesenchymal Cells With Chloroquine on the Secretion of Glycoconjugates

M. Moczar

Laboratoire de Biochimie du Tissu Conjonctif, Faculté de Médecine, Université Paris, 94010 Creteil, France

The binding of plasma low density lipoproteins (LDL) to the specific surface receptors (1,4) of cultured fibroblasts is regulated by the lipoprotein concentration of the medium (1). The LDL taken up by the mesenchymal cells in tissue culture is rapidly metabolized (2,13). It was demonstrated that intracellular lipid accumulation occurs in cultured fibroblasts when the lysosomal enzymes are inhibited with chloroquine (14). Chloroquine, like other lysosomotropic amines, inhibits the receptor-mediated uptake of lysosomal enzymes into normal fibroblasts (10). The molecular mechanisms of the alterations of the extracellular matrix during early phase hypercholesterolemia are not well understood. To gain insight into this problem, we investigated the biosynthesis of glycoconjugates by cultured human skin fibroblasts with cytoplasmic lipid deposition induced by chloroquine and homologous LDL (14).

MATERIAL AND METHODS

Confluent cultures of human skin fibroblasts were enriched with free and esterified cholesterol by treating the cells with chloroquine and homologous plasma LDL for 6 hr, according to Stein et al. (14). The cholesterol-enriched cells were further incubated with 0.1 μCi 1-^{14}C-glucosamine (59 mCi/mM) at 37°C up to 36 hr. Control cells and cells exposed for 6 hr to LDL without chloroquine were also incubated for 36 hr with labeled glucosamine. After incubation, the medium was removed, the cell layer washed with PBS buffer, and the cells dispersed with trypsin (2). The cells were centrifuged, and the cell pellet was hydrolyzed with 1 M NaOH for determination of protein (6) and radioactivity.

Incorporation of ^{14}C-Glucosamine into Macromolecules

Lyophilized samples of the dialyzed culture medium were hydrolyzed with 4 N HCl at 100°C *in vacuo*. The hexosamines were purified on cation exchange column and separated by paper chromatography (8).

Separation of Macromolecules Secreted Into the Medium

The macromolecules were reduced with dithiothreitol, alkylated with iodacetamide and fractionated by exclusion chromatography on BioGel A5m column (11).

Proteins were hydrolyzed with trypsin, reduced with 2-mercaptoethanol in the presence of SDS, and applied to Biogel P30 column with 0.2 M Tris-HCl 0.1% SDS, pH 7.4 elution buffer (11).

Enzymatic Assays

The aliquots of the excluded peak on BioGel P30 column (from trypsin digests of the macromolecules in the medium) were hydrolyzed with chondroitinase AC at pH 7.3 and chondroitinase ABC at pH 8.0 in Tris chloride-acetate buffer (3). The hydrolysates were fractionated on BioGel P30 column under conditions described above.

RESULTS AND DISCUSSION

The incorporation of ^{14}C-glucosamine into macromolecules was investigated in cultures of normal skin fibroblasts and in cultures of cells preincubated with LDL, chloroquine, and the mixture of chloroquine and LDL. The results on the metabolic fate of the radioactive label of cells and of the glycoconjugates excreted into the incubation medium are presented in Table 1. The inhibition of the lysosomal enzymes with chloroquine in the absence or presence of LDL resulted in an increased secretion of labeled macromolecules into the medium. The ^{14}C-label of the cell layer and of the pericellular matrix (trypsinate) was similar for the different cell culture systems.

The radioactive hexosamines purified after partial hydrolysis and cochromatographed with D-glucosamine and D-galactosamine accounted for 70% recovery of the radioactivity from the medium. The ^{14}C-glucosamine to ^{14}C-galactosamine ratio was 3:1 in control cells. Increased amount of radioactivity was incorporated into galactosamine by the cells treated with chloroquine.

TABLE 1. *Incubation of human skin fibroblast cultures with ^{14}C-glucosamine for 18 and 36 hr[a]*

Addition to incubation medium	Cells		Trypsinate		Medium		Total	
	18 hr	36 hr	18 hr	36 hr	18 hr	36 hr	18 hr	36 hr
None	17.8	19.3	15.3	19.6	45.7	92.9	78.8	131.8
LDL	16.2	20.8	12.9	20.9	40.7	77.0	69.8	118.7
Chloroquine	19.0	22.9	16.0	19.0	75.9	131.0	110.9	172.9
Chloroquine + LDL	19.6	22.4	14.9	16.0	66.1	120.0	100.6	159.3

[a] cpm/μg cell protein.

In experiments to investigate the nature of macromolecules excreted into the medium, the exclusion chromatography was carried out on reduced and S-carboxamidomethylated samples. A typical radioactive elution diagram is given in Fig. 1. The major radioactive peak was excluded from the column with a

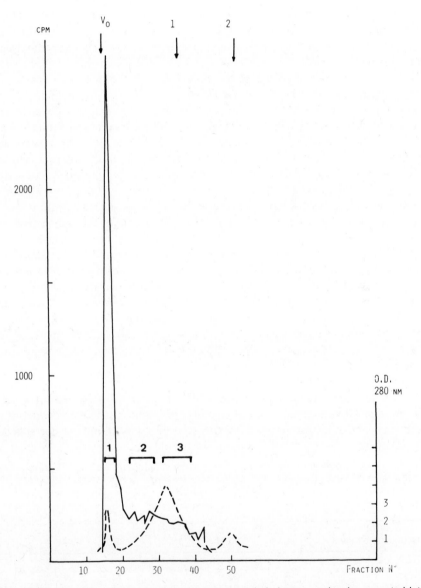

FIG. 1. Exclusion chromatography of ^{14}C-hexosamine-labeled macromolecules excreted into the culture medium by normal fibroblasts incubated in the presence of ^{14}C-glucosamine for 36 hr. BioGel A5m column. Elution buffer; 0.2 M; Tris-HCl-0.1% SDS; pH 7.4 The elution position of the standards: 1, bovine gamma globulin; 2, myoglobin; V_o, void volume; *solid line*, cpm; *dashed line*, O.D. 280 nm.

molecular weight $\geqq 5.10^6$. The incorporation of ^{14}C-hexosamines into the excluded fraction was about 2.5 times higher for cells preincubated with chloroquine (Table 2). The ^{14}C-labels of the minor retarded fractions were similar in the different culture systems.

In further experiments to determine whether the high molecular weight peak contained proteoglycans or glycoproteins, the macromolecules released into the medium were hydrolyzed with trypsin and fractionated by gel chromatography. Proteoglycans are hydrolyzed to relatively high molecular weight peptidoglycans, and hyaluronic acids are not digested (5,7). Glycoproteins excreted by human skin fibroblasts are degraded with trypsin to fragments with an apparent molecular weight $< 2.10^4$ (11). When the proteins in the medium were hydrolyzed with trypsin and reduced with mercaptoethanol, the major radioactive peak was excluded from the BioGel P30 column with an exclusion limit of 3.10^4.

The appearance of the high molecular weight ^{14}C-hexosamine-labeled peak from the trypsin digests suggests that this fraction is derived from proteoglycans or hyaluronic acid. For further characterizations, the excluded fraction from BioGel P30 column was hydrolyzed with chondroitinase AC and chondroitinase ABC. The hydrolysates with chondroitinase AC were separated into two fractions on BioGel P30 chromatography. The most prominent radioactive peak was eluted at the position of low molecular weight oligosaccharides derived from chondroitin-4 sulfate and chondroitin-6 sulfate with chondroitinase AC. The minor peak emerged in the void volume of the BioGel P30 column for control cells and for both type of chloroquine-treated cultures. About 90% of radioactivity in the chondroitinase AC-resistant peak were degraded with chondroitinase ABC to a retarded fraction of molecular weight < 300. The gel filtration data of the degradation products obtained with chondrotinase AC and chondroitinase ABC indicate that the excluded peak from the trypsin digest contain galactosaminoglycans: chondroitin-4 sulfate, chondroitin-6 sulfate, and dermatan sulfate (12).

To obtain some preliminary information on the ratio of glycosaminoglycans to glycoproteins excreted into the medium, the radioactivities recovered in the excluded and retarded peaks from the trypsinized medium are correlated in

TABLE 2. Incorporation of ^{14}C-hexosamines into macromolecules secreted by fibroblasts into the culture medium; incubation of cells in the presence of ^{14}C-glucosamine for 18 and 36 hr; gel filtration of the S-carboxamidomethyl proteins on BioGel A5m column (Fig. 1)[a]

Addition to incubation medium	Fraction 1		Fraction 2		Fraction 3	
	18 hr	36 hr	18 hr	36 hr	18 hr	36 hr
None	18.6	34.4	9.2	17.3	10.0	17.9
LDL	19.5	38.0	9.7	14.3	8.0	16.8
Chloroquine	50.4	79.7	7.8	20.6	11.2	16.3
Chloroquine + LDL	48.2	74.2	9.9	16.8	9.7	15.4

[a] cpm/μg cell protein.

FIG. 2. Hydrolysis with trypsin of ^{14}C-hexosamine-labeled macromolecules excreted by fibroblasts into the culture medium. Ratio of the radioactivity cpm/µg cell protein recovered in the excluded and retarded fraction on BioGel P30 column. Incubation of the cell cultures with ^{14}C-glucosamine for 18 hr **(A)** and 36 hr **(B)**. Treatment of cell cultures: *open bars*, none (control cells); *solid bars*, LDL; *horizontally striped bars*, chloroquine + LDL; *vertically striped bars*, chloroquine.

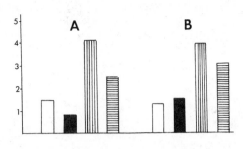

Fig. 2. The highest radioactive ratio was obtained from fibroblast cultures preincubated with chloroquine. The ratio decreases when lipids have been accumulated in the chloroquine-treated cells. The findings shown in Fig. 2 suggest that interiorization of lipids in fibroblasts by the action of chloroquine modifies the excretion of glycosaminoglycans and glycoproteins.

The defect of the processing of the endogenous hydrolytic enzymes induced by chloroquine (10) associated with interiorization of lipids in tissue culture resulted in an increased radioactive label of the glycosaminoglycans in the culture medium.

As the incorporation of ^{14}C-glucosamine into fibroblasts and in the pericellular glycoconjugates was found similar in the control and chloroquine-treated cultures, the increased radioactive label of the medium seems to arise from decreased catabolism (9) rather than an increase in synthesis.

ACKNOWLEDGMENTS

Thanks are extended to Drs. O. and Y. Stein, Hadassah Medical School, Jerusalem, who provided their laboratory facilities and advice during the performance of the experiments. The investigation was supported by grants from the CNRS, the Fondation Simone, and Cino del Duca, and by grant no. 78–7–2600 from DGRST.

REFERENCES

1. Bierman, E. L., and Albers, F. (1977): Regulation of low density lipoprotein receptor activity by cultured human arterial smooth muscle cells. *Biochem. Biophys. Acta,* 488:152–160.
2. Bierman, E. L., Stein, O., and Stein, Y. (1974): Lipoprotein uptake and metabolism by rat aortic smooth muscle cells in tissue culture. *Circ. Res.,* 35:136–150.
3. Breen, M., Weinstein, H. G., Blacik, L. F., Borcherding, M. S., and Sittig, R. A. (1976): Microanalysis and characterization of glycosaminoglycans from human tissue via zone electrophoresis. In: *Carbohydrate Chemistry,* edited by R. L. Whistler and J. M. Be Miller, pp. 101–115. Academic, New York.
4. Goldstein, J., and Brown, M. S. (1974): Binding and degradation of low density lipoproteins by cultured human fibroblasts. *J. Biol. Chem.,* 249:5153–5162.
5. Heinegård, D., and Hascall, V. C. (1974): Characterization of chondroitin-sulfate isolated from trypsin-chymotrypsin digests of cartilage proteoglycans. *Arch. Biochem. Biophys.,* 165:427–441.

6. Lowry, O. H., Rosebrough, N. J., Farr, A. L., and Randall, R. J. (1951): Protein measurement with Folin phenol reagent. *J. Biol. Chem.,* 193:265–275.
7. Mathews, M. B. (1971): Comparative biochemistry of chondroitinsulfate proteins of cartilage and notochord. *Biochem. J.,* 125:37–46.
8. Montreuil, J., and Spik, G. (1968): Méthodes chromatographiques et électrophorétiques de dosage des glucides constituant les glycoprotéines. *Monogr. Lab. Chim. Biol. Fac. Sci. Lille,* 199–219.
9. Prinz, R., Schwerman, J., Buddecke, E., and Von Figura, K. (1978): Endocytosis of sulphated proteoglycans by cultured skin fibroblasts. *Biochem. J.,* 176:671–676.
10. Sando, G. N., Titus Gillon, P., Hall, C. W., and Neufeld, E. F. (1979): Inhibition of receptor mediated uptake of a lysosomal enzyme into fibroblasts by chloroquine, procaine and ammonia. *Exp. Cell Res.,* 199:359–364.
11. Sear, H. J., Grant, E. M., and Jackson, D. S. (1977): Biosynthesis and release of glycoproteins by human skin fibroblasts in culture. *Biochem. J.,* 168:91–103.
12. Sjöberg, I., and Fransson, L. A. (1977): Synthesis of glycosaminoglycans by human embryonic lung fibroblasts. *Biochem. J.,* 167:383–392.
13. Stein, O., and Stein, Y. (1975): Surface binding and interiorization of homologous and heterologous serum lipoproteins by rat aortic smooth muscle cells in culture. *Biochem. Biophys. Acta,* 398:377–384.
14. Stein, O., Vanderhoek, J., Friedman, G., and Stein, Y. (1976): Deposition and mobilization of cholesterol ester in cultured human skin fibroblasts. *Biochem. Biophys. Acta,* 450:367–378.

Diet and Drugs in Atherosclerosis,
edited by G. Noseda, B. Lewis, and R. Paoletti.
Raven Press, New York © 1980.

Lipofundin Administration and Vessel Damages

H. Jellinek, J. Hársing, Sz. Füzesi, and M. Bihari-Varga

Second Department of Pathology, Semmelweis Medical University, Budapest, Hungary

Colloidal iron (Ferrlecit, Nattermann, Köln) was used to study permeability changes of the vessel wall in various model experiments. This method proved to be excellent since the blue-colored Prussian-blue reaction was easily detected by light microscopy. The intravenously administered iron, however, was not detectable in any layer of a normal vessel of the animals killed 1 hr after treatment. The transport of iron through the damaged cell wall was easily visualized in the endothelium, subintimal space, and media (1). The route of transport became masked by the presence of iron granules in the endothelium of the adventitial capillary network.

The colloidal iron method appeared to be useful also in electron microscopic studies. In preparations contrasted only by uranylacetate, the iron granules appeared as black, electron-dense structures.

To detect the exact route and mechanism of adventitial material transport under the conditions of exalted permeability, a new method has been developed. We added an equal amount of lipofundin (Braun, Melsungen) to the colloidal iron preparation (2). Neither the iron nor the lipofundin was ever seen to penetrate any normal vessel wall. In vessels damaged by hypoxia, hypertension, or acid treatment, the presence of lipofundin was detectable by Sudan staining in the endothelial cells and in the media 1 hr after the intravenous administration of the lipofundin-iron mixture (3). The colloidal iron was adsorbed at the surface of the lipofundin granules, as shown by electron microscopy. The *in vitro* formation of a lipofundin-iron complex was also demonstrated by chemical methods (4). The lipofundin chylomicron coated with iron was well detectable in every step of its transport through the vessel wall.

In these studies, it became clear that the chylomicra transported through the vessel wall were drained through the adventitial lymph vessels. The entrance of the lipofundin-iron complex into the endothelial cells and the lumen was easily detectable in these studies.

To shed more light on the possible underlying mechanism, we examined the effect of the administration of lipofundin alone in rats.

MATERIALS AND METHODS

Lipofundin (1 ml), an oil extract of soybeans stabilized to form a suspension of chylomicra of 1 μm diameter, was administered intravenously to the animals three times a day for a total of 8 days. On the following day, the animals were given an equal mixture of lipofundin and iron and were killed 1 hr later. Preparations for light- or electron-microscopic studies were obtained from the animals. For light microscopy, the preparations were stained with Prussian-blue or with Sudan IV, or in frozen section both with Prussian-blue and Sudan IV.

RESULTS AND DISCUSSION

The light-microscopic studies have shown that the prolonged lipofundin administration affected the vessel wall permeability, as revealed by the presence

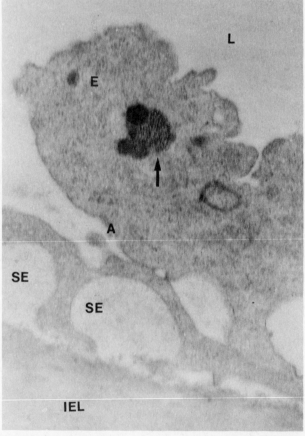

FIG. 1. Endothelial cell in preparation (contrasted only with uranylacetate) from a specimen obtained from an animal treated with lipofundin for 8 days. The endothelial cell (E) is bulging toward the lumen (L); it contains many iron granules *(arrow)*. Some endothelial cells are elevated from the internal elastic lamina (IEL). In the subendothelial space (SE), granular material is seen.

of Prussian-blue reaction. In the Sudan stained preparations, the presence of lipofundin was demonstrable not only in the endothelial cells but also in the media. Thus light microscopy showed the damage of the vessel walls and the appearance of Sudan-positive material.

Under the electron microscope, we examined preparations contrasted only with uranylacetate. These revealed the presence of considerable amounts of colloidal iron in the endothelial cells (Fig. 1). The presence of lipid-like droplets was also observed. On the surface of these droplets, we occasionally saw some adsorbed iron granules.

In uranyl-contrasted preparations, enlargement of the subendothelial space was seen. In this space, there first appeared some granular material, which later developed into a granular basement membrane-like material (Fig. 2). In some of the contrasted preparations, we saw the extension into the subendothelial space of slightly edematous processes of smooth muscle cells. The latter caused the endothelial cells to bulge toward the lumen (Fig. 3).

Changes were seen also in the media. Basement membrane-like material accu-

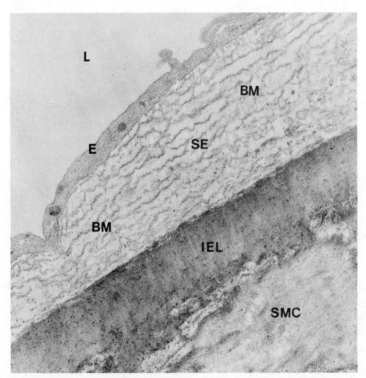

FIG. 2. Subendothelial space (SE) between the endothelial cell (E) and the internal elastic lamina (IEL) is dilated and contains basement membrane-like material (BM). *L*, lumen; SMC, smooth muscle cell of the media. The preparation was contrasted only with uranylacetate.

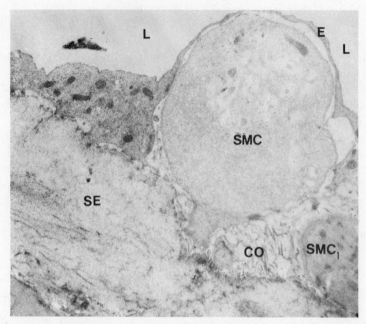

FIG. 3. Part of the endothelial cell (E) bulges into the lumen (L). There is a smooth muscle cell (SMC) present below it. The subendothelial space (SE) is enlarged. Accumulation of collagen fibers (CO) is seen between the first elastic fiber and the cells. SMC_1, part of another smooth muscle cell migrated into the subendothelium; Weibel-Palade granules in the endothelial cells. The preparation was contrasted only with uranylacetate.

mulated in the intracellular space between the smooth muscle cells. The latter contained lipofundin droplets surrounded by iron granules (Fig. 4). Also in the adventitial fibroblasts and between the collagen fibers, granules of the lipofundin-iron complex appeared. In some cases, the presence of large amounts of lipofundin in the lumens of the lymph vessels suggested the drainage of this material via the lymph circulation.

These data favor the idea that the extensive administration of lipofundin for 8 days produced permeability changes, subendothelial basement membrane-like material accumulation, and smooth muscle cell mobilization similar to those seen in cholesterol-fed experimental animals.

Biochemical analysis of the aortas of lipofundin-treated animals showed that neither the total lipid nor the total glycosaminoglycan content had changed. Nevertheless, there was a demonstrable decrease in the amount of loosely bound, saline-extractable lipoproteins relative to that of the saline-insoluble, firmly bound lipoproteins. These changes are similar to those seen in the initial phase of atherosclerosis.

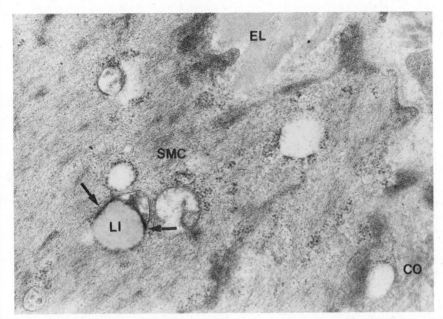

FIG. 4. A smooth muscle cell (SMC) from the media containing lipofundin chylomicron (LI) coated with iron granules *(arrow)*. EL, elastic lamella; CO, collagen fibers. The preparation was contrasted only with uranylacetate.

SUMMARY

Lipofundin-S is an emulsion of oily soybean extract. This material was administered to rats in 1-cm doses 3 times daily for 8 days. The last dose was given together with the same amount of a colloidal iron preparation. The animals were killed 1 hr after the last injection. Light microscopy was used to detect permeability changes by Berlin-blue reaction and to localize the appearance of sudanophilic areas by Sudan staining. Uncontrasted preparations were used for the electron-microscopic detection of material transport through the vessel wall. The exalted permeability and the appearance of sudanophilia were assessed. The role of the adventitial drainage was demonstrated by registering the presence of lipofundin in the lymph vessels. Alterations in the lipid content and composition of the vessel wall has been measured by chemical methods. Structural changes in the aortic proteoglycans and fibrillar proteins were studied by means of biochemical and thermoanalytical methods.

REFERENCES

1. Jellinek, H. (1974): *Arterial Lesions and Arteriosclerosis.* Plenum, London.
2. Jellinek, H. (1977): The use of a twin tracer technique for the study of the movement of exogenous

particles through the hypoxic arterial wall and their uptake by adventitial lymphatics. *Fol. Angiol.*, 25:156.

3. Jellinek, H. (1977): Evidence of the specificity of the colloidal iron tracer technique and demonstration of partial injury of the aortic wall by twin tracer technique. *Fol. Angiol.*, 25:261.

4. Jellinek, H., and Bihari-Varga, M. (1978): Further investigations on the use of a twin tracer technique for the study of the movement of exogenous particles through the arterial wall. *Fol. Angiol.*, 26:150.

Diet and Drugs in Atherosclerosis,
edited by G. Noseda, B. Lewis, and R. Paoletti.
Raven Press, New York © 1980.

Tolerance of One Year's Treatment With Bezafibrate in Patients With Hyperlipoproteinemia

Paul Dieter Lang, Heinz Dieter Holler, and Joachim Vollmar

*Department of Medical Research, Boehringer Mannheim GmbH,
6800 Mannheim, West Germany*

Dietary as well as drug treatment of hyperlipoproteinemia in most instances must be instituted on a long-term basis. It is necessary, therefore, to examine a drug not only for long-term efficacy but also for long-term safety.

MATERIALS AND METHODS

There were 1,091 patients with primary hyperlipidemia (cholesterol > 260 mg/100 ml and/or triglycerides > 200 mg/100 ml) who were treated in a multicenter field study with bezafibrate (200 mg t.i.d.) for 1 year. Examination dates were 1, 2, 4, 6, 8, 10, and 12 months after determination of pretreatment values. Dietary habits were kept unchanged.

Body weight, blood pressure, hemoglobin, white cell counts, and urinary glucose and protein were determined in the individual laboratories of the investigators. All other laboratory parameters were determined from deep-frozen serum samples in the clinical chemistry laboratories of Boehringer Mannheim.

From the 1,091 patients who entered the study, 783 (72%) could be included in the evaluation of safety laboratory parameters, body weight, and blood lipids. Reasons for exclusion were as follows: lack of cooperation in 150 cases, intercurrent diseases in 41 cases, change of location or physician in 27 cases, and various nondrug-related events in nine cases. In 34 patients, pretreatment values were missing or were not obtained according to the trial plan. Ten patients died during or after the treatment phase. No relationship between death and treatment with bezafibrate was seen by any investigator; most patients died from preexisting diseases. In 37 cases, side effects led to discontinuation of treatment.

The characteristics of 783 patients included in the statistical evaluation of the safety laboratory parameters were as follows. The relationship of men and women was 59 to 41%; median age was 58 years; median relative body weight was 1.23 in relation to ideal weight (1); and 70% of the patients were on a lipid-lowering diet prior to entry into the study. Concomitant medication for other preexisting diseases or those necessary intercurrently did not include drugs known to affect lipid metabolism to a significant degree.

Statistical analysis of the data was carried out with the nonparametric Wilcoxon test for matched samples, comparing pretreatment and treatment values. All statistical comparisons were based on a probability of error of the first kind of $\alpha=0.01$.

RESULTS AND DISCUSSION

The side effects leading to discontinuation of treatment in 37 cases (3.4% of the 1,091 patients) are listed in Table 1. The majority occurred early in the study. Most frequently, upper abdominal symptoms were observed, consisting of nausea, lack of appetite, feeling of pressure or pain in the gastric area, and acid sensation in the stomach. Reduction of potency was observed in five patients. Giddiness and pressure in the head were probably not drug-related. Itching and exanthema occurred in three and two cases, respectively. Increased appetite was recorded without associated weight gain. Myositis-like syndrome with moderate increase in CPK, as has been described for clofibrate (6), occurred once. A rise in creatinine was seen in a patient who, because of increased initial creatinine levels, was not eligible for the study. His value increased from 1.7 to 2.8 and returned to pretreatment value upon withdrawal of the drug. More recent studies in patients with impaired renal function have led to the recommendation of lower doses according to the degree of impairment of renal function in these patients (4). Cholestasis was the investigator's diagnosis in a patient with jaundice. No clinical chemical evidence was present for intra- or extrahepatic cholestasis. This side effect, as well as 15 others, were considered only suspected side effects due to bezafibrate by the respective investigators. In 10 patients, verification of the side effects was obtained by reexposition to the drug.

TABLE 1. *Number of patients excluded because of side effects*

| Side effect | Number of patients per time of occurrence (months) | | | | | | | Total |
	1	2	4	6	8	10	12	
Upper abdominal symptoms	7	3	2		4		1	17
Reduction of potency		1	2	1		1		5
Giddiness, pressure in head	1	2	1					4
Itching	2	1						3
Exanthema		1			1			2
Increased appetite			1					1
Myositis-like syndrome			1					1
Rise in creatinine in serum						1		1
Cholestasis			1					1
Noncharacteristic symptoms	2							2
Total	12	8	8	1	5	2	1	37

Blood pressure remained constant during the course of the study. Hemoglobin decreased by 0.3 to 0.4 g/100 ml. White cell count showed a minor reduction. No change occurred in the glucose or protein excretion in urine. CPK values were higher by 4 U/liter at the end of the treatment period. Creatinine levels increased by 0.1 mg/100 ml. There are no indications thus far that these and the small changes in hemoglobin and white cell count, although statistically significant, are of clinical importance.

Liver parameters are shown in Fig. 1. SGOT remained constant during the

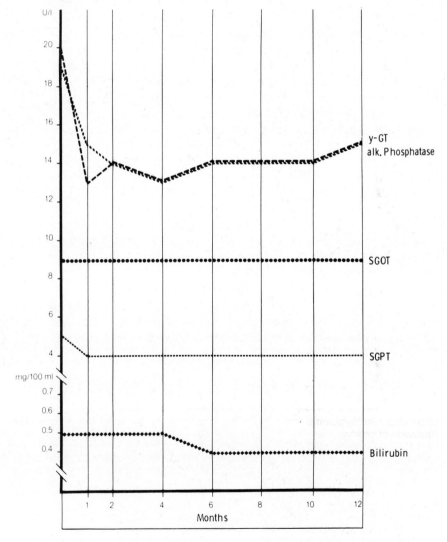

FIG. 1. Median values for SGOT, SGPT, γ-GT, alkaline phosphatase, and bilirubin.

course of the study. SGPT values were reduced by 1 U/liter. For both γ-GT and alkaline phosphatase, bezafibrate treatment caused a reduction by ~ 5 U/ liter. Bilirubin decreased slightly but significantly. No signs of liver toxicity were found. Examination of the percentages of patients above the accepted normal levels for SGOT, SGPT, γ-GT, and bilirubin (Table 2) shows a decrease during the 1-year treatment. This indicates that even patients with increased levels at study entry give no indication for liver toxicity of bezafibrate.

In other studies designed to evaluate effectiveness and safety in patients with defined lipid disorders, similar changes in safety laboratory parameters have been observed. In all instances, they had been reversible upon termination of treatment (5,8).

Figure 2 shows that body weight did not change during the 12 months of treatment. Cholesterol decreased significantly during the entire treatment period, reductions ranging between 7 and 11% at the various examination dates. Triglycerides also decreased significantly, ranging between 31 and 36%. The continued lowering of blood lipids indicates the lack of any escape phenomenon, as well as good compliance of the patients to bezafibrate treatment.

Since hyperlipidemia in the patients studied was not typed according to Fredrickson, interpretation of the lipid data must be done with caution. Separate analysis of the 171 patients with hypercholesterolemia (> 260 mg/100 ml) and normal triglycerides (< 200 mg/100 ml) showed an 18% decrease in cholesterol after 2 months of treatment, a degree of reduction corresponding to studies with properly classified type IIa patients (2,3,7). Cholesterol reduction was somewhat smaller (−12%) in patients with increases in both lipids ($N = 323$), but triglyceride reduction was marked (−46%). In patients with increases in triglycerides only ($N = 189$), this parameter declined by 37%. These results are also in agreement with those in properly typed IIb or IV patients (2,3,9).

The change in cholesterol and triglycerides was not related to relative body weight at the start of the trial, indicating that bezafibrate was effective also in patients with moderate or marked overweight. The degree of cholesterol and triglyceride reduction was dependent on the pretreatment level, as higher concen-

TABLE 2. *Percentage of patients with values above accepted normal limits for SGOT, SGPT, γ-GT, and bilirubin*

| | | Patients (%) | | | | | | |
| | | Bezafibrate (200 mg t.i.d.) (months) | | | | | | |
Liver parameter	Pre-treatment	1	2	4	6	8	10	12
SGOT (>12 U/liter)	20	16	18	19	19	17	13	13
SGPT (>12 U/liter)	7	3	2	3	4	3	4	3
γ-GT (>28 U/liter)	34	18	18	17	20	21	19	24
Bilirubin (>1.0 mg/100 ml)	6	2	3	2	1	1	1	1

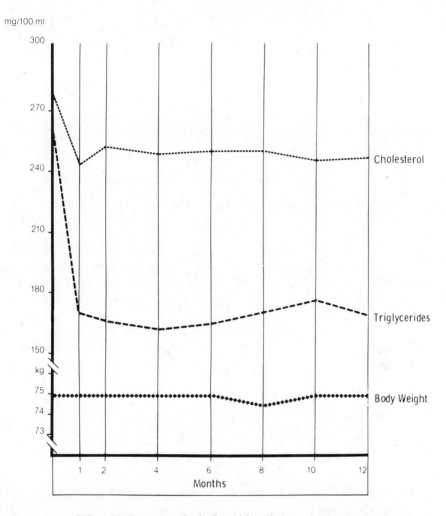

FIG. 2. Median values for body weight, cholesterol, and triglycerides.

trations were lowered to a greater degree. This was true for absolute changes or those expressed in relative terms.

In summary, bezafibrate was effective and well tolerated in a 1-year field trial in more than 1,000 patients with primary hyperlipidemia.

REFERENCES

1. Anonymous (1959): New weight standards for men and women. *Stat. Bull. Metropol. Life Ins. Co.*, 40:2.
2. Arntz, H. R., Klemens, U. H., Lang, P. D., and Vollmar, J. (1978): Vergleich von Clofibrat und Bezafibrat bei Hyperlipoproteinämie Typ II a und Typ II b. *Med. Klin.*, 73:1731–1737.

3. Kaffarnik, H., Schneider, J., Schubotz, R., Mühlfellner, O., Mühlfellner, G., Hausmann, L., and Zöfel, P. (1978): Long-term results with bezafibrate, a new derivative of clofibrate. In: *International Conference on Atherosclerosis,* edited by L. A. Carlson, R. Paoletti, C. R. Sitori, and G. Weber, pp. 129–133. Raven Press, New York.

4. Kösters, W., Abshagen, U., Lang, P. D., and Endele, R. (1979): Pharmakokinetik und Metabolismus von Bezafibrat bei Patienten mit eingeschränkter Nierenfunktion. In: *Lipoproteine und Herzinfarkt. Neue Aspekte in Diagnostik und Therapie von Hyperlipämien,* edited by H. Greten, P. D. Lang, and G. Schettler. Verlag G. Witzstrock, Baden-Baden, pp. 113–116.

5. Lageder, H. (1980): Vergleichende Doppel-Blinduntersuchung von Bezafibrat und Clofibrat bei Patienten mit primärer Hyperlipoproteinämie. *Wein. Klin. Wochenschr.,* 92:95–101.

6. Langer, T., and Levy, R. I. (1968): Acute muscular syndrome associated with administration of clofibrate. *N. Engl. J. Med.,* 279:856–858.

7. Olsson, A. G. (1979): Effect of bezafibrate on lipids and lipoproteins in patients with hyperlipoproteinaemia type II a and IV on long term treatment. In: *Lipoproteine und Herzinfarkt. Neue Aspekte in Diagnostik und Therapie von Hyperlipämien,* edited by H. Greten, P. D. Lang, and G. Schettler. Verlag G. Witzstrock, Baden-Baden, pp. 173–174.

8. Olsson, A. G., and Lang, P. D. (1978): Dose-response study of bezafibrate on serum lipoprotein concentrations in hyperlipoproteinaemia. *Atherosclerosis,* 31:421–428.

9. Olsson, A. G., Rössner, St., Walldius, G., Carlson, L. A., and Lang, P. D. (1977): Effect of BM 15.075 on lipoprotein concentrations in different types of hyperlipoproteinaemia. *Atherosclerosis,* 27:279–287.

Diet and Drugs in Atherosclerosis,
edited by G. Noseda, B. Lewis, and R. Paoletti.
Raven Press, New York © 1980.

Pharmacology of Probucol

David Kritchevsky

The Wistar Institute of Anatomy and Biology, Philadelphia, Pennsylvania 19104

Probucol [4,4'-(isopropylidenedithio)*bis*(2,6-di-t-butylphenol)] was initially studied by Barnhart et al. (2), who reported lower cholesterol levels in mice fed at a level of 0.06% of the diet. Serum cholesterol levels fell from 166 ± 8 to 72 ± 5 mg/dl ($p < 0.001$). Further studies in mice (1) indicated a dose-response effect with a dietary level of 0.125%, causing a 73% fall in serum cholesterol levels, and a level of 0.075% leading to a 22% reduction (Table 1). The influence of 0.25% probucol was tested in fasted and nonfasted rats for 2 weeks, and its effect was compared with clofibrate. As seen in Table 2, the drug is effective in either case.

Kritchevsky (9) reported that probucol exerted a significant hypolipidemic effect when administered to Wistar rats as 0.3% of the diet. In contrast to the findings of Barnhart et al. (2), the drug appeared to lead to hepatic enlargement (Table 3).

Probucol was shown to have a significant hypocholesteremic effect in monkeys. The drug (200 mg/kg/day) was administered to normocholesteremic cynomolgus monkeys and caused a 27% reduction in cholesterol levels ($p < 0.05$) (2). When probucol was fed to hypercholesteremic monkeys (300 mg/kg/day) for 9 weeks, serum cholesterol levels fell from 983 ± 98 to 469 ± 65 mg/dl ($p < 0.01$).

Probucol is also hypocholesteremic in man. Colmore [quoted by Heel et al. (8)] fed various levels of probucol to 31 healthy volunteers whose serum choles-

TABLE 1. *Influence of dietary probucol on serum cholesterol levels in mice[a,b]*

Probucol in diet (%)	Reduction of serum cholesterol (%)[c]
0.125	73
0.06	74
0.03	40
0.015	31
0.0075	22

[a] After Barnhart et al. (1).
[b] Twelve mice per group; 4-week feeding.
[c] All reductions statistically significant ($p < 0.01$).

143

TABLE 2. *Influence of probucol and clofibrate on serum and liver lipids in fasted and fed rats*[a]

Parameter	Treatment		
	Probucol	Clofibrate	Control
Fasted			
Serum cholesterol (mg/dl)	57 ± 5.7[b,c]	79 ± 3.9[b]	78 ± 3.5[c]
Serum triglyceride (mg/dl)	34 ± 4.9[d]	20 ± 2.8[d,e]	45 ± 4.9[e]
Liver cholesterol (mg/g)	2.8 ± 0.07[f]	2.3 ± 0.1[f,g]	2.7 ± 0.1[g]
Liver triglyceride (mg/g)	5.4 ± 0.5[h]	4.8 ± 0.4[i]	7.3 ± 0.6[h,i]
Liver weight (g)	3.8 ± 0.1[j]	4.7 ± 0.2[j,k]	3.8 ± 0.07[k]
Fed			
Serum cholesterol (mg/dl)	57 ± 3.9[l]	50 ± 1.11	82 ± 3.5[l,m]
Serum triglyceride (mg/dl)	25 ± 2.1	18 ± 1.1	25 ± 3.9
Liver cholesterol (mg/g)	2.1 ± 0.04[n]	1.7 ± 0.07[n,o]	2.0 ± 0.04[o]
Liver triglyceride (mg/g)	5.9 ± 0.07	4.9 ± 0.5[q]	4.4 ± 0.3[q]
Liver weight (g)	5.2 ± 0.1[s]	7.1 ± 0.2[s,t]	4.6 ± 0.3[t]

[a] After Barnhart et al. (2). Eight male rats per group; drugs fed as 0.25% of diet.
[b-t] Values bearing same letter are significantly different.

terol levels were either elevated or in the high normal range. At a dosage of 375 mg/day, there was a 24% reduction after 6 weeks. Reductions on doses of 750, 1,500, and 3,000 mg/day were 29, 29, and 32%, respectively. All trials lasted 6 weeks.

Heel et al. (8) have summarized the results of a number of human trials in which the dose was usually 1 g/day; the duration ranged from 6 to 88 weeks in controlled trials to 0.5 to 5 years in open trials. Serum cholesterol levels

TABLE 3. *Influence of 0.3% probucol on lipid metabolism in rats*[a]

Parameter	Probucol	Control
No.	5/6	6/6
Weight gain (g)	92 ± 6	70 ± 9
Liver weight (g)	9.4 ± 0.6	6.8 ± 0.5[b]
Liver (% of body weight)	3.93 ± 0.14	3.13 ± 0.08[c]
Serum Lipids (mg/dl)		
Cholesterol	20 ± 1	44 ± 5[c]
Triglyceride	42 ± 5	75 ± 8[c]
Phospholipids	49 ± 7	38 ± 5
Liver lipids (mg/100 g)		
Cholesterol	140 ± 19	104 ± 12
Triglyceride	412 ± 2	417 ± 6
Phospholipids	145 ± 6	183 ± 9[c]
Serum plus liver pool (mg)		
Cholesterol	15	10
Triglycerides	42	33
Phospholipids	17	15

[a] Drug fed for 21 days. All values $\pm$ SEM.
[b] $p < 0.01$; [c] $p < 0.001$.

TABLE 4. *Influence of probucol on serum cholesterol: Controlled series*

Study	No.	Dose (g/day)	Duration (weeks)	Percent change	Authors
1[a]	19	1.0	12	−23	Brown and deWolfe (1974)
2	10	0.75	6	−17	Brusco et al. (1971)
3	10	1.0	21–38	−17	Davignon (1974)
4[a]	30	1.0	12	−13	LeLorier et al. (1977)
5	15	1.0	26	−21	Miettinen and Toivonen (1975)
6	24	1.0	12–88	−14	Nash (1975)
7	57	1.0	12–52	−23	Polachek et al. (1973)
8[a]	11	1.0	12	−18	Salel et al. (1976)

[a] Patients on fat-restricted diets.

were reduced in every instance. In the open studies, the reduction ranged from 9 to 29% and in the controlled trials from 13 to 23%. The data are summarized in Tables 4 and 5. Miettinen (12) administered probucol (2 g/day) to five subjects with familial hypercholesteremia and was able to effect a 27% reduction in serum cholesterol levels.

The mechanism of action of probucol is unclear. Barnhart et al. (2) found that when probucol-treated rats or mice were given labeled mevalonic acid, there was no effect on liver lipids; compared to controls, however, the animals showed significantly less radioactivity in their serum.

In a later study, Barnhart et al. (1) tested the effects of probucol on the utilization of intravenously administered [^{14}C]acetate. Mice were fed 0.06% probucol for 3 days and then given an intravenous dose of [1-^{14}C]acetate. There was 50% less radioactivity in the liver nonsaponifiable fraction of the treated mice and about 48% less radioactivity in the liver sterols. Rats were fed 0.125% probucol or clofibrate for 2 weeks and then injected intravenously with sodium [1,2-^{14}C]acetate. Serum cholesterol levels were reduced significantly ($p < 0.05$) by both drugs. Liver cholesterol levels were significantly lower in the clofibrate-treated rats but were unchanged in rats given probucol. The specific activity of the liver sterols was reduced by 65% ($p < 0.05$) in rats fed clofibrate but

TABLE 5. *Influence of probucol on serum cholesterol: Open studies*

Study	No.	Dose (g/day)	Duration (years)	Percent change	Authors
1	20	1	0.5	−15	Brusco et al. (1972)
2	117	1	1–4	−14	Canosa et al. (1975)
3	15	1	3	−15	Davignon (1974)
4	50	1	1	−19	Harris et al. (1974)
5	56	1	5	−29	McCaughan (1976)
6	23	1–2	0.67	−9	Miettinen and Toivonen (1975)
	15	1–2	0.5	−15	
7	61	1	1	−16	Parsons (1972)
8	50	1	2	−15	Parsons (1978)

only by 9% in rats fed probucol. Using the double isotope technique (15), Barnhart et al. (1) investigated the effect of probucol on cholesterol absorption in rats fed 0.25% clofibrate or probucol for 12 days. The percent absorption in the control rats was 63.1 ± 4.3, in probucol-treated rats 50.6 ± 4.0 ($p < 0.05$), and in clofibrate-treated rats 53.9 ± 3.2

Fecal steroids were determined in hypercholesteremic cynomolgus monkeys for 21 days before they were given 300 mg/kg/day probucol for 36 days. Fecal steroids were also determined during the drug treatment period. Fecal neutral steroid excretion averaged 0.63 ± 0.10 g/3 days before drug administration and 0.44 ± 0.02 g/3 days during treatment. The difference was not significant. Fecal bile acid excretion averaged 2.81 ± 0.22 mg/3 days prior to drug adminis-tration and 4.31 ± 0.37 during treatment ($p < 0.01$). Miettinen (12) administered 2 g/day probucol for 4 weeks to five patients with familial hypercholesteremia. He determined fecal steroid patterns and serum methylsterol levels to assess cholesterol synthesis and found a significant reduction in methylsterol levels during the first 24 days of treatment. During the treatment period, Miettinen found a significant increase in fecal fat, a slight increase in fecal neutral steroids, and a pronounced increase in fecal bile acids (Table 6). The hypocholesteremic action of probucol seems to involve a reduction in cholesterol absorption and synthesis and increased excretion of fecal bile acids.

Another possible mode of action of probucol might involve redistribution of cholesterol from serum and liver to other tissues. Duncan et al. (6) found that hyperthyroid rats had a higher total body cholesterol content than hypothy-roid rats but that the sterol was mostly in muscle and skin. Hypercholesteremic monkeys were given 300 mg/kg/day probucol for 9 weeks; the cholesterol levels of 19 tissues from each monkey were determined. Data from some of the more important tissues are given in Table 7. Both increases and decreases in cholesterol content were noted. When one considers the weight of organs involved, however, the overall effect is one of decreased cholesterol content (4).

Although probucol has been tested extensively vis-a-vis its effects on lipid metabolism, there are few data concerning its effects in atherosclerosis. We

TABLE 6. *Influence of probucol on sterol metabolism in man*[a]

| | Fecal steroids $\pm$ SEM (mg/g) | | |
| | Neutral | | |
Period[b] (days)	Dietary	Endogenous	Bile acids
Pretreatment (9)	218 ± 27	491 ± 45	164 ± 23
Transitional (15–21)	256 ± 25	517 ± 124	304 ± 48
Stable (9–13)	274 ± 31	392 ± 69	233 ± 48

[a] After Miettinen (12). Data from five subjects with familial hypercholesteremia.
[b] *Transitional*, period when serum cholesterol was decreasing; *stable*, period when serum cholesterol was at new low level.

TABLE 7. *Tissue cholesterol levels of hypercholesteremic monkeys with and without probucol treatment[a]*

Tissue	Cholesterol (mg/g ± SD)	
	Control	Drug
Liver	54.6 ± 27.7	28.8 ± 11.9
Spleen	7.4 ± 1.8	20.8 ± 12.9
Aorta	10.8 ± 10.3	8.0 ± 9.3
Skin	6.4 ± 1.9	6.2 ± 1.8
Lung	6.6 ± 1.0	5.9 ± 0.8
Testes	2.6 ± 0.4	3.6 ± 0.8
Ovary	27.0 ± 14.4	37.6 ± 5.0
Fat	2.7 ± 0.7	2.1 ± 0.7
Intestine	3.2 ± 0.4	3.0 ± 0.5
Heart	2.0 ± 0.2	2.1 ± 0.3

[a] (Ref. 4).

(10) have tested the effects of probucol (0.3 and 1.0% of diet) on atherosclerosis in rabbits fed cholesterol (2%) in corn oil (6%) for 8 weeks.

When probucol was fed at a level of 0.3%, it (a) had no effect on serum or liver cholesterol levels, (b) increased serum triglycerides by 57%, and (c) decreased liver triglycerides by 25%. There was no effect on the average atherosclerosis (graded on a 0 to 4 scale), which was about 11% lower in the test group. When probucol was administered as 1% of the diet, it lowered serum and liver cholesterol levels by 32 and 28%, respectively. In the test group, serum triglycerides were elevated by 18%, but liver triglycerides were 24% lower. Atherosclerosis in the rabbits fed 1% probucol was significantly less severe (by 28%). Aortas were graded on a 0 to 4 scale. Of the test rabbits, only 36% showed atherosclerosis in the arch of severity 2+ or higher, and only 7% of thoracic aortas exhibited this severity. In contrast, severity of atherosclerosis of 2+ or higher was observed in 59% of the control aortic arch and 24% of control thoracic aorta (Table 8).

The disposition of probucol has been studied in the rat, dog, monkey, and man. In rats fed ¹⁴C-labeled probucol, about 70% of the dose appeared in the feces within 30 hr. In general, about 3% of an oral dose and 4.5% of an intravenous dose of probucol was found in the carcass, skin, and adipose tissue (4). In dogs, 1.63% of an oral dose of probucol was found in the liver and 1.47% in the blood 16 hr after administration of labeled probucol. In monkeys, 0.85% of the ¹⁴C appeared in the plasma 16 hr after administration. A die-away curve revealed four plasma components with half-times of 0.5, 2, 10, and 51 days. The first two components accounted for most of the radioactivity (4).

In humans fed 3 g probucol, the average peak plasma level was seen at 24 hr (4.3 μg/ml). Up to 93% of the probucol appeared in the feces in 96 hr. Plasma disappearance curves revealed two components with half-times of 1 and 23 days, respectively (4).

Studies in rats fed 0.25% probucol for 2 weeks showed no changes in liver

TABLE 8. *Effect of 1% probucol in rabbits fed an atherogenic diet[a]*

Parameter	Group	
	Probucol	Control
No.	28/30	29/30
Weight gain (g)	231	230
Liver weight (g)	143	132
Serum lipids (mg/dl)		
Cholesterol	1,283	1,889
Triglyceride	224	190
Liver lipids (g/100 g)		
Cholesterol	4.01	5.56
Triglyceride	0.65	0.86
Average atheromata		
Arch	1.57	2.07
Thoracic	0.93	1.41

[a] Summary of three experiments; 2% cholesterol and 6% corn oil fed for 8 weeks.

glycogen levels. Among the liver enzymes tested, only glutamic dehydrogenase showed significant elevation (Table 9). In contrast, a number of enzyme activities, especially catalase, were elevated in clofibrate-fed rats (1). The livers of probucol-fed rats showed normal morphology.

Neither rats nor mice show evidence of toxicity following large single doses of probucol or chronic doses (100 to 800 mg/kg/day) for 2 years (13). Dogs tolerate large doses for short periods of time; in longer studies (3 to 24 months), however, about 33% of the dogs died suddenly, probably due to ventricular fibrillation. Studies in dogs, rats, mice, and monkeys suggest that probucol sensitizes the canine myocardium to epinephrine-induced ventricular fibrillation. This effect is not seen in other species (11,13).

In man, probucol (1 g/day) fed for 12 to 24 weeks produces few changes in baseline values for most biochemical indices (enzymes, thyroid, renal, and hepatic function, urinary and plasma steroids, glucose tolerance). Minor changes in serum CO_2, aldolase, and growth hormone were seen (3). Increases in serum uric acid levels have been observed (5).

TABLE 9. *Influence of probucol and clofibrate on rat liver enzymes[a]*

Enzyme	Probucol	Clofibrate
Catalase	1.07	8.34[b]
Lactic dehydrogenase	1.02	1.58[b]
Glutamic dehydrogenase	1.32[b]	1.62[b]
Glucose-6-phosphatase	1.00	1.05
Glutamate-pyruvate transaminase	1.26	1.59[b]

[a] After Barnhart et al. (1). Control = 1.00.
[b] Statistically different from control, $p < 0.05$.

The drug has been found to cause mild, transient eosinophilia (7), but the usual adverse side effects are gastrointestinal in nature (8,14).

In summary, probucol is a drug that lowers serum cholesterol levels (about 17% on the average) but has variable effects on serum triglycerides. The precise mechanism of action of probucol is not yet clear. In man, no serious side effects have been reported to date.

ACKNOWLEDGMENTS

This work was supported by grant HL 03299 and by Research Career Award HL 0734 from the National Institutes of Health.

REFERENCES

1. Barnhart, J. W., Rytter, D. J., and Molello, J. A. (1977): An overview of the biochemical pharmacology of probucol. *Lipids,* 12:29–33.
2. Barnhart, J. W., Sefranka, J. A., and McIntosh, D. D. (1970): Hypocholesteremic effect of 4,4'-(isopropylidenedithio)bis(2,6-di-t-butylphenol) (Probucol). *Am. J. Clin. Nutr.,* 23:1229–1233.
3. Danowski, T. S., Vester, J. W., Sunder, J. H., Gonzalez, A. R., Khurana, R. C., and Jung, Y. (1971): Endocrine and metabolic indices during administration of a lipophilic bis-phenol, probucol. *Clin. Pharmacol. Ther.,* 12:929–934.
4. Dow Chemical Co. (1979): *Personal communication.*
5. Drake, J. W., Bradford, R. H., McDearmon, M., and Furman, R. H. (1969): The effect of 4,4'-(isopropylidenedithio)bis(2,6-di-t-butylphenol) (DH581) on serum lipids and lipoproteins in human subjects. *Metabolism,* 18:916–925.
6. Duncan, C. H., Best, M. M., and Lubbe, R. J. (1964): Effects of L- and D-thyroxine and thyroidectomy on tissue weights and cholesterol content of the rat. *Metabolism,* 13:1–7.
7. Harris, R. S., Gilmore, H. R., Bricker, L. A., Kiem, I. M., and Ruben, E. (1974): Long-term oral administration of probucol 4,4'-(isopropylidenedithio)bis(2,6-di-t-butylphenol) (DH-581) in the management of hypercholesterolaemia. *J. Am. Geriatr. Soc.,* 22:167–175.
8. Heel, R. C., Brogden, R. N., Speight, T. M., and Avery, G. S. (1978): Probucol: a review of its pharmacological properties and therapeutic use in patients with hypercholesterolaemia. *Drugs,* 15:409–428.
9. Kritchevsky, D. (1971): Newer hypolipidemic agents. *Fed. Proc.,* 30:835–840.
10. Kritchevsky, D., Kim, H. K., and Tepper, S. A. (1971): Influence of 4,4'-(isopropylidenedithio)bis(2,6-di-t-butylphenol) (DH-581) on experimental atherosclerosis in rabbits. *Proc. Soc. Exp. Biol. Med.,* 136:1216–1221.
11. Marshall, F. N., and Lewis, J. E. (1973): Sensitization to epinephrine-induced ventricular fibrillation produced by probucol in dogs. *Toxicol. Appl. Pharmacol.,* 24:594–602.
12. Miettinen, T. A. (1972): Mode of action of a new hypocholesteraemic drug (DH-581) in familial hypercholesteraemia. *Atherosclerosis,* 15:163–176.
13. Molello, J. A., Gerbig, C. G., and Robinson, V. B. (1973): Toxicity of 4,4'-(isopropylidenedithio)bis(2,6-di-t-butylphenol), probucol, in mice, rats, dogs and monkeys. Demonstration of a species-specific phenomenon. *Toxicol. Appl. Pharmacol.,* 24:590–593.
14. Taylor, H. L., Nolan, R. B., Tedeschi, R. E., and Maurath, C. J. (1978): Combined results of the study of probucol at 1 gm/day in eight centers. *Clin. Pharmacol. Ther.,* 23:131.
15. Zilversmit, D. B. (1972): A single blood sample dual isotope method for the measurement of cholesterol absorption in rats. *Proc. Soc. Exp. Biol. Med.,* 140:862–865.

Diet and Drugs in Atherosclerosis,
edited by G. Noseda, B. Lewis, and R. Paoletti.
Raven Press, New York © 1980.

Toxicologic Studies on Probucol and Comparison of Liver Morphology in Rats Given Probucol, Fenofibrate, or Clofibrate

J. A. Molello, S. D. Barnard, and J. LeBeau

Health and Consumer Products Department, The Dow Chemical Company, Indianapolis, Indiana 46268

Probucol was given orally to 40 male and female rhesus monkeys at doses of 0, 60, 125, 250, or 500 mg/kg/day. Fourteen monkeys were killed at 18 and 24 months; 21 remained on test for 8 years. Observations included growth rate, hematology, clinical chemistry, urinalysis, organ weights, and gross, histopathologic, and electron-microscopic studies. Five unscheduled deaths occurred, none demonstrably related to treatment. No significant differences were observed between treated and control animals in regard to these observations.

Sprague-Dawley rats were given daily doses of approximately 500 mg/kg probucol, 250 mg/kg clofibrate, or 100 mg/kg fenofibrate in their diets for periods of up to 91 days to assess effects on liver cell ultrastructure. Control rats were given untreated basal rations. All compounds reduced serum cholesterol levels significantly. Liver tissues from probucol-treated rats were comparable to those from untreated control animals.

Clofibrate and fenofibrate caused hepatocytomegaly, an increase in the number of peroxisomes, and a mild alteration of the smooth and rough endoplasmic reticulum and mitochondria.

Early studies in animals indicated that probucol lowered serum cholesterol levels without discernible changes in the liver and without evidence of toxicity (2). Subsequent studies, however, showed that a species-specific phenomenon sometimes occurred (5). A review of toxicologic and related studies is the subject of this chapter.

Probucol is a dithiobisphenol with the chemical name 4,4'-(isopropylidene-dithio)bis(2,6-di-t-butylphenol). It is also known as DH-581, Lurselle, and Lorelco. The compound is a white, lipophilic substance.

PROBUCOL STUDIES

The LD_{50} for probucol to the mouse and rat is greater than 5,000 mg/kg/day (5). No evidence of toxicity was observed in a 91-day dietary study in rats, the highest daily average treatment level being 3,000 mg/kg/day (5). The compound was administered in the daily ration of beagle dogs for 91 days, the highest treatment level being 3,000 mg/kg/day. No lesions indicative of toxicity were observed (5). The 91-day test was repeated in another group of dogs with the test material administered in gelatin capsules, the highest dose being 3,000 mg/kg/day. No lesions related to treatment were observed (5).

Chronic studies were conducted in the rat with treatment levels up to and including 800 mg/kg/day. Probucol was administered as a suspension via orogastric intubation daily for 2 years. An adequate number of rats, 50 per gender per group, one control and four treatment groups, were tested. Survival was good, and at no time was there evidence of toxicity or of tumorigenicity (5). A 2-year study was also conducted in beagle dogs. Probucol was administered in the daily ration at individual doses up to and including 600 mg/kg/day. During this study, some treated dogs died. Special studies revealed that some dogs developed sensitization of the myocardium to epinephrine (4). Not all dogs became sensitized, nor did rhesus monkeys similarly treated. This type of response has not been observed in any other species given probucol. The manifestation is considered to be species-specific.

There was no evidence of adverse effect on fertility or length of gestation, pre- or postnatal survival, and other investigated parameters in male and female rats treated with probucol at doses up to and including 1,000 mg/kg/day (6).

Treatment of pregnant rats during periods of organogenesis was free of embryo- or fetotoxicity. Treatment of female rats prior to breeding and through day 15 of gestation and of female rabbits prior to breeding and through day 18 of gestation at dosage levels of 1,000 mg/kg/day was also free of any indication of teratogenicity and was without untoward effects (5). Probucol was nonmutagenic by the Ames test (3).

A number of studies have been conducted with probucol to explore its action in animals with cardiac myopathies. Animals under severe stress were not affected adversely by probucol.

Two studies were conducted by Davidson, Innes, and Weisman at the University of Manitoba in rats affected with cardiac myopathies caused by aortic constriction, cobalt chloride, or isoprenaline. In the first study, 90 rats were treated with 150 mg probucol/kg body weight i.p. twice daily for 21 days after the cardiac insult without adverse effect related to probucol. In the second study, 392 rats were treated once daily with 300 mg probucol/kg body weight for 10 days before and 21 days after the cardiac insult without an adverse effect related to probucol. Additional studies were then conducted in nonrodent species. In studies conducted by Litton-Bionetics, Kensington, Maryland, rhesus and cynomolgus monkeys were given 500 mg probucol/kg daily orally starting 14 days before and continuing 90 days after ligation of the left anterior descending coronary artery. No probucol-related adverse effect was observed.

A similar study was conducted in minipigs (Food Drug Research Laboratories, Waverly, New York); 500 mg/kg probucol was given orally for 10 to 14 days before and for 72 to 79 days following ligation of the left anterior descending coronary artery. Before each animal was submitted to necropsy, it was challenged five consecutive times with intravenous epinephrine bitartrate. Electrocardiograms for each pig revealed no changes indicative of a probucol-related aberration during and after each challenge.

EIGHT-YEAR STUDIES ON MONKEYS

Additional data on the safety of probucol were obtained during the chronic study in rhesus monkeys initiated in the early 1970s. The study started with 40 rhesus monkeys *(Macaca mulatta)* of both sexes.

The animals, approximately 2.5 years of age, were conditioned to our laboratory environment and were negative to the intradermal tuberculin test. These monkeys were assigned to one of five groups, each group consisting of three to five per gender, to be treated with probucol at levels of 0, 60, 125, or 500 mg/kg/day. Probucol was administered initially as a suspension via nasogastric intubation. When mixed with an orange-flavored liquid, the monkeys began to accept treatment without need for restraint, so that nasogastric intubation was gradually discontinued. Originally intended as an 18-month study, duration of the text was repeatedly extended until the monkeys had been on daily treatment, 7 days a week, for more than 8 years (6).

Frequent monitoring of many parameters was conducted throughout the study. Observations included clinical data, ophthalmoscopy, hematology, bone marrow cytology, clinical chemistries, urinalysis, and organ weights. Gross examination at necropsy and histopathologic evaluation of tissues were made of each monkey. At no time was there any indication of a treatment-related deleterious effect. Five unscheduled deaths occurred during the 8-year test; none was related to probucol treatment (Table 1). Electron microscopic examinations on liver tissue from monkeys treated for more than 8 years revealed comparable ultrastructural appearance in control and treated monkeys (Figs. 1 and 2).

RAT LIVER ULTRASTRUCTURE

Treatment of rats and mice with many lipid-lowering compounds causes liver cell alterations. Proliferation and enlargement of peroxisomes with enzymatic

TABLE 1. *Unscheduled deaths during 8-year study with probucol in rhesus monkey*

Probucol (mg/kg/day)	Sex	Years on test	Diagnosis
0	M	0.75	Tuberculosis
0	M	8.26	Adrenal cortical adenoma
60	M	1.63	Hypovolemia, shock
250	F	0.67	Autoimmune hemolytic anemia, pneumococcus infection
250	F	7.76	Asphyxiation due to aspiration

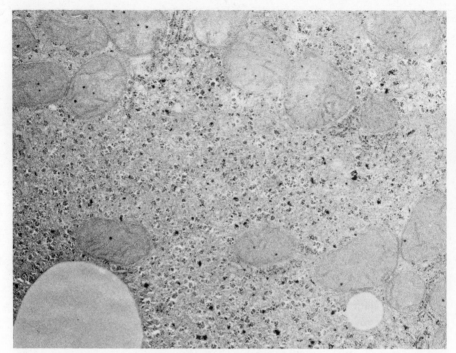

FIG. 1. Normal hepatocellular ultrastructure for untreated control monkey on 8-year test with probucol. Micrograph is representative of untreated monkeys.

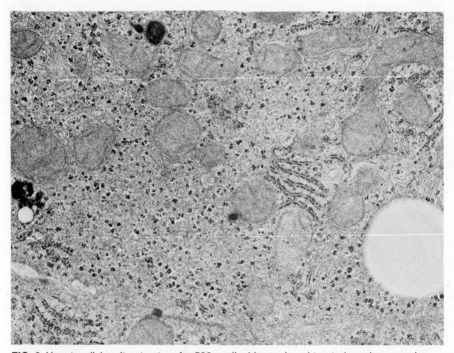

FIG. 2. Hepatocellular ultrastructure for 500 mg/kg/day probucol-treated monkey reveals morphology comparable to that for control animals. Micrograph is representative for treated monkeys.

TABLE 2. *Comparative studies of livers from rats after treatment with probucol, clofibrate, and fenofibrate*

Treatment	Liver (g) (mean)	Liver/body weight ratio (mean)
Control	13.7 ± 0.9	39.2 ± 2.0
Probucol (500 mg/kg)	14.4 ± 1.6	43.8 ± 5.3
Clofibrate (250 mg/kg)	$19.3^a \pm 2.2$	$59.2^a \pm 2.9$
Fenofibrate (100 mg/kg)	$22.2^a \pm 3.7$	$71.6^a \pm 5.4$

$^a p < 0.05$.

changes occur in these organelles. Although there was no indication that probucol induced similar changes in the rodent, specific studies had not been conducted to investigate this possible effect. These studies have now been conducted to determine the effect of probucol on the ultrastructure of the rat liver cell. Comparisons were made with effects elicited by clofibrate and fenofibrate. Liver tissue from the test animals was examined by light and electron microscopy (1).

A statistically significant increase in liver weights and in liver/body weight ratios was effected by clofibrate and fenofibrate; little if any change occurred in probucol-treated rats (Table 2).

Liver tissues of control and probucol-treated animals were comparable when examined by light microscopy, whereas hepatocytomegaly and cytoplasmic eosinophilia and granularity were discernible in liver cells from clofibrate- and fenofibrate-treated rats. Liver tissues from animals treated with probucol, except for possible increases in smooth endoplasmic reticulum, were determined by electron microscopy to have cellular morphology comparable to that of untreated controls. Clofibrate and fenofibrate, however, elicited an increase in the smooth endoplasmic reticulum, a decrease in rough endoplasmic reticulum accompanied by ribosomal detachment, and a slight depletion of glycogen (Figs. 3–10).

Additionally, there were alterations in the mitochondria characterized by pleomorphism, an increase in matrical dense granules, and slightly swollen cristae, which occasionally contained paracrystalline inclusions. The absence of peroxisomal increase in livers from probucol-treated animals has been corroborated by biochemical studies that show no change in liver catalase concentration after treatment. Whether peroxisomal increase is an adaptive response rather than an indication of cell injury or an indication of potential tumorigenicity remains to be resolved.

SUMMARY

The results of these and other experiments indicate that probucol is well tolerated over the short and long term by mice, rats, rabbits, monkeys, and minipigs maintained under conventional laboratory conditions or when subjected

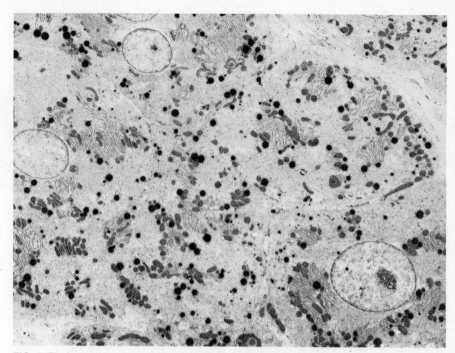

FIG. 3. Electron micrograph of hepatocytes from untreated control rat. *Dark spherical bodies,* peroxisomes.

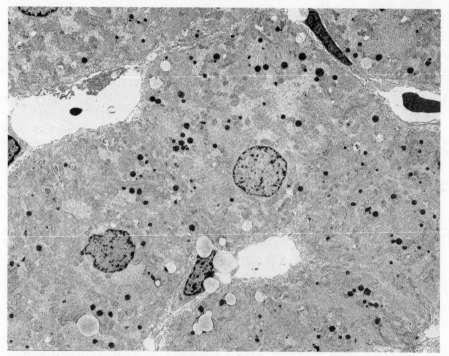

FIG. 4. Electron micrograph of hepatocytes from probucol rat (500 mg/kg/day). There is a normal frequency and size to the peroxisomes.

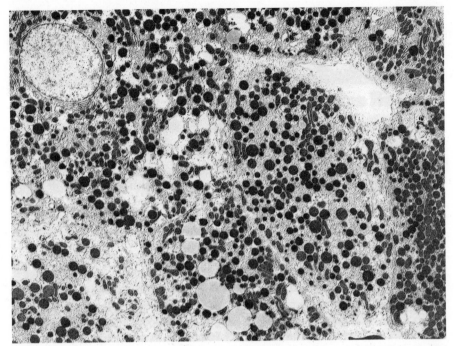

FIG. 5. Electron micrograph of hepatocytes from clofibrate rat (250 mg/kg/day). Peroxisomes are increased in number.

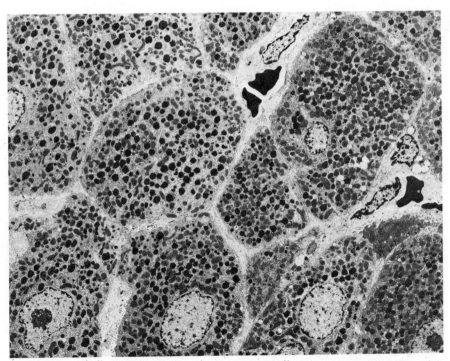

FIG. 6. Electron micrograph of hepatocytes from fenofibrate rat (100 mg/kg/day). There is a marked increase in peroxisomes.

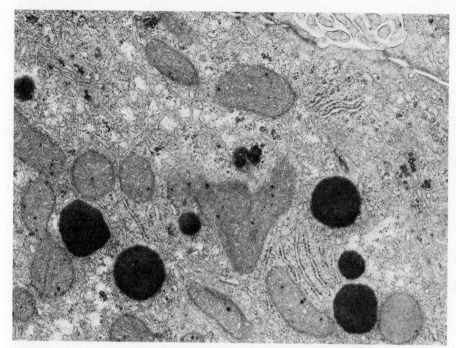

FIG. 7. Electron micrograph, higher magnification, of hepatocellular ultrastructure in untreated control rat.

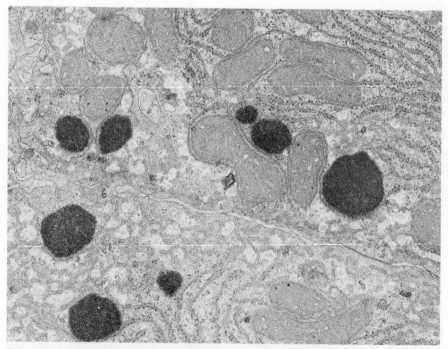

FIG. 8. Electron micrograph, higher magnification, of hepatocellular ultrastructure in probucol rat. Cellular appearance is comparable to that for untreated control except for possible slight increase in the smooth endoplasmic reticulum.

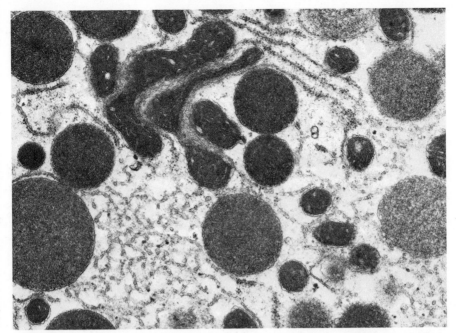

FIG. 9. Electron micrograph, higher magnification, of hepatocellular ultrastructure in clofibrate rat. Peroxisomes are increased, enlarged, and exhibit variable matrix densities. Mitochondria are elongated and occasionally contain paracrystalline inclusions in the cristae; smooth and rough endoplasmic reticulum are altered.

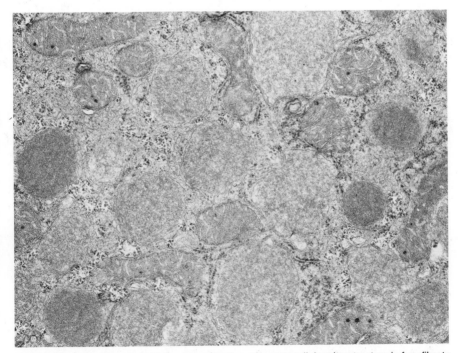

FIG. 10. Electron micrograph, higher magnification, of hepatocellular ultrastructure in fenofibrate rat. There is a marked increase in peroxisomes with greater variability in matrical densities. Mitochondria are pleomorphic and contain increased matrical dense granules. Smooth and rough endoplasmic reticulum are altered.

to severe cardiovascular stress. Dogs, on the other hand, are unique and develop myocardial sensitization to epinephrine. Additionally, unlike some cholesterol-lowering agents, probucol does not cause liver weight increase nor alter hepato-cellular morphology of the rodent and subhuman primate. Therefore, data from toxicologic and related studies suggest that probucol is a safe compound.

REFERENCES

1. Barnard, S. D., and Molello, J. A. (1979): Comparative evaluation of probucol versus fenofibrate and clofibrate when administered to rats for 28 days. *Unpublished data.*
2. Barnhart, J. W., Sefranka, J. A., and McIntosh, D. D. (1970): Hypocholesterolemic effect of 4,4'-(isopropylidenedithio)bis(2,6-di-t-butylphenol) (Probucol). *Am. J. Clin. Nutr.,* 23:1229.
3. Chandler, A. D., Jr. (1978): Mutagenicity evaluation of DH-581 (Probucol) with the salmonella/mammalian-microsome test (Ames test). *Unpublished data.*
4. Marshall, F. N., and Lewis, J. E. (1973): Sensitization to epinephrine-induced ventricular fibrillation produced by probucol in dogs. *Toxicol. Appl. Pharmacol.,* 24:594.
5. Molello, J. A., Gerbig, C. G., and Robinson, V. B. (1973): Toxicity of 4,4'-(isopropylidene-dithio)bis(2,6-di-t-butylphenol), probucol, in mice, rats, dogs and monkeys. Demonstration of a species-specific phenomenon. *Toxicol. Appl. Pharmacol.,* 24:590.
6. Molello, J. A., Thompson, D. J., and LeBeau, J. E. (1979): Eight year toxicity study in monkeys and reproduction studies in rats and rabbits treated with probucol. Presented at Society of Toxicology, New Orleans.

Diet and Drugs in Atherosclerosis,
edited by G. Noseda, B. Lewis, and R. Paoletti.
Raven Press, New York © 1980.

Effect of Probucol and Other Drugs on Sterol Synthesis in Human Lymphocytes

A. Anastasi, D. J. Betteridge, and D. J. Galton

*Diabetes and Lipid Research Laboratory, St. Bartholomew's Hospital,
London EC1 England*

Current therapeutic measures to treat hypercholesterolemia are unsatisfactory, and new hypocholesterolemic drugs are required. The human lymphocyte is a useful model in which to study the effects of potential hypocholesterolemic drugs on sterol synthesis, since there is an active pathway that is regulated in a manner similar to other mesenchymal cells (fibroblasts, smooth muscle cells). Several sites of drug inhibition are possible, either at transcription, translation, or direct pathway inhibition (Fig. 1).

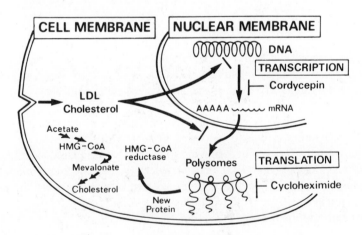

FIG. 1. Scheme of the regulation of sterol synthesis by LDL and possible sites of inhibition by drugs.

TRANSCRIPTION

The pathway for sterol synthesis can be induced by incubation of cells in a lipid-depleted medium or suppressed by incubation of cells in complete serum containing low density lipoprotein (LDL) (2). It is not yet known whether LDL suppresses the pathway by regulating synthesis of messenger RNA for the enzyme or by inhibiting at a posttranscriptional level, e.g., by controlling the translation of existing specific messenger RNA templates. We therefore studied the effect of cordycepin (12 to 50 μg/ml), an inhibitor of messenger RNA synthesis, on the induction of HMG-CoA reductase (4). Although cordycepin inhibited messenger RNA synthesis in lymphocytes by more than 50%, it had no inhibitory effect on the induction of activity of HMG-CoA reductase mediated by lipid-depleted serum. Assuming that cordycepin inhibits the synthesis of messenger RNA for the enzyme to a similar extent as total messenger RNA synthesis, our results indicate that the induction of HMG-CoA reductase by lipid-depleted serum does not require newly synthesized messenger RNA.

From the time course of the induction of HMG-CoA reductase in the presence of cordycepin (50 μg/ml), it appears that messenger RNA for HMG-CoA reductase is relatively stable. Thus inhibition of messenger RNA synthesis by cordycepin for up to 40 hr, which should significantly reduce the level of messenger RNA with a short half-life, did not impair the subsequent induction of HMG-CoA reductase when cells were transferred from complete to lipid-depleted serum. Therefore, the suppression of the enzyme by LDL, which occurs with a half-life of about 3 hr, may not be accounted for by a decrease in the synthesis of messenger RNA. This suggests that potential therapeutic drugs acting at transcription may not be of use for the treatment of hypercholesterolemia, even if they could be made specific for the enzyme HMG-CoA reductase.

TRANSLATION

The rise in activity of HMG-CoA reductase mediated by lipid-depleted serum was totally prevented by cycloheximide (20 μg/ml), a translational inhibitor of protein synthesis (5). The half-life of enzyme decay in the presence of cycloheximide was similar in lymphocytes with repressed or induced enzyme activities. This suggests that the increase in HMG-CoA reductase activity mediated by lipid-depleted serum is due to increased *de novo* synthesis of the enzyme and not to activation of preformed enzyme molecules or decreased degradation of the enzyme. The fact that LDL had an effect on the enzyme similar to that of cycloheximide in reducing the activity, with a half-life of about 3 hr, suggests that lipoprotein acts by rapidly inhibiting the synthesis of HMG-CoA reductase at a posttranscriptional level.

DIRECT PATHWAY INHIBITION

Several drugs have been found to directly inhibit sterol synthesis in human lymphocytes.

Compactin

Compactin is a fungal metabolite isolated from pencillium brevicompactum (3) and has been shown to be a potent competitive inhibitor of HMG-CoA reductase in microsomal enzyme preparations of rat liver (3). We found that compactin (0.2 μM) inhibited the incorporation into sterol of acetate (0.5 mM) but not of mevalonate (1 mM), the product of the HMG-CoA reductase reaction, indicating that the compound specifically inhibits the activity of HMG-CoA reductase (1). Compactin also inhibited sterol synthesis to the same degree in lymphocytes from heterozygous patients with familial hypercholesterolemia.

Probucol

Probucol has been reported to be an effective hypocholesterolemic agent in the mouse, rat, and dog, and in man. Its mechanism of action is incompletely identified; it could increase excretion of fecal bile acids or inhibit cholesterol synthesis. The drug is sparingly soluble in organic solvents. Difficulty was experienced in testing the drug on human lymphocytes *in vitro*. Probucol (19 μM), however, when dissolved in ethanol (10 μl), did not appear to inhibit sterol synthesis from ^{14}C-acetate. When dissolved in dimethylsulfoxide, probucol (0.1 mM) produced a 20% inhibition of sterol synthesis from acetate, but the solvent damaged the cells. Probucol at high concentrations (up to 1 mM), emulsified with bovine serum albumin, produced a $37 \pm 12\%$ ($N = 11$) inhibition of sterol synthesis from ^{14}C-acetate. It is possible, therefore, that some of the hypocholesterolemic action of probucol may be mediated by inhibition of sterol synthesis if other cells respond in the same manner.

REFERENCES

1. Betteridge, D. J., Krone, W., Reckless, J. P. D., and Galton, D. J. (1978): Compactin inhibits cholesterol synthesis in lymphocytes and intestinal mucosa from patients with familial hypercholesteremia. *Lancet*, ii:1342–1343.
2. Brown, M. S., Dana, S. E., and Goldstein, J. L. (1973): Regulation of 3-hydroxy-3-methylglutaryl coenzyme A reductase activity in human fibroblasts by lipoprotein. *Proc. Natl. Acad. Sci. USA*, 70:2162–2166.
3. Endo, A., Tsujita, Y., Kuroda, M., and Tanzawa, K. (1976): Inhibition of cholesterol synthesis *in vitro* and *in vivo* by ML-236A and ML-236B competitive inhibitors of 3-hydroxy-3-methylglutaryl coenzyme A reductase. *Eur. J. Biochem.*, 77:31–36.
4. Krone, W., Betteridge, D. J., and Galton, D. J. (1979): Regulation of sterol synthesis in human lymphocytes: evidence for post-transcriptional control by LDL. *Biochim. Biophys. Acta*, 574:361–365.
5. Krone, W., Betteridge, D. J., and Galton, D. J. (1979): Mechanism of regulation of 3-hydroxy-3-methylglutaryl coenzyme A reductase activity by LDL in human lymphocytes. *Eur. J. Clin. Invest.*, 9:405–410.

Diet and Drugs in Atherosclerosis,
edited by G. Noseda, B. Lewis, and R. Paoletti.
Raven Press, New York © 1980.

Hypolipidemic Effect and Mechanism of Action of Probucol in Mice and Rabbits

R. Infante and D. Petit

Liver Research Unit, I.N.S.E.R.M., 75571 Paris Cedex 12 France

The hypocholesterolemic effect of probucol was originally observed by Barnhart *et al.* in 1970 (1). A consistent decrease in the plasma cholesterol level was obtained in normal mice after 2 weeks of administration of the drug mixed with a standard diet. Further studies (2,6,8,13) have described the hypocholesterolemic action of probucol in rats, rabbits, dogs, and monkeys, and clinical studies have confirmed the efficacy of the drug in the treatment of hypercholesterolemic patients (3–5,7,10,11,13–15).

Few data have been reported on the bioavailability, biotransformation and mechanism of action of the drug (12). The present experiments deal with the pharmacological effect of probucol on plasma and tissue lipids in mice and rabbits after acute or chronic administration of the drug in association with standard, fat-free or high cholesterol and fat diets. Cholesterol synthesis *in vivo* from radioactive mevalonate was also studied.

PROCEDURES

Swiss strain male mice (25 g) and male white rabbits (2.5 to 3 kg) were fed standard or synthetic diets with or without a supplement of probucol. In acute experiments, probucol was first dissolved in purified coconut oil and then emulsified by sonication in an aqueous solution of dextrose-lecithin containing a small amount of a nonionic detergent. The micellar solution was stable for several hours. Control groups of mice and rabbits were injected with the same micellar solution of lecithin without probucol.

In some experiments, ^{14}C-mevalonolactone (C.E.A., Saclay, France) was injected intravenously 1 hr before sacrifice.

Liver and plasma lipids were extracted (16) and fractionated by thin layer chromatography on silica gel. Lipid analysis (17–19) was performed by conventional methods, and radioactivity was measured by liquid scintillation spectrometry.

RESULTS

Effect of Probucol on Plasma and Liver Lipid in Mice

Probucol administration (0.06% of diet) to mice results in a sharp decrease of plasma cholesterol (−33%) and triglyceride (−44%) after 7 days, which is even more pronounced after 21 days of treatment. NEFA concentration is significantly lowered by the drug (Tables 1 and 2). Liver weight and liver lipid concentrations do not change with treatment.

The rapid and substantial decrease in plasma cholesterol could be the expression of a redistribution of cholesterol between plasma and tissue compartments. To investigate this possibility and to estimate endogenous cholesterol synthesis, groups of mice were fed a synthetic diet devoid of fat and cholesterol and to which 1% linoleic acid had been added. After 10 days, the animals were divided in two groups; one received the synthetic diet alone, whereas the diet of the second group was supplemented with probucol. Two weeks later, ^{14}C-mevalonate was injected intravenously 1 hr before sacrifice. Unexpectedly, plasma cholesterol levels were not affected by probucol under these conditions. Indeed, liver, intestine, and carcass cholesterol content and the distribution of *de novo* synthesized ^{14}C-cholesterol were identical in the treated and control mice.

To explain these results, it was assumed that in the absence of a normal amount of alimentary fat, the bioavailability of the drug would be below the minimum required for a pharmacological effect. This hypothesis was tested in a series of experiments in which four groups of mice were fed a synthetic diet (delipidated caseine-sucrose-cellulose-salts-vitamins and linoleic acid). This basic diet, free of fat and cholesterol, was supplemented with lard and vegetable oil in amounts sufficient to give a range in fat concentration from 0 to 10% (isocaloric amounts of sucrose were subtracted from the mixture). To this latter diet (10% fat), 1% cholesterol and 0.5% Na cholate were added in order to induce a moderate alimentary hyperlipemia. One batch of each type of diet was supplemented with 0.06% probucol.

Probucol administration was ineffective in lowering plasma cholesterol when

TABLE 1. *Effect of probucol (0.6 g/kg diet) on liver and plasma lipids in mice*[a]

Parameter	Control (7 days)	Probucol (7 days)
Body weight gain (g)	8.0	7.0
Liver weight (g)	1.17 ± 0.05	1.13 ± 0.03
Liver cholesterol (mg/g)	3.48 ± 0.17	3.72 ± 0.23
Liver triglycerides (mg/g)	10.7 ± 1.30	12.50 ± 1.7
Plasma cholesterol (mg/100 ml)	63.0 ± 2.10	42.0 ± 3.0[a]
Plasma triglycerides (mg/100 ml)	50.0 ± 5.00	28.0 ± 1.4[a]
Plasma NEFA (μmol/100 ml)	71.0 ± 2.30	44.0 ± 2.0[a]

[a] Mean ± SE from 10 mice per group. Initial body weight, 25 g.
[b] $p < 0.001$.

TABLE 2. *Effect of probucol (0.6 g/kg diet) on liver and plasma lipids in mice[a]*

Parameter	Control (21 days)	Probucol (21 days)
Body weight gain (g)	13.8	17.0
Liver weight (g)	1.28 ± 0.04	1.37 ± 0.04
Liver cholesterol (mg/g)	3.64 ± 0.10	3.69 ± 0.30
Liver triglycerides (mg/g)	14.3 ± 3.40	16.6 ± 1.10
Plasma cholesterol (mg/100 ml)	99.0 ± 5.20	40.0 ± 4.20 [b]
Plasma triglycerides (mg/100 ml)	138.0 ± 14.0	50.0 ± 6.00 [b]
Plasma NEFA (μmol/100 ml)	100.0 ± 6.0	54.0 ± 4.00 [c]

[a] Mean $\pm$ SE from 10 mice per group. Initial body weight, 25 g.
[b] $p < 0.001$.
[c] $p < 0.05$.

it was associated with fat-free or low-fat (1%) diets (Table 3). When the drug was administered together with a normal diet (3% fat), however, significant decreases in plasma cholesterol and triglyceride were obtained (60 and 50%, respectively).

The hypolipidemic effect of probucol was also observed in mice maintained on a diet enriched in fat and cholesterol. In the control animals, plasma cholesterol and triglyceride were raised to more than twice normal levels. Probucol completely prevented the hypercholesterolemia and maintained triglyceride at a slightly higher level than normal. Mice receiving a high-fat diet developed liver steatosis; triglyceride and cholesterol accumulation in the liver was not prevented by probucol administration, thus indicating a selective effect of the drug on plasma lipids and lipoproteins.

Effect of Probucol on Plasma and Liver Lipid in Rabbits

Two groups of rabbits were fed a standard diet supplemented with 0.1 or 0.25 probucol, respectively. Blood samples were collected 10 and 21 days after initiation of the experiment.

Probucol significantly decreased plasma cholesterol (Table 4) when administered at the 1% level; no further decrease was obtained with the higher dose (2.5%). For each dose, however, plasma cholesterol continued to fall after 10 and up to 21 days, at which time decreases of 44 and 56%, respectively, were observed. Plasma triglyceride and NEFA did not change significantly; but a significant decrease in plasma phospholipid concentration was obtained with both doses of probucol.

Plasma and liver protein contents and liver lipids were in the range of normal values.

The protective effect of probucol against the development of hyperlipemia in rabbits was studied in animals receiving a standard diet (6% fat) supplemented with 7% melted lard and 1% cholesterol, added with or without probucol (either 0.1 or 0.25%), for 15 days.

TABLE 3. Effect of probucol (0.6 g/kg diet) on plasma lipids in mice under different diets[a]

Lipid	0% Fat		1% Fat		3% Fat		10% Fat[b]	
	Control	Probucol	Control	Probucol	Control	Probucol	Control	Probucol
Cholesterol (mg/100 ml)	86 ± 7	92 ± 7	75 ± 4	87 ± 8	78 ± 4	31 ± 3[c]	164 ± 11	74 ± 6[c]
Triglycerides (mg/100 ml)	19 ± 4	21 ± 4	42 ± 8	32 ± 5	55 ± 9	25 ± 4[e]	134 ± 12	79 ± 10[d]
NEFA (μmol/100 ml)	168 ± 13	220 ± 10	220 ± 8	230 ± 12	96 ± 8	110 ± 2	100 ± 5	81 ± 6

[a] Mean ± SE from 10 animals per group.
[b] Added with 1% cholesterol and 0.1% Na cholate.
[c] Significantly different from controls, $p < 0.001$.
[d] Significantly different from controls, $p < 0.005$.
[e] Significantly lower from controls, $p < 0.01$.

TABLE 4. *Effect of probucol on plasma lipids in rabbits fed a standard diet*[a]

Lipid	Probucol (1 g/kg diet)			Probucol (2.5 g/kg diet)		
	Before	10 days	21 days	Before	10 days	21 days
Cholesterol (mg/100 ml)	43.8 ± 4	27.1 ± 5 ($p < 0.05$)	24.6 ± 4 ($p < 0.01$)	44.8 ± 7	26.5 ± 2 ($p < 0.05$)	19.7 ± 3 ($p < 0.01$)
Triglycerides (mg/100 ml)	82.0 ± 19	104 ± 15	56 ± 5	118 ± 11	143 ± 17	107 ± 14
Phospholipids (mg/100 ml)	123.6 ± 9	106.8 ± 9	69 ± 5.6 ($p < 0.001$)	121.3 ± 9	115.4 ± 10	68 ± 7 ($p < 0.001$)
NEFA (µmol/100 ml)	47.3 ± 1		65 ± 16	47.3 ± 1		53.8 ± 6

[a]Mean ± SE from 10 animals per group. In parenthesis, significance compared to control values.

The control group developed a marked hyperlipemia involving all lipid classes, and particularly cholesterol, which was raised 30-fold higher than the initial level (Table 5). Although probucol did not prevent the hyperlipemia, a much lower increase in cholesterol and phospholipid levels was observed at both concentrations of the drug. As in the rabbit fed a normal diet, probucol has a negligible effect on plasma triglyceride levels. Liver lipid content was significantly increased in all animals; probucol did not protect against fatty liver.

Effect of Intravenous Administration of Probucol on Plasma Lipids in Mice and Rabbits

Mice injected with the excipient solution developed a moderate and transient hypertriglyceridemia (Fig. 1). Probucol produced a significant decrease of plasma cholesterol at 6 hr, which remained for as long as 10 days after injection. Phospholipid levels rapidly decreased after drug injection and remained far lower than the initial values some 10 days later.

After injection of the triglyceride-phospholipid emulsion, control rabbits showed a sharp increase in all plasma lipid fractions (Fig. 2). Cholesterol was increased to almost five times the normal values. Probucol remarkably protected the animals against this type of hyperlipemia. In fact, cholesterol and phospholipid levels were significantly lower than those found before injection. These effects remained 10 days after injection, presumably because of the long lifetime of probucol in the body.

Studies on the Mechanism of Action of Probucol

Cholesterol synthesis has been studied in mice receiving a standard diet either supplemented or not with 0.06% probucol for 1 or 3 weeks. The animals received an intravenous injection of ^{14}C-mevalonolactone 1 hr before they were anesthetized and exsanguinated by aortic puncture.

Plasma cholesterol decreased in the animals receiving probucol for 1 or 3 weeks to 44 and 47%, respectively, of control values. The cholesterol contents of liver, intestine, and carcass were similar in treated and control groups. The specific radioactivity of tissue cholesterol was similar in control and probucol-treated animals. Plasma ^{14}C-cholesterol in the animals fed probucol for 21 days (40.276 ± 1.375 cpm/ml) was about half that of controls (91.708 ± 2.988 cpm/ml), thus suggesting a decrease in lipoprotein-cholesterol secretion.

DISCUSSION

Probucol has a definite hypocholesterolemic effect in mice fed a standard diet. Plasma triglycerides are also lowered, and NEFA levels are below control values after 7 days of treatment. Barnhart *et al.* (2) have described the hypocho-

TABLE 5. *Plasma lipid composition in rabbits fed a cholesterol-rich diet supplemented or not with probucol*[a]

Lipid	Control		Probucol (1 g/kg diet)		Probucol (2.5 g/kg diet)	
	Before	15 days	Before	15 days	Before	15 days
Cholesterol (mg/100 ml)	40.5 ± 3.9	1.375 ± 57	57.5 ± 8	860 ± 80 ($p < 0.001$)	45.7 ± 5.3	1.052 ± 105 ($p < 0.05$)
Triglycerides (mg/100 ml)	81.6 ± 8.5	214 ± 26	87.0 ± 9.7	148 ± 36	119 ± 21.0	180 ± 30
Phospholipids (mg/100 ml)	108.6 ± 8.7	600 ± 39	128.7 ± 8.0	403.5 ± 44	136.2 ± 9.5	434 ± 39 ($p < 0.02$)
NEFA (µmol/100 ml)	47.3 ± 1.4	104 ± 10.7		84 13.7		65.8 ± 4.8 ($p < 0.02$)

[a]Mean ± SE from 10 animals per group.
Standard diet (6% fat) enriched with 1% cholesterol and 7% lard. In parentheses, statistical significance of values in probucol-treated animals compared to corresponding controls (15 days).

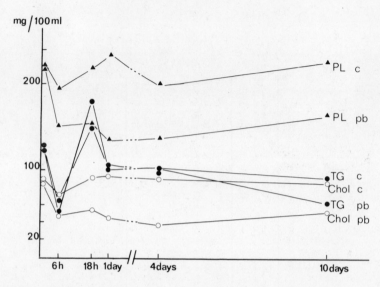

FIG. 1. Effect of a single dose (80 mg/kg b.w. i.v.) of probucol (pb) on plasma lipid concentration in mice. Control animals (c) were injected with the excipient used to dissolve probucol. *Triangles*, phospholipid; *open circles*, cholesterol; *solid circles*, triglycerides. Mean values from 10 animals per group.

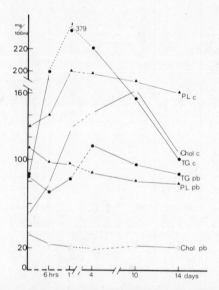

FIG. 2. Effect of a single dose (80 mg/kg b.w. i.v.) of probucol (pb) on plasma lipid concentration in rabbits. Control animals (c) were injected with the coconut oil-lecithin-dextrose micellar solution used to dissolve probucol. *Triangles*, phospholipid; *open circles*, cholesterol; *solid circles*, triglycerides. Means from 10 animals per group.

lesterolemic effect of probucol in mice, which is grossly proportional to the administered dose with a maximal response at 0.6 g probucol/kg diet.

In addition to the effect on "basal" lipid levels, the drug partly prevents the development of an alimentary-induced hyperlipemia, although it fails to modify cholesterol and triglyceride storage in the liver.

As in mice, administration of probucol to rabbits produces a significant fall in plasma cholesterol levels in normal or cholesterol-fed animals. Plasma NEFA and triglycerides, however, are not affected by probucol in this species. Furthermore, liver steatosis that developed with a cholesterol-rich diet is not prevented by the drug. Of particular interest is the acute effect of probucol after a single intravenous administration to mice and rabbits.

From these experiments, one may speculate on the mechanism of action of probucol. Any effect on cholesterol intestinal absorption can be discarded. It is unlikely that a marked decrease of plasma cholesterol and phospholipid levels in 6 hr could be obtained through an inhibition of cholesterol synthesis. This seems to be unaffected by the drug, as far as it could be estimated by acetate (2) or mevalonate incorporation into cholesterol of liver, intestine, and other tissues.

The fact that not only plasma cholesterol but also phospholipid (and in mice triglyceride) levels are depressed by the drug without any effect on tissue lipid concentration suggests that probucol develops its pharmacological effect by inhibiting lipoprotein synthesis or by enhancing their catabolism.

Preliminary experiments in our laboratory have shown that in mice treated with probucol for 3 weeks, lipoprotein synthesis *in vivo,* as assessed by ^{3}H-leucine and ^{14}C-glycerol incorporation, is inhibited. Very low density lipoprotein (VLDL) triglyceride synthesis is decreased to one-third of the control values, and a less marked but significant decrease of ^{3}H-leucine incorporation into VLDL apoprotein has been observed. Cholesterol-lipoprotein synthesis and release in treated and control animals are currently under investigation.

Besides the apparent lack of effect of probucol in animals on liver cholesterol synthesis, intestinal absorption, cholesterol catabolism, and fecal sterol or bile acid excretion, some results suggest a moderate effect of the drug on neutral sterol and bile acids output in man (11) and in cynomolgus monkeys (2). Thus some inhibition of cholesterol synthesis, as estimated by the fall in plasmatic methylsterol levels, has been described by Miettinen (11) in human volunteers. Other studies in humans (9), however, have failed to confirm any effect of probucol on the later stages of cholesterol synthesis. At present, there is a lack of information on the effect of probucol on lipoprotein metabolism in man.

Probucol is probably not absorbed by the intestinal mucosa in the absence of alimentary fat. Presumably, this hydrophobic compound is solubilized in the micellar phase of the intestinal content formed by fat, the products of lipolysis, cholesterol, and bile acids. It should be noted, however, that the drastic conditions used in our experiments in mice (synthetic diet of low fat content), although useful for evaluation of the bioavailability of the drug, are not found in patients even when the drug is administered in association with a low-fat diet.

REFERENCES

1. Barnhart, J. W., Sefranka, J. A., and McIntosh, D. D. (1970): Hypocholesterolemic effect of [4,4'-(isopropylidenedithio)-bis(2,6, di-t-butylphenol)] (Probucol). *Am. J. Clin. Nutr.*, 23:1229–1233.
2. Barnhart, J. W., Rytter, D. J., and Molello, J. A. (1977): An overview of the biochemical pharmacology of Probucol. *Lipids*, 12:29–33.
3. Brown, H. B., and De Wolfe, V. G. (1974): The additive effect of Probucol on diet in hyperlipidemia. *Clin. Pharmacol. Ther.*, 16:44–50.
4. Davignon, J. (1974): Clofibrate and DH 581 in the long-term treatment of primary hyperlipoproteinemia. In: *Third International Symposium on Atherosclerosis*, edited by G. Scheltler and A. Weizer, pp. 794–797. Springer Verlag, Berlin.
5. Drake, J. W., Bradford, R. H., McDearmon, M., and Furman, R. H. (1969): The effect of [4,4'-(isopropylidenedithio)-bis(2,6-di-t-butylphenol)] (DH 581) on serum lipids and lipoproteins in human subjects. *Metabolism*, 18:916–925.
6. Duncan, C. H., and Best, M. M. (1973): The additive effects of clofibrate and probucol (DH 581) on rat serum cholesterol. *Atherosclerosis*, 17:161–166.
7. Harris, R. S., Gilmore, H. R., Bricker, L. A., Kiem, I. M., and Rubin, E. (1974): Long-term oral administration of Probucol [4,4'-(isopropylidenethio)-bis(2,6-di-t-butylphenol)] (DH 581) in the management of hypercholesterolemia. *J. Am. Geriatr. Soc.*, 22:167–175.
8. Kritchevsky, D., Kim, H. K., and Tepper, S. A. (1971): Influence of [4,4'-(isopropylidenedithio)-bis(2,6-di-t-butylphenol)] (DH 581) on experimental atherosclerosis in rabbits. *Proc. Soc. Exp. Biol. Med.*, 136:1216–1221.
9. Le Lorier, J., Du Breuil, S., Lussier, S., Huang, Y. S., and Davignon, J. (1977): Diet and Probucol in lowering cholesterol concentrations. *Arch. Int. Med.*, 137:1429–1437.
10. McCaughan, D. (1974): Long-term use of Probucol in patients with hypercholesterolemia. In: *Fifth International Symposium on Drugs Affecting Lipid Metabolism*, p. 70. Milan.
11. Miettinen, T. A. (1972): Mode of action of a new hypocholesteraemic drug (DH 581) in familial hypercholesterolemia. *Atherosclerosis*, 15:163–176.
12. Molello, J. A., Gerbig, C. G., and Robinson, V. B. (1973): Toxicity of [4,4'-(isopropylidenedithio)-bis(2,6-di-t-butylphenol)] (Probucol), in mice, rats, dogs and monkeys: Demonstration of a species-specific phenomenon. *Toxicol. Appl. Pharmacol.*, 24:590–593.
13. Nash, D. T. (1974): Safety and efficacy of Probucol during one year administration. *J. Clin. Pharmacol.*, 14:470–475.
14. Nash, D. T. (1975): Probucol. A new cholesterol lowering drug. *J. Med.*, 6:305–315.
15. Salel, A. F., Zelis, R., Sodhi, H. S., Price, J., and Mason, D. T. (1976): Probucol: A new cholesterol-lowering drug effective in patients with type II hyperlipoproteinemia. *Clin. Pharmacol. Ther.*, 20:690–694.
16. Folch, J., Lees, M., and Sloane-Stanley, G. H. (1957): A simple method for the isolation and purification of total lipids from animal tissues. *J. Biol. Chem.*, 226:19.
17. Delsal, J. L., and Manhouri, H. (1955): Etude comparative des dosages colorimétriques du phosphore. Recherche d'une méthode de haute sensibilité applicable au dosage du phosphore organique dans les spots aprés chromatographie. *Bull. Soc. Chim. Biol.*, 37:1041–1054.
18. Kessler, G., and Lederer, H. (1965): Fluorometric measurement of triglycerides. In: *Automation and Analytical Chemistry*, edited by L. T. Sreegs, pp. 341–344. Technicon Symposia, New York.
19. Roschlau P., Bernt, T., and Gruber, W. (1974): Test combination cholesterol (enzymatic colorimetric method). *Z. Klin. Chem. Klin. Biochem.*, 12:403.

Diet and Drugs in Atherosclerosis,
edited by G. Noseda, B. Lewis, and R. Paoletti.
Raven Press, New York © 1980.

Probucol in the Long-Term Management of Hypercholesterolemia

D. McCaughan

Department of Medicine, Veterans Administration Medical Center, The Peter Bent Brigham Hospital and Harvard Medical School, Boston, Massachusetts 02115

One hundred eighteen male patients with serum cholesterol levels greater than 250 mg/dl (determined from three pretreatment cholesterol determinations) were randomized in a double-blind study. Eighty-eight patients received probucol (500 mg b.i.d.) and 30 received placebo. At the end of 1 year, the majority of the probucol-treated patients were treated for further periods of up to 9 years. The selection of patients for entry into the study was based on serum cholesterol levels; many had significant cardiovascular disease (Table 1). Of the treated group, 60% had abnormal electrocardiograms (ECGs), 40% had a history of angina pectoris, and 34% had a history of myocardial infarction; 41% were receiving antihypertensive medication, 32% an antianginal drug, and 14% digitalis. Similar findings were present in the placebo group. The average ages at entry (Table 2) were 49.4 years (probucol) and 51 years (placebo). The pretreatment mean serum cholesterol levels were 305 mg/dl (probucol) and 307 mg/dl (placebo). All patients were male, and all but two were white (Table 2).

Data were available for 1 year on 103 patients (78 probucol and 25 placebo). The probucol group showed a significant lowering of serum cholesterol at 1 month of 8.4%, compared with a placebo effect of 0.7% ($p < .01$). After 6 months of probucol treatment, the mean serum cholesterol reduction was 17.2%, compared with a placebo effect of 5.7%. For the remainder of the first year, serum cholesterol levels in the probucol-treated group remained at significantly lower levels than the placebo-treated patients (Table 3).

After the initial 6 months, the placebo-treated patients began to exhibit a reduction of serum cholesterol levels that did not significantly affect the overall results. This may be attributed to regression to the mean and the effect of heightened awareness of dietary considerations. At the end of 1 year, 61 patients in the probucol group elected to continue long-term probucol therapy. Many of these patients are now entering their tenth year of treatment. Serum cholesterol levels have remained lowered, with a mean value 23 to 28% below baseline values. Significant cholesterol lowering was shown in different lipoprotein phenotypes (types IIa, IIb, and IV). No subjects with types I, III, or V were studied. No consistent or significant effect was seen on serum triglyceride levels.

175

TABLE 1. *Percentage of patients with various findings at entry*[a]

Finding	Probucol (N = 88)		Placebo (N = 30)	
	No.	%	No.	%
ECG				
Normal	53	60	18	60
Abnormal	35	40	12	40
Angina				
Yes	35	40	9	30
No	53	60	21	70
Myocardial infarction				
Yes	30	34	10	33
No	58	66	20	67
Cerebrovascular accident				
Yes	1	1	1	3
No	87	99	29	97
Arterial thrombosis				
Yes	0	0	0	0
No	88	100	30	100
Peripheral vascular insufficiency				
Yes	3	3	3	10
No	85	97	27	90
Cardiomegaly				
Yes	2	2	3	10
No	86	98	27	90
Cardiac murmur				
Yes	5	6	1	3
No	83	94	28	94
Unknown			1	3
Smoker				
Yes	46	52	7	23
No	42	48	22	74
Unknown			1	3
Blood pressure (mmHg)				
Diastolic				
>90	25	28	10	33
≤90	63	72	20	67
Systolic				
>140	24	27	11	37
≤140	64	73	19	63

[a] One-year, double-blind, placebo-controlled trial.

TABLE 2. *Demographic data*[a]

Parameter	Probucol	Placebo
Male patients (N = 118)	88	30
Caucasian	87	29
Negro	1	1
Average age ± SD	49.4 ± 6.7	51.0 ± 5.6
Average serum cholesterol (mg/dl ± SD)	304.7 ± 36.4	306.6 ± 34.8
Average serum triglycerides (mg/dl ± SD)	260.4 ± 141.9	204.0 ± 111.6

[a] Double-blind trial.

TABLE 3. Cholesterol level response to probucol therapy[a]

Month	Total patients	Response level					
		>0	0 to -4.9	-5 to -9.9	-10 to -14.9	-15 to -19.9	>-19.9
12	77	9 (11.7)[b]	4 (5.2)	4 (5.2)	11 (14.3)	13 (16.9)	36 (46.8)
24	61	5 (8.2)	9 (14.7)	5 (8.2)	6 (9.8)	4 (6.6)	32 (52.4)
36	58[c]	1 (1.7)	1 (1.7)	5 (8.6)	3 (5.1)	10 (17.2)	38 (65.6)
48	59	0 (0)	0 (0)	2 (3.4)	8 (13.6)	8 (13.6)	41 (69.5)
60	55	1 (1.8)	3 (5.4)	5 (9.0)	3 (5.4)	6 (10.9)	37 (67.3)
72	55	0 (0)	1 (1.8)	6 (10.9)	7 (12.7)	5 (9.0)	36 (65.5)
84	47	2 (4.2)	0 (0)	5 (10.6)	7 (14.9)	6 (12.8)	27 (57.4)

[a] Long-term open trial. Probucol was supplied by Medical/Clinical Investigation group of the Human Health and Consumer Products Department, The Dow Chemical Company, Indianapolis, Indiana.
[b] Number of patients (%) showing indicated change in serum cholesterol.
[c] Value for 36 months missing for one patient.

All patients were examined every 2 months for 5 years and at 3-month intervals thereafter. Blood counts, blood urea nitrogen, SGPT, and urinanalysis showed no deviation from normal values. Ophthalmologic and slit lamp examination of the eyes at 6-month intervals showed no deviations from baseline for 5 years. ECGs at yearly intervals showed no deviations from baseline, except in cases in whom myocardial infarctions developed. Three patients developed atrial fibrillation, one with a history of paroxysmal atrial fibrillation at entry, one with multifocal premature atrial contraction at entry, and the third with coronary heart disease. Two were converted to normal sinus rhythm, which has been maintained; one had chronic atrial fibrillation controlled by digitalis. Ten patients had submaximal exercise tolerance tests without developing arrhythmias.

A D-xylose absorption test was performed during the first year on 21 patients (16 on probucol, five on placebo). No difference was observed in the 5-hr excretion between treated patients and controls. Side effects were limited to the gastrointestinal tract. During the first year, 17 of 88 patients on probucol (19%) complained of diarrhea, compared with three of 30 on placebo (10%); diarrhea was usually intermittent. After the first year, the incidence of diarrheal episodes decreased to 5% or less. No patients discontinued therapy because of side effects.

As expected in a high risk population, the causes of death (Table 4) were primarily cardiovascular. During the first year, two patients on probucol died of coronary heart disease (2%) compared with three deaths in the placebo group (10%). Two of these were cardiovascular and one due to cancer. At the end of the first year, two additional deaths occurred in the probucol group; one of a fractured neck suffered in an automobile accident 1 month after stopping probucol, and one of multiple injuries following an automobile accident.

The cumulative 5-year mortality by life table analysis was 10.3% . The 5-year incidence of coronary heart disease deaths and definite nonfatal myocardial

TABLE 4. *Causes of death[a]*

Parameter	Probucol	Placebo
No. of patients	88	30
No. of deaths (all causes)	11	3
Coronary heart disease	9[b]	2
Automobile accident	1[c]	—
Pneumonia	1	—
Cancer	0	1

[a] Patients treated with probucol over a period of about 7.5 years. Placebo period was 1 year. Causes of death over 8 years, 9 months.

[b] One of these patients died of a myocardial infarction 12 days after resection of an abdominal aneurysm. This patient had a pretreatment history of angina pectoris with left anterior hemiblock on ECG and had hypertension.

[c] This patient had been off probucol 1 month before the accident.

infarction was 14%. At 8 years 9 months of follow-up, 11 patients had died (nine coronary heart deaths). No patients in the treatment group had developed cancer.

The total incidence of definite nonfatal myocardial infarction was six incidents in five patients; one patient with a history of myocardial infarction at entry has survived two additional infarctions. Four minor cerebrovascular episodes without sequelae have occurred. Two patients exhibited congestive heart failure responding to appropriate therapy during the course of the trial.

SUMMARY

In summary, probucol has been shown to be an effective and safe agent for the long-term treatment of hypercholesterolemia with type II and type IV phenotypes. The reduction of serum cholesterol levels was greater than 25%; this is maintained with continuing therapy.

The mortality and new cardiovascular event rates in the small group of patients is encouraging and warrants further investigation in a larger controlled trial. The experience in the Coronary Drug Project (1) placebo group that serum cholesterol level is directly related to mortality in a straight line manner (slope 0.45) and is independent of all 40 other baseline variables, including triglyceride level, which was not shown to be a risk factor after myocardial infarction, makes such a trial virtually mandatory. The Coronary Drug Project (1) experience would indicate that a 10% reduction of serum cholesterol level in postmyocardial infarction patients would save six lives/1,000/yr in the group; a 25% reduction would save 12 lives/1,000/yr. Considering the large population at risk, such a reduction in mortality would be highly desirable.

REFERENCE

1. The Coronary Drug Project Research Group (1975): *JAMA*, 231:4.

Diet and Drugs in Atherosclerosis,
edited by G. Noseda, B. Lewis, and R. Paoletti.
Raven Press, New York © 1980.

Effect of Probucol and Diet on Serum Lipids and Lipoprotein Fractions in Primary Hypercholesterolemia

R. Mordasini, M. Keller, and W. F. Riesen

Lipid Research Laboratory and Institute for Clinical and Experimental Cancer Research (Tiefenauspital) of the University of Bern, 3004 Berne, Switzerland

A fat-modified, low-cholesterol diet reduces serum cholesterol concentration by about 10% (3,17). New regimens, such as soya protein and high fiber diets, are being tested and show promise in reducing cholesterol levels (18). At present, however, the reduction of increased cholesterol levels resulting from dietary measures alone is often insufficient. Thus the administration of cholesterol-lowering drugs may be necessary. Anion exchange resins are considered to be the most effective cholesterol-lowering substances, but their use is limited by their bulk and by side effects, such as constipation and nausea, leading to problems with drug compliance. High doses of nicotinic acid and its derivatives may cause flushing and diarrhea, limiting use in many patients. The synthetic antioxidant probucol is a promising agent acting on cholesterol but not on serum triglyceride concentrations (1,13).

In the present study, effectiveness, side effects, and tolerance of probucol were tested in patients with primary hypercholesterolemia. Special attention was paid to high density lipoproteins (HDL) since they have been proved to be of major importance as predictors of coronary heart disease risk (4,10). Twenty-seven patients (11 females and 16 males) were studied (mean age, 51 years; range, 27 to 71 years). Secondary hyperlipoproteinemias were excluded. Medications that might influence lipid metabolism were discontinued. The entire study was completed by 13 patients receiving probucol and by 10 patients receiving a placebo.

Cholesterol and triglycerides were measured in whole plasma and in the individual lipoprotein fractions after ultracentrifugation. Measurement of apo-B was performed on commercial plates (Behringwerke) by radial immunodiffusion. Apo-AI and apo-AII were determined by radioimmunoassay (14). Standard biochemical and hematological observations were made. The patients received an isocaloric, fat-reduced, and fat-modified diet for at least 3 months. This phase was followed by a 6-week period in which placebo was administered in addition to the diet. In the subsequent double-blind study, the patients received either diet and placebo (4 tablets per day) or diet and probucol (4 250-mg

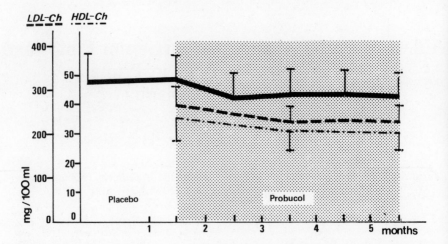

FIG. 1. Total serum cholesterol, LDL-, and HDL-cholesterol content before and during probucol treatment ($N = 13$).

tablets per day) for 4 months. The subjects were ambulant; blood analyses were performed monthly.

Compared with the mean value in the placebo period, total cholesterol concentration was reduced by probucol by an average of 41 mg% (13%). This effect was fully manifest after 1 month. The reduction of cholesterol was significant ($p < 0.05$) (Fig. 1). No significant changes in the serum cholesterol levels were seen in the placebo group at any time (Fig. 2). The low density lipoprotein (LDL)-cholesterol content was reduced by probucol, parallel to that of total cholesterol, from a mean of 265 ± 35 to 223 ± 27 mg/100 ml (16%, $p < 0.0025$). A slight, statistically nonsignificant decrease occurred in HDL-choles-

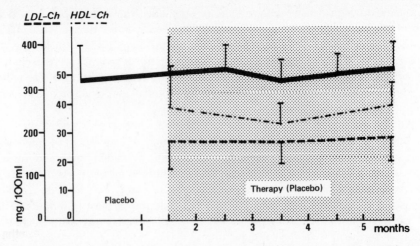

FIG. 2. Total serum cholesterol, LDL- and HDL-cholesterol before and during placebo ($N = 10$).

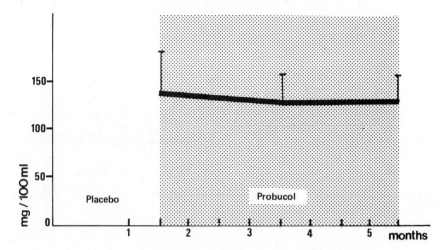

FIG. 3. Apo-B before and during probucol treatment ($N=13$).

terol levels (Fig. 1). In the placebo group, no significant changes of the LDL- and HDL-cholesterol content were observed (Fig. 2). Apo-B was reduced by probucol from 143 ± 31 to 126 ± 30 mg%. This decrease was not statistically significant ($p < 0.15$) (Fig. 3). In the placebo group, apo-B remained almost unaltered (Fig. 4).

In the probucol and placebo groups, serum triglyceride concentrations (Figs. 5 and 6), as well as the VLDL- and LDL-triglyceride content, were almost unchanged. A reduction in levels of apo-AI and apo-AII was seen in placebo and probucol groups (Figs. 7 and 8). With probucol, AI was reduced from an average of 104 ± 17 to 76 ± 16 mg/100 ml ($p < 0.0005$), while AII fell from

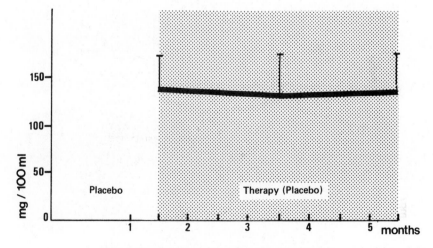

FIG. 4. Apo-B before and during placebo ($N=10$).

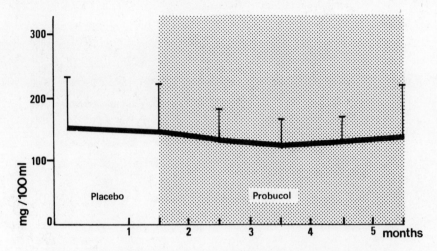

FIG. 5. Serum triglycerides before and during probucol treatment (*N* = 13).

31 ± 10 to 14 ± 2 mg/100 ml ($p < 0.0005$). In the placebo group, the decrease of AI was limited and not significant, whereas the reduction of AII (from 35 ± 9 to 26 ± 2 mg/100 ml) was statistically significant ($p < 0.005$).

In general, the drug was well tolerated. In four patients, the study had to be discontinued because of subjective side effects. Three of these were receiving placebo and one probucol. In this patient, after approximately 4 weeks of treatment, severe aphthous stomatitis occurred, which promptly subsided after interrupting probucol intake. This side effect cannot be attributed to probucol therapy with absolute certainty, although no other cause could be detected. In two other patients, we noted slight epigastric pain during the first week of probucol

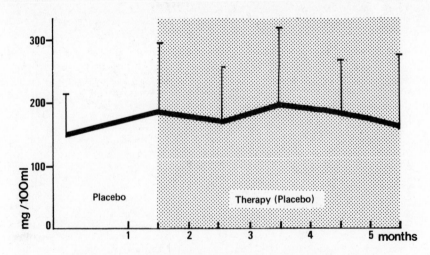

FIG. 6. Serum triglycerides before and during placebo (*N* = 10).

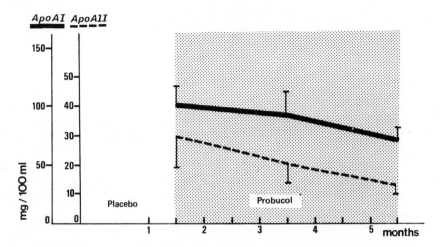

FIG. 7. Apo-AI and apo-AII before and during probucol treatment ($N = 13$).

treatment. Without interrupting therapy, these complaints ceased at later examinations. No other side effects of probucol were observed. Red and white blood cell counts and liver and renal function showed no alterations.

According to the results of the present study, probucol can be considered a cholesterol-lowering substance with good subjective and objective tolerance. When administered in addition to an adequate diet reviewed at frequent intervals, probucol shows a significant cholesterol-lowering effect, with a mean reduction of 13% in total cholesterol and a decrease of 16% in LDL-cholesterol. HDL-cholesterol levels remain nearly unchanged under probucol treatment; plasma

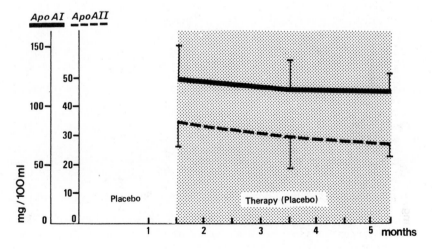

FIG. 8. Apo-AI and apo-AII before and during placebo ($N = 10$).

triglyceride levels do not show remarkable changes. These data largely confirm those obtained in earlier studies with probucol (2,5,9,16).

The cholesterol-lowering effect of probucol corresponds approximately—with considerably fewer side effects—to that of high dose treatment with nicotinic acid derivatives (6,11). It is probable that probucol is less potent than the anion exchange resins in reduction of total and LDL-cholesterol, but compliance and tolerance are definitely better. The major apoproteins of the HDL-fraction, apo-AI and apo-AII, in particular former, showed a significant decrease under probucol.

Similar findings for apo-I are reported by Miettinen et al. (8). However, a small reduction could also be demonstrated in the patients receiving placebo, which suggests that the degree of the reduction might in part be due to technical problems. Fresher sera produce higher apo-AI and apo-AII values; all the samples were determined in one batch at the end of the study. Nevertheless, it cannot be excluded that reduction of apo-AI may be a disadvantageous feature of the use of probucol in prevention of atherosclerotic lesions.

In summary, it can be stated that probucol is a well-tolerated cholesterol-lowering substance. Even if the effect of probucol on total serum cholesterol and on the LDL-cholesterol fraction is only moderate, the substance is useful because there are no major problems with drug compliance. Probucol acts only on serum cholesterol but not on the serum triglyceride and triglyceride-rich lipoproteins. While the HDL-cholesterol levels remain practically unchanged under probucol, there is a significant decrease in the major apoproteins of HDL, apo-AI and apo-AII. The clinical significance of this finding remains uncertain.

ACKNOWLEDGMENT

This work was supported by a grant from the Schweizerischer Nationalfonds zur Förderung der wissenschaftlichen Forschung.

REFERENCES

1. Barnhart, J., Ryter, D., and Molello J. (1977): An overview of the biochemical pharmacology of probucol. *Lipids,* 12:29.
2. Brown, H., and De Wolfe, V. (1974): The additive effect of probucol on diet in hyperlipidemia. *Clin. Pharmacol. Ther.,* 16:44.
3. Dayton, S., Pearce, M., Hashimoto, S. et al. (1969): A controlled clinical trial of a diet high in unsaturated fat in preventing complications on atherosclerosis. *Circulation [Suppl.],* 39:2.
4. Gordon, T., Castelli, W., Hjortland, M., Kannel, W., and Dawber, T. (1977): High density lipoprotein as a protective factor against coronary heart disease. *Am. J. Med.,* 62:707.
5. Harris, R. S., Gilmore, H. R., Bricker, L. A., Kiem, I. M., and Rubin, E. (1974): Long-term oral administration of probucol in the management of hypercholesterolemia. *J. Am. Geriatr. Soc.,* 22:167.
6. Klose, R., Mordasini, R., Middelhoff, G., Augustin, J., and Greten, H. (1978): Medikamentöse Behandlung primärer Hyperlipoproteinämien. *Klin. Wochenschr.,* 56:99.
7. Lipid Research Clinic Program (1974): *Manual of Laboratory Operations, Vol. 1.* U.S. Government Printing Office, Washington, D.C.

8. Miettinen, T., Huttunen, J., Kumlin, T., Naukkarinen, V., Mattila, S., and Enholm, C. (1980): *This volume.*
9. Miettinen, T., and Toivonen, I. (1975): Treatment of severe and mild hypercholesterolemia with probucol and neomycin. *Postgrad. Med. J.,* 51:71.
10. Miller, G., and Miller, N. (1975): Plasma-high-density lipoprotein concentration and development of ischaemic heart disease. *Lancet,* I:16.
11. Mordasini, R., Schlumpf, E., Nobile, P., Brun Del Re, G., and Riva, G. (1978): Hochdosierte Behandlung mit Beta-Pyridylcarbinol: Ergebnisse bei Patienten mit Hypercholesterinämie. *Schweiz. Med. Wochenschr.,* 108:533.
12. Nash, D. (1974): Safety and efficacy of probucol during one year of administration. *J. Clin. Pharm.,* 14:470.
13. Nash, D. (1975): Probucol, a new cholesterol lowering drug. *J. Med.,* 6:305.
14. Riesen, W., Mordasini, R., and Middlehoff, G. (1978): Quantitation of the two major apoproteins of human high-density lipoproteins by solid phase radioimmunoassay. *FEBS Lett.,* 91:1–35.
15. Salel, A. F., Fong, A. Zelis, R., Miller, R., Borhani, N., and Mason, D. T. (1977): Accuracy of numerical coronary profile. *N. Engl. J. Med.,* 296:1447.
16. Salel, A. F., Zelis, R., Sidhi, H. S., Price, J., and Mason, D. T. (1976): Probucol: A new cholesterol-lowering drug effective in patients with type II hyperlipoproteinemia. *Clin. Pharmacol. Ther.,* 20:690.
17. Schlierf, G., Vogel, G., Heuck, C. et al. (1980): Zur Diätherapie der familiären Hypercholesterinämie bei Kindern und Jugendlichen. *Monatsschr. Kinderheilkd. (in press).*
18. Sirtori, C., Agradi, E., Conti, F., and Mantero, O. (1977): Soybean-protein diet in the treatment of type II hyperlipoproteinemia. *Lancet,* I:275.
19. Technicon Clinical Method No. 24 (1972): Technicon Instruments, Tarrytown, New York.

Diet and Drugs in Atherosclerosis,
edited by G. Noseda, B. Lewis, and R. Paoletti.
Raven Press, New York © 1980.

High Density Lipoprotein Levels During a Five-Year Multifactorial Intervention Against Coronary Heart Disease Risk Factors

T. A. Miettinen, J. K. Huttunen, T. Kumlin, V. Naukkarinen, S. Mattila, and C. Ehnholm

Second Department of Medicine, University of Helsinki, and Central Public Health Laboratory, Helsinki, Finland

Epidemiological evidence (6,9) indicates that low serum concentration of high density lipoprotein (HDL) is inversely related to the risk of coronary heart disease (CHD). Dietary measures, when successful, appear to increase HDL cholesterol in some multifactorial trials of CHD prevention (4,5), while antihypertensive drugs may decrease HDL cholesterol (3). No information is available on the long-term effects of hypolipidemic agents on serum HDL levels or its composition. The interim results of our multifactorial intervention trial suggested that antihypertensive treatment does not influence the HDL level or composition, while hypolipidemic drugs, clofibrate and probucol in particular, may decrease the HDL level and its relative cholesterol content (7,8). This chapter presents our final results on serum lipids and HDL in the first 206 men who have completed the 5-year intervention program.

The series includes three main groups. Group I comprises 50 of 589 men (45 to 60 years old) who had no risk factors at entry. They received no treatment or advice. Group II (50 men) originates from the high-risk control group of 610 men. Group III is from the high-risk intervention group of 612 men. The control and intervention groups were matched at entry, and all the individuals had one or more risk factors, e.g., hypertension, hyperlipidemia, smoking, obesity, and abnormal glucose tolerance. The control group received no treatment or advice, whereas the intervention group visited us three times a year and received oral and written instructions to stop smoking, reduce body weight, increase physical activity, and to follow a lipid-lowering diet. If after 4 months on the program the subjects were still hypertensive or hyperlipidemic or if these abnormalities developed later during the trial, antihypertensive drugs (β-blocking agents alone or combined with diuretics and/or hydralazin when necessary) and lipid-lowering agents were used. Group III was divided according to treatment into subgroups, as shown in Table 1.

During the follow-up of 5 years, the subjects in group I (low risk) increased significantly in body weight and serum cholesterol, while in group II (high

TABLE 1. Body weight and serum lipids in subjects prior to and after a 5-year follow-up with and without different intervention measures[a]

Group[b]	Treatment	No. of subjects	Weight		Cholesterol		Triglycerides	
			Before	After	Before	After	Before	After
I	None	50	108 ± 1	110 ± 1[c]	6.0 ± 0.1	6.3 ± 0.1[c]	1.16 ± 0.06	1.19 ± 0.06
II	None	50	118 ± 2[d]	118 ± 1[d]	7.0 ± 0.2[d]	7.2 ± 0.2[d]	1.68 ± 0.10[d]	1.67 ± 0.11[d]
IIH	None	18	120 ± 3	121 ± 2	7.6 ± 0.3	7.7 ± 0.3	2.15 ± 0.19	2.51 ± 0.05
IIL	None	32	116 ± 2	115 ± 2	6.7 ± 0.2	6.8 ± 0.2	1.42 ± 0.09	1.20 ± 0.05
III	Intervention	106	116 ± 1[d]	114 ± 1[d,e]	7.1 ± 0.1[d]	6.7 ± 0.1[c,d,e]	1.83 ± 0.09[d]	1.43 ± 0.06[c,d]
IIIN	Diet, no drugs	26	114 ± 2	112 ± 2	6.5 ± 0.2	6.3 ± 0.2	1.43 ± 0.08	1.24 ± 0.06[c]
IIID	Diet + Ah-drugs	20	120 ± 3	116 ± 3[c]	6.6 ± 0.3	6.7 ± 0.2	1.99 ± 0.27	1.34 ± 0.12[c]
IIIC	Diet + clofibrate	15	115 ± 3	115 ± 3	7.3 ± 0.2	6.8 ± 0.3[c]	2.41 ± 0.26	1.45 ± 0.11[c]
IIIP	Diet + probucol	36	115 ± 2	113 ± 2[c]	7.6 ± 0.2	6.7 ± 0.2[c]	1.68 ± 0.14	1.38 ± 0.09[c]
IIICP	Diet + clofibrate + probucol	9	122 ± 7	121 ± 5	8.1 ± 0.3	7.5 ± 0.3	2.26 ± 0.35	2.32 ± 0.41

[a] Mean ± SE (mmoles/liter).

[b] Group I, no risk factors initially; group II, nontreated control group; group III, matched intervention group with one or several risk factors in two initial examinations; group IIL, cases from group II with final serum triglycerides less than 1.8 mmoles/liter; and group IIH, more than 1.7 mmoles/liter. Ah, antihypertensive; weight, relative body weight.

[c] Statistically significant change; [d] difference of groups II and III from I; [e] difference between II and III at 5% level at least.

risk), no consistent changes were observed. In group III (high risk), body weight and serum lipids were decreased during the intervention period as compared with baseline values and with those in the nontreated control group II, but the levels of group I were not attained. Serum triglycerides were decreased significantly in all the subgroups of group III, with the exception of the subjects treated with a combination of clofibrate and probucol. Serum cholesterol was decreased by clofibrate (–7%) and probucol (–12%), the final values being similar to those in group I.

Since our interim results indicated that the HDL cholesterol and apo AI levels had decreased markedly during the storage of sera frozen at –18° C for almost 4 years (7,8), no accurate follow-up study could be made of HDL cholesterol and AI. Therefore, HDL values could only be compared between the different groups, as shown in Table 2. HDL cholesterol, phospholipids, apo-AI, and apo-AII were measured after heparin manganese precipitation. The HDL cholesterol levels of groups II and III were similar, but they were lower than in group I. In agreement with the earlier observations (1,7,8), HDL cholesterol was negatively correlated with serum triglycerides ($r = -0.386$ for group I and -0.374 for group II). Thus the reduction of triglycerides by dietary measures in groups IIIN and IIID to the group I level during the follow-up of 5 years was accompanied by an increase in the HDL levels of these groups, so that their final HDL cholesterol equaled that in group I. In fact, HDL cholesterol of group IIID is higher than that of IIH, despite similar initial body weights and serum triglyceride levels. The low HDL cholesterol level in group IIIC may partly have occurred in clofibrate-resistant hypertriglyceridemic individuals; as compared with groups IIIN and IIID, however, the expected final value should have been higher. Groups IIIP and especially IIICP had the lowest HDL cholesterol levels not explainable by the serum triglycerides. HDL cholesterol of IIICP was insignificantly lower than that of the control group IIH matched for body weight and serum lipids. As in our interim results (7,8), the HDL cholesterol was negatively correlated with duration of the probucol treatment ($r = -0.331$).

The percentage esterification of HDL cholesterol was similar in all groups, although in IIIC the value was slightly lower than in group I. The percentage esterification showed a significant correlation with the HDL cholesterol level in group IIICP only ($r = 0.749$).

As compared with group II, the intervention measures of group III did not increase the fraction of serum total cholesterol transported by HDL; especially in group IIICP, the fraction remained very low. In groups IIIN and IIID, it was within the group I range.

HDL phospholipids were strongly correlated with HDL cholesterol (r-value range, 0.430 to 0.891 in the different groups) but not with serum triglycerides. The mean phospholipid levels of group II and III were equal; but in group III, it was slightly lower than in group I because the concentrations were low in the subgroups treated with probucol. The ratio of HDL cholesterol/HDL

TABLE 2. HDL cholesterol, phospholipids, and apoproteins in subjects after a 5-year follow-up with and without different intervention measures[a]

| Group[b] | Cholesterol | | | PL | AI | AII | 10 × | Cholesterol/Apo | | 10² × | 10² × |
	mmoles/liter	Ester %	% of Total	(mmoles/liter)	(mg/100 ml)		AI/AII	AI × 10⁵	AII × 10²	Cholesterol/PL	PL/AI
I	1.17 ± 0.04	81.5 ± 0.6	18.9 ± 0.7	1.11 ± 0.03	105 ± 2	43 ± 1	25 ± 1	111 ± 3	28 ± 1	105 ± 2	106 ± 2
II	1.06 ± 0.04	80.2 ± 0.5	15.1 ± 0.7[c]	1.03 ± 0.03	96 ± 2[c]	32 ± 1[c]	31 ± 1[c]	111 ± 4	34 ± 1[c]	103 ± 3	107 ± 3
IIH	0.92 ± 0.07[c]	80.6 ± 0.9	11.8 ± 0.8[c]	0.99 ± 0.05[c]	90 ± 3[c]	31 ± 2[c]	31 ± 1[c]	102 ± 7	30 ± 2	93 ± 6	110 ± 6
IIL	1.13 ± 0.04	80.0 ± 0.7	16.9 ± 0.7[c]	1.05 ± 0.03	100 ± 3	33 ± 1	32 ± 1	116 ± 4	36 ± 1	108 ± 4	106 ± 3
III	1.01 ± 0.03[c]	80.2 ± 0.3	15.3 ± 0.4[c]	1.02 ± 0.02[c]	101 ± 2	39 ± 1[c,d]	27 ± 1[c,d]	101 ± 3[c,d]	27 ± 1[d]	98 ± 2	102 ± 3
IIIN	1.14 ± 0.05	80.0 ± 0.8	18.0 ± 0.7	1.08 ± 0.05	100 ± 4	36 ± 2[c]	28 ± 1[c]	117 ± 2	32 ± 1[c]	106 ± 2	111 ± 6
IIID	1.13 ± 0.05	80.7 ± 0.9	17.1 ± 0.8	1.12 ± 0.05	108 ± 4	39 ± 2	28 ± 1[c]	106 ± 5	30 ± 1	102 ± 4	107 ± 7
IIIC	0.99 ± 0.05[c]	79.1 ± 0.9[c]	14.9 ± 1.3[c]	1.04 ± 0.05	109 ± 3	47 ± 2	24 ± 1	92 ± 8[c]	22 ± 3	93 ± 4[c]	96 ± 6
IIIP	0.94 ± 0.05[c]	80.7 ± 0.5	14.0 ± 0.7[c]	0.95 ± 0.04[c]	97 ± 3[c]	37 ± 2[c]	26 ± 1	95 ± 5[c]	25 ± 1[c]	97 ± 3[c]	98 ± 4
IIICP	0.73 ± 0.08[c]	80.0 ± 1.0	9.8 ± 1.0[c]	0.85 ± 0.05[c]	94 ± 4[c]	38 ± 2[c]	25 ± 1	76 ± 6[c]	19 ± 2[c]	84 ± 7[c]	90 ± 3[c]

[a] Mean ± SE.
[b] Groups and treatments as in Table 1. PL, phospholipids.
[c] Statistically different from I; [d] difference between II and III at 5% level at least.

phospholipids exhibited a positive correlation with HDL cholesterol (e.g., $r =$ 0.659 in group II) and a negative one with serum triglycerides (e.g., $r = -0.645$ in group II), indicating that in hypertriglyceridemic subjects and at the low HDL levels in general, HDL becomes rich in phospholipids in relation to cholesterol.

Apo-AI and apo-AII were lower, and the ratio AI/AII was higher in group II than in group I. In the intervention group III, the values were almost similar to those in group I. In agreement with earlier observations (1,7,8), the apoproteins were not correlated with serum triglycerides. The mean ratio of HDL cholesterol/AI or AII in group II was similar to or higher than that in group I, whereas the HDL of group III was poor in cholesterol. In general, the HDL fraction of hypertriglyceridemic subjects was poor in cholesterol but not in phospholipids. As compared with the normolipidemic controls (group IIL), the diet group (IIIN) had similar apo-AI and apo-AII levels. In the subjects treated with diet and antihypertensive drugs or clofibrate, the apoproteins, AII in particular, were high. Since HDL_3 has been suggested to be richer in apo-AII than HDL_2 (2), the finding suggests, in agreement with our interim results (7,8), that clofibrate increases HDL_3 levels. Fairly low apo-AI levels were found in the two probucol-treated groups, but the means tended to be higher than in the hyperlipidemic control group IIH. Non-HDL apo-AI (i.e., the apo-AI precipitated by heparin-manganese) varied in parallel with HDL apo-AI in our interim results (8). The cholesterol and phospholipid contents of the HDL fraction were lowest in the groups treated with hypolipidemic drugs, suggesting that the ratio of HDL_2/HDL_3 had decreased.

SUMMARY

A 5-year multifactorial intervention program aimed at reduction of CHD risk factor levels significantly lowered serum cholesterol and triglyceride levels as compared with the values at entry or with those of matched controls. However, the levels of an initially low-risk control group were not achieved. The serum HDL cholesterol, phospholipids, apo-AI, and apo-AII concentrations, measured at the end of the 5-year period from fresh sera after heparin manganese precipitation, were lower in the two matched high-risk groups than in the low-risk group. In the intervention group, the concentrations of HDL lipids were similar to those in the matched controls because in the subgroups treated with clofibrate, probucol, and their combination, the HDL cholesterol and to a lesser extent the HDL phospholipids were fairly low. The apoprotein levels, AII in particular, were high, especially in subjects treated with clofibrate. In individuals treated with probucol, apo-AI levels were similar to those of the matched controls. Thus multifactorial prevention measures failed to normalize the HDL concentration and may even have decreased it in subgroups treated with hypolipidemic drugs. On the other hand, the HDL cholesterol/protein ratio decreased.

ACKNOWLEDGMENT

This work was supported by the National Council for Medical Research, Finland.

REFERENCES

1. Albers, J. J., Cheung, M. C., and Hazzard, W. R. (1978): High-density lipoproteins in myocardial infarction survivors. *Metabolism,* 27:479.
2. Cheung, M. C., and Albers, J. J. (1977): The measurement of apolipoprotein A-I and A-II levels in men and women by immunoassay. *J. Clin. Invest.,* 60:43.
3. Helgeland, A., Hjermann, I., Leren, P., Enger, S. C., and Holme, I. (1978): High-density lipoprotein cholesterol and antihypertensive drugs: the Oslo study. *Br. Med. J.,* 2:403.
4. Hjermann, I., Enger, S. C., Helgeland, A., Holme, I., Leren, P., and Trygg, K. (1979): The effect of dietary changes on high density lipoprotein cholesterol. The Oslo Study. *Am. J. Med.,* 66:105.
5. Hulley, S., Ashman, P., Kuller, L., Lasser, N., and Sherman, R. (1979): HDL-cholesterol levels in the multiple risk factor intervention trial (MRFIT). *Lipids,* 14:119.
6. Kannel, W. B., Castelli, W. P., and Gordon, T. (1979): Cholesterol in the prediction of atherosclerotic disease. *Ann. Intern. Med.,* 90:85.
7. Miettinen, T. A., Huttunen, J. K., Kumlin, T., Naukkarinen, V., Mattila, S., and Ehnholm, C. (1979): High density lipoprotein cholesterol and apolipoproteins AI and AII during long-term treatment with clofibrate and probucol. *Eur. J. Clin. Invest.,* 9:II:141.
8. Miettinen, T. A., Huttunen, J. K., Kumlin, T., Naukkarinen, V., Mattila, S., and Ehnholm, C. (1980): Effect of long-term antihypertensive and hypolipidemic treatment on HDL cholesterol and apolipoproteins AI and AII. *Atherosclerosis (in press).*
9. Miller, N. E., Tholle, D. S., Førde, O. H., and Mjøs, O. D. (1977): The Tromsø heart study. High density lipoprotein and coronary heart disease: a prospective case control study. *Lancet,* 1:965.

Diet and Drugs in Atherosclerosis,
edited by G. Noseda, B. Lewis, and R. Paoletti.
Raven Press, New York © 1980.

Efficacy and Tolerance of Probucol and Clofibrate

J. L. De Gennes and J. Truffert

*Service d'Endocrinologie et Métabolisme Groupe Hospitalier Pitié-Salpêtrière
75013 Paris, France*

To evaluate hypolipidemic action of clofibrate and probucol, 38 patients were selected from subjects with primary hypercholesterolemia. Patients with evident coronary insufficiency during the past months, those with abnormal hepatic or renal function, those with hematologic abnormalities, and women of childbearing age were excluded.

On the basis of baseline total cholesterol levels exceeding 300 mg/100 ml, triglyceride levels under 170 mg/100 ml, and predominant increase of beta-lipoprotein band on agarose or polyacrylamide gel electrophoresis, the 38 patients were selected and randomized into equal groups for double-blind study on either probucol (500 mg b.i.d.) or clofibrate (1,000 mg b.i.d.). Before drug treatment, all patients started a low cholesterol (<300 mg daily), low saturated, high polyunsaturated fat (P/S ratio > 1) diet. A 2-month diet and placebo period preceded the 2-month probucol or clofibrate period. Blood was obtained monthly after a 12-hr fast. Total cholesterol and triglyceride levels were determined by an autoanalyzer technique and total lipids by the Chabrol and Charonnat manual method.

RESULTS

Probucol Group

In the probucol group, 19 patients (nine females and 10 males) with a mean age of 46 years and a mean weight of 67 kg (mean height, 167 cm) have completed the study. Final lipid levels in each experimental period were compared. The decrease of total cholesterol averaged −13%, from a mean of 376 ± 70 mg/100 ml at the end of the placebo period to 329 ± 72 mg/100 ml at the end of the probucol period (Fig. 1) ($p < 0.05$). The simultaneous decrease of triglycerides averaged −11% (from 123 ± 53 to 109 ± 38 mg/100 ml). The decrease was not statistically significant (Fig. 2).

Regarding hypocholesterolemic effects, it is important to distinguish good responders from nonresponders on an individual basis. One patient showed an increased cholesterol level of +12% at the end of the probucol period; two

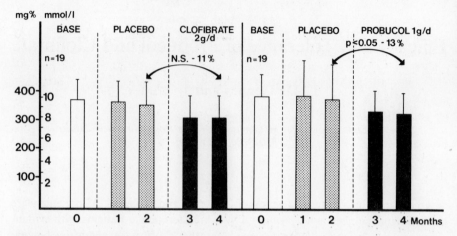

FIG. 1. Serum cholesterol. Comparative response of clofibrate or probucol in 38 cases of essential familial hypercholesterolemia. The statistical significance of the cholesterol decrease in the two groups has been measured by the Student's *t*-test on the values at the end of the placebo period and the active treatment period.

other patients exhibited a decrease of less than -5%. On the other hand, six patients exhibited a marked decreases of cholesterol ($-20, -21, -22, -22, -24,$ and -27%), respectively. Mean SGPT activity was 10 IU during the placebo period and 11 IU at the end of probucol period.

Clofibrate Group

In the clofibrate group, 19 patients (12 females and seven males) with a mean age of 50 years and a mean weight of 64 kg (mean height, 165 cm)

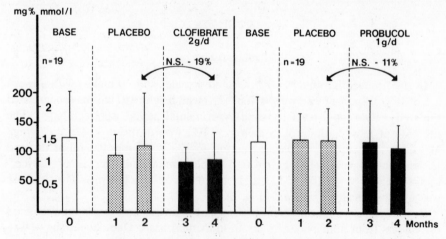

FIG. 2. Serum triglycerides. See legend to Fig. 1.

completed the study. The decrease of total cholesterol averaged −11%, falling from a mean of 347 ± 80 mg/100 ml at the end of the placebo period to 310 ± 74 mg/100 ml at the end of the clofibrate period (Fig. 1); this is not statistically significant on the Student's *t*-test. The simultaneous decrease of triglyceride averaged −19% (from 113 ± 93 to 92 ± 43 mg/100 ml) (Fig. 2). Although more consistent than that observed after probucol, this is also not statistically significant.

Two patients exhibited an increase of cholesterol during the clofibrate period of +14 and +33%, while two patients showed a cholesterol fall of less than −5%. Four patients exhibited rather good responses, with individual changes in cholesterol of −20, −23, −33, and −36%. Mean SGPT activity was 12 IU during the control period and 11 IU at the end of the clofibrate period.

No intolerance occurred during the 2 months of drug therapy with probucol or clofibrate.

CONCLUSION

The results we have obtained with probucol are in agreement with those of other investigators (5,6). In this short-term study, probucol was an effective cholesterol-lowering drug. The significant decrease of 13% compares well with that of clofibrate. Other studies have shown that this effect can increase with prolonged treatment (1). Studies of HDL cholesterol by Miettinen and co-workers (4) have shown a slight decrease of HDL cholesterol and a relative fall in cholesterol saturation of HDL.

As probucol has no obvious effect on triglycerides, it appears to have a more specific action than clofibrate and other derivatives on cholesterol metabolism and pure hypercholesterolemia. On the other hand, as it does not have potential lithogenic effects (2), and since it does not increase neutral sterols in bile (3), it could be safer by these criteria than clofibrate and derivatives for long-term treatment of many cases of familial hypercholesterolemia.

Probucol is a useful addition to hypolipidemic agents, e.g., for treatment of hypercholesterolemia responding poorly to clofibrate and its derivatives, in patients on anticoagulants, and in patients not accepting or tolerating other drugs, e.g., cholestyramine or colestipol.

REFERENCES

1. Heel, R. C., Brogden, R. N., Speight, T. M. et al. (1978): Probucol: A review of its pharmacological properties and therapeutic use in patients with hypercholesterolemia. *Drugs*, 15:409.
2. Mareček, M., Jirsa, M., and Kordač, V. (1980): *This volume.*
3. Miettinen, T. A. (1972): Mode of action of a new hypocholesterolemic drug (DH-581) in familial hypercholesterolemia. *Atherosclerosis*, 15:163.
4. Miettinen, T. A., Huttunen, J. K., Kumlin, T., Naukkarinen, V., Mattila, S., and Enholm, C. (1980): *This volume.*
5. Nash, D. T. (1975): Probucol. A new cholesterol-lowering drug. *J. Med.*, 6:(5–6)305.
6. Polachek, A. A., Katz, H. M., Sack, J. et al. (1973): Probucol in the long-term treatment of hypercholesterolemia. *Curr. Med. Res. Opin.*, 1:(6)323.

Diet and Drugs in Atherosclerosis,
edited by G. Noseda, B. Lewis, and R. Paoletti.
Raven Press, New York © 1980.

Clinical Experience of the Safety and Cholesterol-Lowering Action of Probucol

R. E. Tedeschi, H. L. Taylor, and B. L. Martz

Health and Consumer Products Department, The Dow Chemical Company,
Indianapolis, Indiana 46268

Probucol was the subject of clinical studies in the United States beginning in 1968 and was approved for marketing as a cholesterol-lowering agent early in 1977. This chapter summarizes the premarketing clinical studies involving approximately 1,000 patients and the continued surveillance of about 450 patients after marketing for a total observation period of approximately 10 years. The data presented were obtained from reports of physician visits at 3-month intervals.

In a placebo-controlled, multiinvestigator trial (five centers) utilizing a common protocol, there was a 10% or greater lowering of serum cholesterol in 58% of patients receiving probucol (1 g/day) ($N = 189$) compared to 16% of placebo ($N = 63$) patients ($p < 0.01$). The mean lowering of serum cholesterol after 3 months was 12% for the probucol-treated patients and 2.9% for the placebo patients. The incidence of side effects was quite low (Table 1).

TABLE 1. *Symptoms and/or side effects[a]*

	Treatment	
Category	Probucol ($N=189$) Reports/man year[b]	Placebo ($N=63$) Reports/man year[c]
Gastrointestinal disturbances	0.33	0.55
Subjective and ill-defined	0.31	0.21
Miscellaneous	0.00	0.07
Skin and hair problems	0.04	0.07
Throat, chest, and respiratory	0.00	0.00
Nervous and special senses	0.00	0.00
Musculoskeletal	0.13	0.07
Eye or visual	0.22	0.07
Kidney, bladder-genitourinary	0.02	0.07
Circulatory	0.00	0.00
Liver and gallbladder	0.00	0.07
	1.05	1.18

[a] Controlled studies, 3 months.
[b] Based on 45.0 man years of probucol experience.
[c] Based on 14.6 man years of placebo experience.

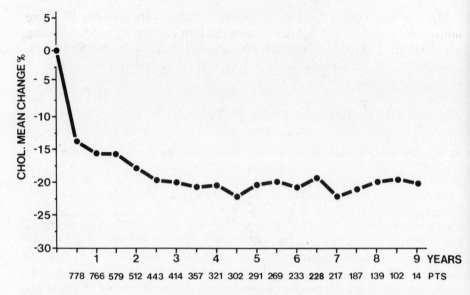

FIG. 1. Probucol long-term therapy. All studies combined. Cholesterol mean percent change.

All other data were derived from open studies. Analysis of the long-term clinical investigative experience with probucol showed a mean fall of serum cholesterol of about 20% (Fig. 1). The average serum cholesterol reduction in absolute terms was from 296 to ~240 mg/dl. Table 2 shows that about 70 to 80% of patients treated with probucol exhibited a 10% or greater lowering of serum cholesterol, and about 60 to 70% showed a lowering of 15% or greater. Probucol was well tolerated in the open studies; the most frequently reported side effect was loose stools and/or diarrhea. Generally, these side effects subsided with time and were not severe enough to discontinue therapy.

TABLE 2. *Percent of patients responding to probucol according to percentage cholesterol response*

Time on probucol	No. of patients	Percentage of patients exhibiting indicated fall in serum cholesterol	
		10% or greater reduction	15% or greater reduction
6 Months	778	66.3	50.5
1 Year	766	70.9	55.4
2 Years	512	77.3	64.6
3 Years	414	82.6	71.0
4 Years	321	83.7	71.6
5 Years	291	81.8	70.5
6 Years	233	83.3	72.1
7 Years	217	86.6	78.3
8 Years	139	82.0	67.6

Many of the patients involved in probucol studies were seriously ill before initiation of treatment. All had one or more risk factors at time of entry, including a history of myocardial infarction (MI), hypertension, smoking, and high serum cholesterol level (see Table 3).

An analysis of morbidity and mortality and dropout status was conducted on the 1,133 patients treated with 1 g/day probucol who were involved in clinical investigative studies. Mortality and morbidity were analyzed, using the life-table method (3). This method has several advantages in calculating cumulative morbidity and mortality rates. First, it makes use of all morbidity and mortality information accumulated up to the closing date of the study. Thus, in computing a 5-year mortality rate, one need not restrict the material only to those patients who entered observation 5 or more years prior to the closing date. Patients who entered observation 4, 3, 2, or even 1 year or less prior to the closing date can contribute useful information. Finally, the life-table method takes into consideration dropouts, mortality due to all causes, patients who completed the study, and those patients still in the study. The present analysis includes patients who were receiving probucol and does not include patients who ceased taking medication. Because of the relatively small number of patients on placebo and the relatively short period of time these patients were on placebo, a life-table analysis of morbidity and mortality was not performed on them. The comparatively small experience with placebo compared with probucol did not permit meaningful comparison of long-term mortality and morbidity.

A total of 42 of 1,133 patients who received probucol treatment died. The causes of death are shown in Table 4. The majority of deaths were cardiovascular. The incidence of nonfatal events, including nonfatal MI, with and without a previous history of MI, or new angina, which occurred during probucol treatment, is shown in Table 5.

A life-table cumulative event rate for dropout patients is shown in Fig. 2. The cumulative 7-year percent dropout rate for probucol-treated patients was 50.7%. The most frequent reasons for discontinuing probucol therapy included: completion of study, patient noncompliance, unrelated health problems, poor response to drug, death, patients moved or transferred, and adverse reactions. Four hundred and seventy-nine (479) patients received probucol for 3 years, and 157 patients received the drug for 7 years. The life-table cumulative event rate for mortality events is shown in Table 6. Analysis of morbidity is shown in Tables 7 and 8.

It was of particular interest to analyze the incidence of total mortality, coronary death, and nonfatal MI in probucol-treated men with a history of MI, and the incidence of biliary tract disease, and to contrast the results with the incidence of mortality and nonfatal MIs reported in the Coronary Drug Project. The patients enrolled in the Coronary Drug Project were males with a history of MI. The number of risk factors recorded at entry into the trial were not as extensive as for the Coronary Drug Project. The percentage of men with risk characteristics at entry for the men treated with probucol and for the placebo-

TABLE 3. *Percentage of patients with various findings at entry: Male patients with a history of MI[a]*

Characteristic at entry	Probucol experience		Coronary drug project	
	Total no. of probucol subjects	%	Total no. of placebo subjects	%
MI, male	228	100	2,789	100
Congestive heart failure				
Yes	11	4.8	446	16
No	217	95.2	2,343	84
Cerebrovascular accident (stroke)				
Yes	14	6.2	56	2
No	213	93.8	2,733	98
Arterial thrombosis peripheral				
Yes			67	2.4
No			2,722	97.6
Arterial thrombosis				
Yes	64	28.2		
No	163	71.8		
Angina				
Yes	152	66.7	1,612	57.8
No	76	33.3	1,177	42.2
Blood pressure				
Diastolic				
<90	132	58.4		
≥90	94	41.6		
Systolic				
<140	118	52.2		
≥140	108	47.8		
Diastolic				
≥85			1,023.6	36.7
Systolic				
≥130			1,433.5	41.5
Smoking				
Yes	72	31.7		
No	155	68.3		
			1,057	37.9
Cigarettes/day, ≥ 1				
Pulse				
<70	46	20.4		
≥70	179	79.6	1,255	45
Age				
<55	124	54.5		57
≥55	104	45.6	1,199	43
Nitroglycerin				
Yes	31	14.6	1,183	42.2
No	182	85.4		
Cardiac glycosides (digitalis)				
Yes	31	13.6	418	15.0
No	197	86.4		
Cardiac size				
Enlarged	27	11.9	508	18.2
Normal	200	78.1		
Serum cholesterol (≥250 mg %)		98.0		46.9

[a] Missing data for certain characteristics not available.

TABLE 4. *Causes of death in patients on probucol[a]*

Fatal event	Total no.
All causes	42
All cardiovascular (coronary death)	32
Sudden[c]	23
Nonsudden	9
All noncardiovascular	8
Sudden	1
Cancer	1[b]
Other noncardiovascular	6
Accidents	1
Cause unknown	2
Following surgery	0

[a] Based on probucol experience in 1,133 patients involving 3,928 patient years.

[b] This patient was inadvertently included as a death among the patients still on medication; the patient died 4 months following cessation of probucol treatment.

[c] Sudden death is defined either as death within 24 hr of being seen alive or as classified and indicated by the attending physician.

treated men in the Coronary Drug Project (1) are shown in Table 3. Examination of the information in this table shows that in some cases (arterial thrombosis), the demarcation points were different. In some cases, the percentage of probucol-treated patients exhibiting certain risk characteristics was about the same as the percentage of placebo-treated patients in the Coronary Drug Project.

In other cases, there were differences between the groups with respect to risk characteristics at entry. One major difference was that 98% of the probucol-treated patients exhibited a serum cholesterol value $\geq$ 250 mg% compared to

TABLE 5. *Nonfatal events: Probucol studies*

Nonfatal events[a]	Number
All patients with definite MI	20
All patients with definite nonfatal MI without previous history of MI	8
All patients with definite nonfatal MI with previous history of MI	12
All patients with new angina, regardless of previous history	32
Pulmonary embolism	5
Cerebral thrombosis	0
Cerebrovascular accident	6
Arterial embolism	1

[a] Based on probucol experience in 1,133 patients involving 3,928 patient years.

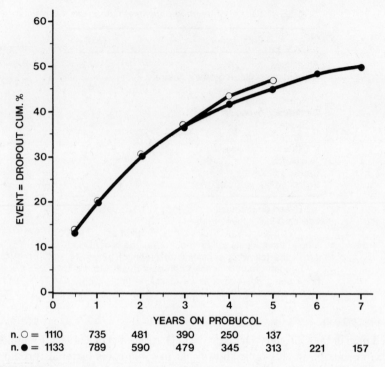

FIG. 2. Life table cumulative rate for dropouts. *Open circles,* Rx to January 1976; *Solid circles,* Rx to June 1978.

TABLE 6. *Cumulative mortality rates: Probucol studies (life table analysis)*

Mortality event	N^a	5-Year rate (%)	7-Year rate (%)
Cumulative total mortality, all subjects	1,133	6.4	8.0
All patients with history of MI	267	16.2	18.0
All patients without history of MI	866	2.4	4.1
Male patients with history of MI	228	17.4	19.3
Arteriosclerotic coronary heart disease with history of MI	267	12.4	14.3
Arteriosclerotic coronary heart disease without history of MI	866	1.8	3.4
Arteriosclerotic coronary heart disease, male patients with history of MI	228	11.6	13.7
Sudden death[b] patients with MI	267	9.0	10.9
Sudden death patients without MI	866	1.0	1.7

[a] Number of patients in each category at entry.

[b] Sudden death is defined either as death within 24 hr of being seen alive or as classified and indicated by attending physician.

TABLE 7. *Cumulative morbidity rates referrable to nonfatal MI:*
Probucol studies (life table analysis)

Nonfatal MI	N^a	5-Year rate (%)	7-Year rate (%)
All patients	1,133	2.9	2.9
Patients with MI	267	6.1	6.1
Patients without MI	866	1.8	1.8
Male patients with MI	228	7.3	7.3

[a] Number of patients in each category at entry.

TABLE 8. *Summary of morbidity referrable to biliary tract disease using*
life-table analyses: Probucol studies

Event	Group 5 (6-Year cumulative percent rate)
Cholecystectomy	
All patients ($N = 1,133$)	2.3
Male patients ($N = 729$)	2.2
Female patients ($N = 404$)	2.7
Other biliary tract disease	
All patients	1.8
Male patients	1.1
Female patients	3.0
Cholecystectomy plus other biliary tract disease	
All patients	4.1
Male patients	3.3
Female patients	5.8

~ 47% of the placebo-treated patients in the Coronary Drug Project. Tables 9 and 10 show the cumulative morbidity and mortality rates (calculated by life-table analysis) for patients from the Coronary Drug Project treated with either clofibrate, niacin, or placebo, compared with the cumulative mortality and morbidity rates for the probucol patients. Of 228 men with a history of MI who were treated with probucol, 116 had been treated for a period of 3 years and 73 for as long as 5 years.

Examination of the data in Table 9 shows that the incidence of total mortality, mortality due to coronary death, and nonfatal MI was less for the probucol-treated group than for the placebo-treated patients in the Coronary Drug Project.

In view of recent concern regarding possible deleterious effects of lipid-lowering regimens on bile composition and on the incidence of biliary tract disease (1,4), special attention was given to analysis of combined biliary tract disease in patients receiving probucol. The data in Table 10 show the incidence (6-year rate) of combined biliary tract disease reported in the Coronary Drug Project (2) for patients taking clofibrate, niacin, and placebo contrasted to the

TABLE 9. *Cumulative mortality and nonfatal MI rates from the Coronary Drug Project[a] and from the probucol experience: Life table analysis of male patients with history of MI[c]*

	Coronary Drug Project[a] (5-year rate %)			Probucol experience[b] 5-year rate (%) (N = 228)
Event	Clofibrate (N = 1,103)	Niacin (N = 1,119)	Placebo (N = 2,789)	
Total mortality	20.0	21.0	20.9	17.4
Coronary death	14.0	16.0	16.5	11.6
Definite Nonfatal MI	12.5	10.0	13.7	7.3

[a] From ref. 1.
[b] Probucol experience in 228 male patients with history of MI.
[c] Because of inherent differences between groups in the Coronary Drug Project and the probucol studies, these trials should not be statistically contrasted.

TABLE 10. *Cumulative incidence of combined biliary tract disease[a] from the Coronary Drug Project and from the probucol experience: Life table analyses of male patients with a history of MI*

	Coronary Drug Project (6-year rate %)			Probucol experience[b] 6-year rate (%) (N = 721)
	Clofibrate (N = 1,103)	Niacin (N = 1,119)	Placebo (N = 2,789)	
Combined biliary tract disease	4.59	3.56	3.02	3.3

[a] Combined biliary tract disease: Cholecystectomy, cholelithiasis, and cholecystitis.
[b] Because of inherent differences between groups in the Coronary Drug Project and the probucol studies, these trials should not be statistically contrasted.

incidence for those receiving probucol. There was no significant increase in the incidence of combined biliary events for nicotinic acid when compared to placebo; however, there was a significant increase in the clofibrate-treated patients. Thus the cumulative 6-year event rate for combined biliary tract disease among males treated with probucol does not appear to be excessive when compared to the Coronary Drug Project patients who received placebo.

In summary, the clinical observations involving 1,133 patients and 3,928 patient years of experience with probucol have shown that it is a well-tolerated and effective cholesterol-lowering agent. The morbidity and mortality of patients treated with probucol are within the expected range. Although a protective action is plausible, the lack of exactly comparable reference groups does not allow statistical analysis of the results.

ACKNOWLEDGMENTS

We are indebted to the following clinical investigators for supplying the clinical data for the probucol studies: S. Altshuler, Philadelphia, PA; R. Batterman,

Berkeley, CA; R. E. Cole, Chelmsford, MA; J. Davignon, Montreal, Canada; R. S. Harris, Jr., Miami, FL; Z. Kalams, Norwich, CT; D. McCaughan, West Roxbury, MA; T. Miettinen, Helsinki, Finland; D. T. Nash, Syracuse, NY; W. Parsons, Jr., Scottsdale, AZ; A. Polachek, Brooklyn, NY; J. A. Rider, San Francisco, CA; and R. W. Robinson, Worcester, MA.

REFERENCES

1. The Coronary Drug Project Research Group (1975): Clafibrate and niacin in coronary heart disease. *JAMA*, 231:4.
2. The Coronary Drug Project Research Group (1977): Gallbladder disease as a side effect of drugs influencing lipid metabolism. *N. Engl. J. Med.*, 296:1185.
3. Cutler, S. J., and Ederer, J. (1958): Maximum utilization of the life table method in analyzing survival. *J. Chronic Dis.*, 8:699.
4. Report from the Committee of Principal Investigators (1978): A cooperative trial in the primary prevention of ischaemic heart disease using clofibrate. *Br. Heart J.*, 40:1069.

Diet and Drugs in Atherosclerosis,
edited by G. Noseda, B. Lewis, and R. Paoletti.
Raven Press, New York © 1980.

Short- and Long-Term Trials of Probucol in Type II Hyperlipoproteinemia

V. Beaumont, J. C. Buxtorf, B. Jacotot, and J. L. Beaumont

*Unité de Recherches sur l'Athérosclérose, I.N.S.E.R.M., Hôpital Henri-Mondor,
Créteil, France*

European and American epidemiological studies have recently produced conflicting results with respect to the efficacy of hypolipidemic drugs for the prevention and therapy of atherosclerotic ischemic diseases (5,16). The occurrence in long-term treatment of side effects which might be related to these drugs, has led to questions about their use (16).

It must be kept in mind that the relationship of serum cholesterol to ischemic disease has been strongly demonstrated, especially in type II hyperlipoproteinemia (HLP), and that cholesterol is a marker of the atherosclerotic lesion. Valuable pharmacological research is needed to find compounds effective not only on serum lipids but also on cholesterol tissue deposition.

Probucol, 4,4'(isopropylidenedithio)*bis*(2,6 di-t-butylphenol), has a chemical structure different from that of any of the usual lipid-lowering drugs. Its hypocholesterolemic effects in mice, rats, and monkeys were first reported in 1970 (1). It has proved remarkably nontoxic in animals.

This study was conducted to test the hypolipidemic effect in type II patients, its maintenance and tolerance in long-term treatment, and its action on cholesterol deposition in tissues.

MATERIAL AND METHOD

Short-Term Trial

Nineteen patients (13 males and six females), aged 19 to 69 years (mean age, 44) whose serum cholesterol level exceeded 300 mg/100 ml were selected for the study. Patients with secondary hyperlipidemia were excluded.

The mean serum lipid values of the 19 patients, determined at the end of a 1-month washout period, were 454 ± 126 mg/100 ml for serum cholesterol and 210 ± 140 for triglycerides. Following serum electrophoretic phenotyping (2), eight patients had a type IIa and 11 a type IIb HLP. Presence of tendon xanthomas was recorded in 13 patients, xanthelasma in two, and ischemic disease in 10.

Following the washout period, each patient received either probucol (250 mg twice daily) or placebo for 1 month in randomized order. No special regimen was given during the study, and the patients were advised to maintain their normal diet. Body weight was controlled. Except for hypolipidemic drugs, usual treatments were not changed. Nine patients were on antivitamin K, and regular controls of prothrombin time were done.

Patients were seen at the end of each month of probucol or placebo for physical examination, determination of fasting cholesterol (7), triglycerides (10), phospholipids, determination of BUN, blood sugar, uric acid, SGOT, SGPT, bilirubin, alkaline phosphatase, complete blood count, and differential. Results obtained at the end of each of the two periods were statistically compared with Student-Fisher paired t-test.

Long-Term Trial

Probucol was tested in a 6-month open trial in 20 type II HLP patients, including 17 patients from the above group and three new patients. The group (14 men and six women; mean age, 44 years) had a mean cholesterol level of 435 ± 100 mg/100 ml and triglyceride level of 216 ± 138 mg/100 ml. Ten had a type IIa and 10 a type IIb HLP, according to electrophoretic patterns. Tendon xanthomas were present in 11 and xanthelasma in four.

The patients were given 500 mg probucol twice daily and maintained on a normal diet. Physical examination and laboratory determinations, as above, were done at the end of every 2 months. Moreover, modifications of the tissue cholesterol content was investigated. Skin biopsies were obtained before and at the end of treatment. Free and esterified cholesterol from the skin lyophilized fragments were separated by thin layer chromatography on Silicagel and measured by gas chromatography (8). Statistical comparison between data of the washout and treatment periods was done with Student-Fisher paired t-test.

RESULTS

Effects of Probucol on Serum Lipids

Short-Term Treatment

Mean serum cholesterol level was 435 mg/100 ml on placebo and 394 mg/100 ml on probucol, a difference of −9% on treatment ($p < 0.001$) (Table 1). Sixteen of 19 patients were reactive to probucol. The decrease exceeded 15% in six patients.

Mean serum triglycerides, respectively, were 196 and 181 mg/100 ml, a difference of −8% on treatment. Individual data showed that triglyceride levels were differently affected: 10 patients had decreased levels from 10 to 60% on probucol; nine were unaffected. Serum phospholipids, respectively, were 350 and 339 mg/100 ml (−3% on treatment).

TABLE 1. *Short-term comparative trial of probucol versus placebo in 19 type II HLPs[a]*

Mean serum lipids (mg/100 ml)	Placebo (1 month)	Probucol (1 month)	Δ %
Total cholesterol	435	394	−9[b]
Phospholipids	350	339	−3[c]
Triglycerides	196	181	−8[c]

[a] Paired *t*-test: [b] $p < 0.001$; [c] NS.
Sequence of placebo and probucol periods in randomized order.

Long-Term Treatment

The decrease observed in serum lipids after 1 month of treatment was confirmed and maintained during the 6-month treatment period (Table 2).

Mean serum cholesterol levels, 435 mg/100 ml at the end of the washout period, were 399, 405, and 391 mg/100 ml, respectively, at the end of 2, 4, and 6 months, a difference of −8.1% ($p < 0.01$); −6.8% ($p < 0.05$); and −9.9% ($p < 0.001$). Phospholipid levels showed a significant decrease of approximately 10%. The mean triglyceride decrease was between 8 and 13%, a statistically nonsignificant difference.

Individual results showed a variable responsiveness to the lipid-lowering effect: Serum cholesterol was unaffected in 25% of cases, decreased from 5 to 10% in 15% of cases, from 11 to 15% in 45% of cases, and more than 15% in 15% of cases. Triglyceride levels were unaffected in 45% of cases, decreased less than 20% in 25% of cases, and from 30 to 50% in 30% of cases. Thus 60% of patients may be considered good responders for cholesterol, 30% for triglycerides.

TABLE 2. *Long-term trial of probucol (1,000 mg/day) in 20 type II HLPs*

Mean serum lipids (mg/100 ml)	Washout period (1 month)	Treatment period (months)		
		2	4	6
Total cholesterol	435	399	405	391
Δ %		−8.1	−6.8	−9.9
p^a		c	b	d
Phospholipids	371	334	330	343
Δ %		−10	−11	−7.6
p^a		c	b	b
Triglycerides	216	187	217	198
Δ %		−13	+0.5	−8
p^a		NS	NS	NS

[a] Paired *t*-test: [b] $p < 0.05$; [c] $p < 0.01$; [d] $p < 0.001$.

Effects of Probucol on Tissue Lipids

As previously reported (8), the free and esterified cholesterol content of skin fragments was statistically different in normal and hyperlipidemic subjects (Table 3). Free cholesterol, expressed in micrograms cholesterol for milligrams dry tissue, was 1.58 in controls and 2.25 in type II patients ($p < 0.001$). Esterified cholesterol content was 0.16 and 0.44 μg/mg dry tissue, respectively ($p < 0.001$). Following a 6-month treatment with probucol, skin free cholesterol content was unchanged, but esterified cholesterol was increased from 0.44 to 0.66 μg/mg dry skin ($p < 0.01$).

In patients with skin deposits, there was no appreciable modification of tendon xanthomas after 6 months of treatment. Xanthelasmas remained unchanged in three of four patients. In the last case, the xanthelasma was almost completely rubbed out, leaving a noninfiltrated scar.

Side Effects and Tolerance

Clinical Tolerance

Few side effects were reported, even during the long-term trial: nausea in the first days of treatment in one case, loose stools in two cases, and gastric pain in a patient with hiatal hernia. Two other side effects were recorded, but their relationship to probucol is doubtful: (a) a hematuria in a patient on antivitamin K and probucol, who took antiinflammatory treatment without advice and lowered his prothrombin time, and (b) gingival hypertrophy and pruritus of the face and head on the 15th day of probucol, for which the treatment was discontinued.

Biological Tolerance

Blood cell count, blood urea, serum bilirubin, and serum alkaline phosphatase remained unchanged. In the long-term study, a progressive increase in SGOT

TABLE 3. *Influence of probucol treatment on tissue cholesterol*

Subjects	N	Age (years)	Skin cholesterol (μg/100 mg dry tissue) Free cholesterol	Esterified cholesterol
Normolipidemic controls	40	48	1.58 ⎤	0.16 ⎤
Type II hyperlipidemias	20	44	⎬ b	⎬ b
Before treatment			2.25 ⎦	0.44 ⎦
After treatment			2.16 ⎤ c	0.66 ⎤ a

$^a p < 0.01$; $^b p < 0.001$; ^{c} NS.

and SGPT was observed. Respective mean values in units for the washout period and the 2-, 4-, and 6-month period were 18.7, 20.1, 24.3, and 26.8 for SGOT; 17.4, 16.6, 19.9, and 23 for SGPT. The increase was significant at 6 months (SGOT, $p < 0.01$; SGPT, $p < 0.05$). However, all individual values remained within the normal range.

Potentialization of Anticoagulant Therapy

Seven patients on long-term anticoagulant therapy were maintained on antivitamin K during the short-term probucol study. The dose of anticoagulant was kept unchanged after the addition of probucol, and routine prothrombin times were done weekly during 1 month. Prothrombin time was unchanged in five cases and decreased in two.

COMMENTS

Our results are in agreement with those previously reported. A significant cholesterol-lowering effect was obtained in 75% of type II HLP patients, with a mean decrease of 9%, similar to the results usually obtained with probucol in type II (3,6,11,13,17) but less than those reported in other types (9,12,14,15). Our patients were on a free or moderately restrictive diet.

A triglyceride-lowering effect was sometimes obtained in individual cases, but the mean triglyceride level was not significantly affected, in agreement with all other studies.

In addition to the serum lipid-lowering effect, probucol mobilizes tissue cholesterol in long-term treatment. Regressions of tendon xanthoma and xanthelasma were reported after 2 years of treatment (4,9). In our 6-month study, there was no apparent modification of tendon xanthoma in any of the 13 xanthomatous patients. However, xanthelasma was completely flattened in one of four cases.

The increase of the skin cholesterol ester content that we observed may reflect an interaction of probucol with one step of the metabolism of cholesterol in the cells. Further research will be necessary to determine if it is related to an increased synthesis of esters by the cells, which would be consistent with an increase of transportable cholesterol. On the other hand, interaction of probucol with the cell receptors of low density lipoproteins will have to be studied.

Probucol was well tolerated. No clinical side effects and minimal laboratory changes occurred. Prothrombin time was not modified in patients with antivitamin K therapy.

Probucol appears to be a safe and efficient therapy for the treatment of type II HLP. Different in its chemical structure, it is also probably different in its mode of action from other lipid-lowering drugs, such as clofibrate and procetofen, which have a potent effect on triglyceridemia. Its action on tissue lipids may be of a major interest.

REFERENCES

1. Barnhart, J. W., Sefranka, J. A., and McIntosh, D. D. (1970): Hypocholesterolemic effect of 4,4'-(isopropylidene-dithio)bis(2,6-di-t-butylphenol) (Probucol). *Am. J. Clin. Nutr.,* 23:1229–1234.
2. Beaumont, J. L., Carlson, L. A., Cooper, G. R., Fejfar, Z., and Fredrickson, D. S. (1970): Classification of hyperlipidemias and hyperlipoproteinemias. *WHO Bull.,* 43:891–915.
3. Brown, H. B., and De Wolfe, V. G. (1974): The additive effect of probucol on diet in hyperlipidemia. *Clin. Pharmacol. Ther.,* 16:44–50.
4. Canosa, F. L., Aparicio, A. M., and Boyle, E. (1974): Reduction of hyperlipidemia in humans with DH.581 (Probucol). In: *Fifth International Symposium on Drugs Affecting Lipid Metabolism,* Milan. Abstr. p. 36.
5. Coronary Drug Project Research Group (1975): Clofibrate and niacin in coronary heart disease. *JAMA,* 231:360–381.
6. Davignon, J. (1974): Clofibrate and DH.581 in the long term treatment of primary hyperlipoproteinemia. In: *Third International Symposium on Atherosclerosis,* pp. 794–797. Springer-Verlag, Berlin.
7. Etienne, G., Papin, J. P., and Renault, H. (1963): Une méthode simple de dosage du cholestérol total par voie automatique. *Ann. Biol. Clin.,* 21:851.
8. Girardet, M., Jacotot, B., Cachera, J. P., and Beaumont, J. L. (1977): Cholestérol cutané dans les maladies coronariennes chez l'homme. Comparison de deux techniques d'extraction. *Arterial Wall,* 4:59–63.
9. Harris, R. S., Gilmore, H. R., Bricker, L. A., Kiem, I. M., and Rubin, E. (1974): Long term oral administration of probucol [4-4'(isopropylidene-dithio)bis(2,6-di-t-butylphenol)] (DH581) in the management of hypercholesterolemia. *J. Am. Geriatr. Soc.,* 32:167–175.
10. Kessler, G., and Lederer, H. (1966): Fluorometric measurement of triglycerides. In: *Automation in Analytical Chemistry,* edited by L. T. Skeggs, pp. 341–344. Mediad, New York.
11. Le Lorier, J., Dubreuil-Quidoz, S., Lussier-Cacan, S., Yung-Sheng Huang, and Davignon, J. (1977): Diet and probucol in lowering serum cholesterol concentrations. *Arch. Intern. Med.,* 137:1429–1434.
12. McCaughan, D. (1976): Probucol in long term management of hyperlipidemias. In: *Fourth International Symposium on Atherosclerosis.* Tokyo, Japan.
13. Miettinen, T. A., and Toivenen, I. (1975): Treatment of severe and mild hypercholesterolemia with probucol and neomycin. *Postgrad. Med. J. [Suppl. 8),* 51:71–75.
14. Nash, D. T. (1974): Safety and efficacy of probucol during one year administration. *J. Clin. Pharmacol.,* 14:470–475.
15. Polachek, A., Katz, H. M., Sack, J., Selig, J., and Littman, M. (1973): Probucol in the long term treatment of hypercholesterolemia. *Curr. Med. Res. Opin.,* 1:323–330.
16. Report from the Committee of Principal Investigators (1978): A cooperative trial in the primary prevention of ischaemic heart disease using clofibrate. *Br. Heart. J.,* 40:1069–1118.
17. Salel, A. F., Zelis, R., Sodhi, H. S., Price, J., and Mason, D. T. (1976): Probucol: A new cholesterol lowering drug effective in patients with type II hyperlipoproteinemia. *Clin. Pharmacol. Ther.,* 20:690–694.

Diet and Drugs in Atherosclerosis,
edited by G. Noseda, B. Lewis, and R. Paoletti.
Raven Press, New York © 1980.

Treatment of Hypercholesterolemia With Probucol

Rafael Carmena and Juan F. Ascaso

Department of Internal Medicine, University of Murcia, Murcia, Spain

Hypercholesterolemia is one of the established risk factors for ischemic heart disease (4). Correction of this state necessitates the use of diets supplemented with polyunsaturated fatty acids, with a low saturated fatty acid content, and, in some cases, with hypolipemic agents. Current treatment of hypercholesterolemia is far from satisfactory. Most drugs show greater effectiveness in correcting high levels of triglyceride than cholesterol levels, while some also have untoward side effects (5). Thus we studied a new agent—probucol (4,4-isopropylidenedithio-*bis*-2,6-di-t-butylphenol)—whose molecular structure is different from that of other drugs, and whose main effect is that of a hypocholesterolemic agent without affecting the triglyceride levels (1,3).

MATERIAL AND METHODS

We studied 20 patients with hyperlipoproteinemia (11 males and nine females) ranging from 33 to 66 years of age. Seven belonged to the IIa phenotype (cholesterol level > 320 mg% and triglyceride level < 200 mg%). Thirteen belonged to the IIb phenotype (cholesterol > 320 mg% and triglycerides > 200 mg%). They were all outpatients and all suffered from primary hyperlipoproteinemia; hyperlipidemia secondary to diabetes, hypothyroidism, renal insufficiency, and nephrotic syndrome were excluded. Patients whose plasma cholesterol levels decreased by more than 40% of the basal value after following an adequate diet for 1 month were also excluded. The experimental design (Fig. 1) was of single-blind crossover type. Cholesterol, triglyceride, total lipids, fasting blood glucose, BUN, bilirubin, alkaline phosphatase, SGOT, SGPT, red and white cell counts, platelet count, and urinalysis were determined for all patients after fasting for 12 hr. Analyses were performed at 4-week intervals for 6 months. The methods used for these determinations have been described elsewhere (6,8).

During the first month, the subjects were given an isocaloric diet with reduced intake of cholesterol and saturated fatty acids and an increase of polyunsaturated fatty acids. Further analyses were made 4 weeks after the start of this diet, and the patients were assigned randomly to two groups. One group received a placebo for 2 months and the other probucol. The diet was continued. The

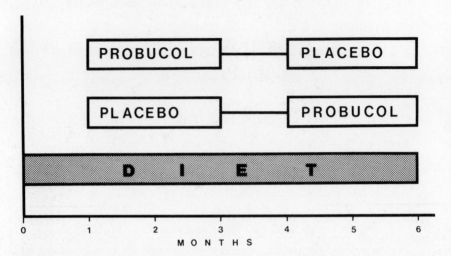

FIG. 1. Experimental design. Single-blind crossover study comparing the effect of probucol and placebo in seven phenotype IIa and 13 phenotype IIb patients.

dosage of both probucol and the placebo was two 250-mg tablets every 12 hr. At the end of 2 months, all patients were kept on dietary treatment for an additional month, and the placebo group was then given probucol in crossover design for 2 months.

RESULTS

No significant drug-related side effects (of clinical or analytical nature) were observed. There were no significant changes in body weight at the end of the 6 months of study (Table 1).

TABLE 1. *Body weight (kg)*

	Baseline	Diet	Placebo	Probucol
X̄	70.2	69.3	69.2	69.0
SD	12.8	12.9	13.7	14.0

[a] $N = 20$.

TABLE 2. *Serum cholesterol: Phenotype IIA*[a]

	Baseline	Diet	Placebo	Probucol
X̄	393.0	366.3	344.8	275.6[b]
SD	71.2	65.0	73.7	56.3
% Fall	—	6.8	12.2	30.0

[a] $N = 7$.
[b] $p < 0.01$.

TABLE 3. *Serum triglycerides: Phenotype IIA[a]*

	Baseline	Diet	Placebo	Probucol
X̄	140.7	157.0	148.6	120.1
SD	42.3	34.9	43.4	54.1
% Fall	—	12.0	5.0	14.0

[a] N = 7.

TABLE 4. *Serum cholesterol: Phenotype IIA[a]*

	Baseline	Diet	Placebo	Probucol
X̄	414.4	384.0	364.1	270.2[b]
SD	96.7	99.9	79.2	65.2
% Fall	—	7.2	12.0	34.7

[a] N = 13.
[b] $p < 0.01$.

TABLE 5. *Serum triglycerides: Phenotype IIA[a]*

	Baseline	Diet	Placebo	Probucol
X̄	330.9	287.3	308.0	265.4
SD	122.8	121.1	102.0	102.2
% Fall	—	13.0	7.0	20.0

[a] N = 13.

A marked fall in levels of cholesterol was seen in the seven patients with type IIa during the probucol treatment period (Table 2). The mean cholesterol level at the end of this period was 276 mg/100 ml, compared with the basal value of 293 mg/100 ml and the 345 mg/100 ml during the placebo period. Triglyceride (Table 3) showed no significant changes during the three periods. Furthermore, a statistically significant fall in cholesterol was seen in the 13 subjects with the IIb phenotype (Table 4) from a basal value of 414 mg/100 ml to 270 mg/100 ml after the period of probucol treatment. As in the previous group, triglyceride did not undergo significant changes (Table 5).

COMMENTS

Probucol is a hypocholesterolemic drug effective in association with a diet low in cholesterol and saturated fats. Its mechanism of action is still not fully known. In patients with familial hypercholesterolemia, probucol can reduce cholesterol levels by inhibiting cholesterol synthesis, increasing excretion of bile acids in the feces, and reducing intestinal absorption of cholesterol (7). Redistribution of cholesterol in the tissues does not take place.

Our results confirm the selective effect of probucol on cholesterol in patients with types IIa and IIb without any significant changes in the values of plasma triglycerides. In combination with diet, probucol causes a fall in cholesterol, which exceeds 30% of basal values. This agrees with previous observations by other authors (1–3,7).

During the 6 months of this study, no important side effects attributable to the drug were observed. As a result, probucol can be considered an effective agent for the treatment of patients with type IIa and IIb hypercholesterolemia placed on a diet low in cholesterol and saturated fats.

REFERENCES

1. Barnhart, J. W., Sefranka, J. A., and McIntosh, D. D. (1970): Hypocholesterolemic effect of 4,4-isopropylidenedithio-bis2,6-di-t-butylphenol (probucol). *Am. J. Clin. Nutr.*, 23:1229.
2. Davignon, J. (1974): Clofibrate and DH-581 in the long-term treatment of primary hyperlipoproteinemia. In: *Third International Symposium on Atherosclerosis*, pp. 794–797. Springer-Verlag, Berlin.
3. Davignon, J., Gattereau, A., Chretien, M., and Collin, R. (1974): The chronic effect of DH-581 (Probucol) on plasma lipid in 20 patients with primary hyperlipoproteinemia. In: *Fifth International Symposium on Drugs Affecting Lipid Metabolism*. Milan, Italy. Abstr. p. 42.
4. Keys, A. (1970): Coronary heart disease in seven countries. *Circulation [Suppl.]*, 41:1.
5. Lees, R. S. (1979): Clofibrate and atherosclerosis. *N. Engl. J. Med.*, 300:491.
6. Leplaideur, F., and Fonty, P. (1962): Dosage du cholesterol de serum sanguin. *Ann. Biol. Clin.*, 20:117.
7. Miettinen, T. A. (1972): Mode of action of a new hypocholesterolemic drug (DH-581) in familial hypercholesterolemia. *Atherosclerosis*, 15:163.
8. Sanchis, J., Carmena, R., and Ascaso, J. (1975): Determinación cuantitativa de los triglicéridos plasmáticos. *Laboratorio (Granada)*, 335:19.

Diet and Drugs in Atherosclerosis,
edited by G. Noseda, B. Lewis, and R. Paoletti.
Raven Press, New York © 1980.

Effect of Probucol in Primary Hypercholesterolemia

A. Gouveia, A. Noronha, I. Dionísio, S. Felix, B. Barros, and M. Carrageta

Department of Cardiology, Almada Medical Centre, Almada, Portugal

The main risk factors for atherosclerotic cardiovascular disease are hypertension, cigarette smoking, and hypercholesterolemia (6,11). These factors contribute to endothelial lesions, platelet activation, proliferation of smooth muscle cells in the intima, and formation of fibrous plaques (10). Control of blood pressure in hypertensive subjects and cessation of smoking both result in a lower incidence of clinical manifestations of atherosclerotic disease (12). The outcome of lowering blood lipids is less rigorously established.

High fat, high cholesterol diets lead to atheroma, which decreases when saturated fats are restricted in the animals' diet (7). In clinical trials, this is more difficult to demonstrate, but some recent papers report a lower incidence of new cases of angina and of nonfatal infarcts in men less than 60 years old after lowering serum lipids (3,5,8,9). In men older than 60 and in women, there is no convincing evidence for the benefits of lowering blood lipids.

Diet is the first choice in the management of hyperlipidemia. Nevertheless, results in patients with pronounced hypercholesterolemia are often disappointing. Therefore, there is a place for effective and well-tolerated drugs that lower cholesterol.

Probucol is a new cholesterol-lowering drug with an incompletely evaluated mechanism of action, although experiments in animals suggest that inhibition of lipoprotein formation and impaired intestinal mucosal transport of cholesterol may be involved (1,2,4,7).

We undertook an open trial to study the activity of probucol on serum levels of cholesterol and triglyceride in patients with primary hypercholesterolemia, and to evaluate the incidence and nature of adverse reactions.

We report on 34 ambulatory patients (16 men and 18 women) between 25 and 65 years of age, with a mean of 47 years for the men and 53 years for the women. Criteria for selection of subjects included a mean of three measurements of serum cholesterol above or equal to 250 mg/dl, with a difference among the three values not greater than 32 mg/dl. Patients followed their usual diets, but body weight was controlled and variations did not exceed 5%. Before recruitment, each candidate had a complete physical examination, chest radio-

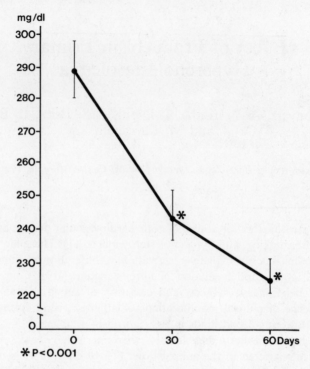

FIG. 1. Serum cholesterol before and at the end of each month of probucol administration. $p < 0.001$ by the Student-Fisher paired t-test.

graph, electrocardiogram, and routine laboratory tests. Blood samples for lipid measurements were drawn at least 12 hr after last intake of food. Every patient received probucol, 500 mg twice daily for 2 months.

As criteria for exclusion we included secondary hypercholesterolemia, serious

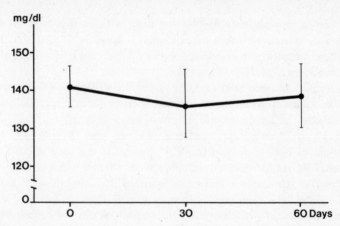

FIG. 2. Serum triglycerides before and at the end of each month of probucol administration.

TABLE 1. *Clinical and laboratory tests*[a]

Item	Before	After 2 months
B.P. (mm Hg)		
Systolic	148 ± 2.9	143 ± 2.5
Diastolic	92 ± 1.8	87 ± 1.5
Hb (g/dl)	14.9 ± 0.3	14.7 ± 0.3
Hematocrit	44 ± 0.7	43 ± 0.7
Erythrocytes ($\times 10^6$)	4.8 ± 0.1	4.7 ± 0.1
WBC ($\times 10^3$)	6.7 ± 0.2	6.5 ± 0.2
Platelets ($\times 10^3$)	246 ± 5.3	238 ± 5.3
SGPT	13 ± 1.3	13 ± 1.0
Alkaline phosphatase	16 ± 2.6	19 ± 3.1
Glucose	90 ± 2.1	86 ± 1.6
BUN	34 ± 1.3	35 ± 1.3
Uric acid	5.2 ± 0.2	5.9 ± 0.3

[a] Mean ± SEM.

and/or chronic illness, diseases of the gastrointestinal tract, abnormal liver function, alcoholism, pregnancy, lactation, and treatment with lipid-lowering drugs in the month preceding the trial.

Patients were evaluated 1 and 2 months after starting therapy with probucol. After 1 month (Fig. 1), mean serum cholesterol levels dropped from 295 to 245 mg/dl ($p < 0.001$). After 2 months, there was a further drop to 228 mg/dl. Mean serum triglyceride levels did not vary significantly (Fig. 2). Physical examination and laboratory tests did not show noteworthy changes (Table 1).

In 32 patients, there were no adverse reactions. Two patients (6%) dropped out in the first week of medication; one had diarrhea and the other constipation.

CONCLUSIONS

After 2 months on probucol, there was a 23% reduction in the mean serum cholesterol levels in 32 patients, confirming that probucol is an effective cholesterol-lowering drug. Probucol does not affect triglyceride levels in a consistent way. We had a 6% incidence of adverse reactions, a higher figure in comparison with previous trials, which may be explained by a chance distribution in our small series of patients.

REFERENCES

1. Barnhart, J. W., Rytter, D. L., and Molello, J. A. (1977): *Lipids,* 12:29–33.
2. Barnhart, J. W., Sefranka, J. A., and McIntosh, D. D. (1970): *Am. J. Clin. Nutr.,* 23:1229–1233.
3. Carlson, L. A. (1977): *Atherosclerosis,* 28:81–85.
4. Colmore, J., Vloedman, D., Schweem, H., and Dubowski, K. (1969): In: *Int. Congress Pharmacol.,* 4:405.
5. Dorr, A. E. (1978): *J. Chronic Dis.,* 31:5–14.

6. Kannel, W. B., Castelli, W. P., Gordon, T., and McNamara, P. M. (1971): *Ann. Intern. Med.*, 74:1–12.
7. Kritchevsky, D., Kim, H. K., and Tepper, S. A. (1971): In: *Proc. Soc. Exp. Biol. Med.*, 136:1216–1221.
8. Miettinen, M. (1972): *Lancet*, 11:835–838.
9. Oliver, M. F. (1978): *N. Engl. J. Med.*, 299:1360–1361.
10. Ross, R., Glomset, J., and Harker, L. (1977): *Am. J. Pathol.*, 86:675–684.
11. Stamler, J., Berkson, D. M., and Lindberg, H. A. (1972): In: *Pathogenesis of Atherosclerosis*, edited by R. W. Wissler and J. C. Geer, p. 41. Williams & Wilkins, Baltimore.
12. Tibblin, G., Wilhelmsen, L., and Werkö, L. (1975): *Am. J. Cardiol.*, 35:514–522.

Diet and Drugs in Atherosclerosis,
edited by G. Noseda, B. Lewis, and R. Paoletti.
Raven Press, New York © 1980.

Clinical Trial of a New Cholesterol-Lowering Agent: Probucol

A. Castro Ribeiro and A. Pereira Viana

Serviço de Patologia Médica, Faculdade de Medicina do Porto, Porto, Portugal

Many epidemiologic studies have shown a highly consistent relationship between ischemic heart disease and levels of serum cholesterol (3,5,6,11,13,15). Although it is not definite that lowering cholesterol results in prolongation of life, preliminary data suggest regression of human atheroma after lowering serum cholesterol (1,2). Moreover, nonfatal myocardial infarct incidence was reduced by 25% in the clofibrate group of the cooperative trial sponsored by the WHO (12). This was achieved after a cholesterol lowering of only 9%. Lowering of cholesterol can be obtained either by dietary means, which is the preferred initial treatment or by drugs when the latter fails. Various trials have shown that probucol is an effective, well-tolerated cholesterol-lowering drug (4,7–10,14). The purpose of our study was to evaluate the efficacy of probucol as a cholesterol-lowering agent in the hypercholesterolemic population of the north of Portugal and to assess the incidence and type of its adverse reactions.

In our double-blind clinical trial, outpatients with serum cholesterol measurements above 240 mg/100 ml in three baseline samples were randomly given probucol, 500 mg twice daily, or placebo for 3 months. We studied 13 patients in each group (Table 1). Subsequent measurements were made after 1, 2, and 3 months, and also 4 months after stopping medication. For cholesterol measurements, we used the enzymatic method, with internal and external quality control.

Participants were instructed to take their usual diet. Variations of body weight

TABLE 1. *Basal characteristics of the patients*

Characteristics	Group of patients	
	Probucol	Placebo
Men	8	5
Women	5	8
Average age	48	47
Age range	36–60	33–65
Body weight (kg)	74	69
Serum cholesterol (mg/100 ml)	297 ± 19	331 ± 22
Serum triglycerides (mg/100 ml)	183 ± 20	227 ± 70

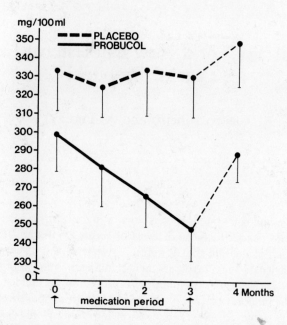

FIG. 1. Serum cholesterol before and during 3 months of treatment with probucol or placebo. Values at the fourth month were determined 1 month after stopping any kind of treatment.

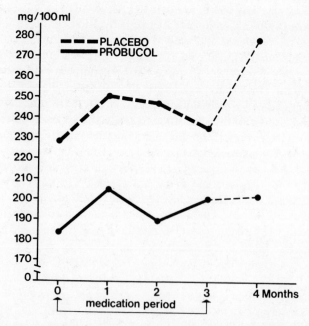

FIG. 2. Serum triglycerides before and during 3 months of treatment with probucol or placebo (see Fig. 1.).

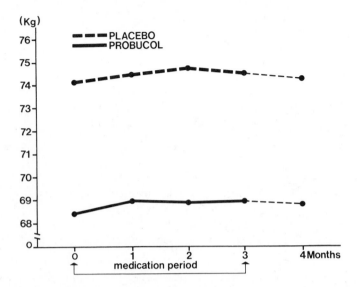

FIG. 3. Body weight before and during 3 months of treatment with probucol or placebo (see Fig. 1.).

greater than 5% were considered a cause for exclusion. No patient had received lipid-lowering drugs in the preceding month.

Figure 1 shows that serum cholesterol trends were different in the two groups. After 3 months on probucol, mean serum cholesterol dropped from 297 to 247 mg/100 ml, a fall of 16.8%. One month after stopping medication, mean serum cholesterol rose to 287 mg/100 ml. In the placebo group, mean serum cholesterol varied from 332 to 329 mg/100 ml during the medication period, and increased to 346 mg/100 ml over 1 month of follow-up.

Analysis of covariance showed a significant difference ($p < 0.05$) between the two groups, in terms of mean serum cholesterol. Moreover, serum cholesterol fell below 250 mg/100 ml in seven patients on probucol and in only 1 patient on placebo (Fisher test $p = <0.008$). Mean serum triglyceride levels (Fig. 2) did not differ significantly between the two groups. Body weight remained practically unchanged (Fig. 3). There were no dropouts due to adverse reactions. Minor digestive disturbances were reported in five patients on probucol and in three patients taking placebo.

Our trial confirms that probucol is an effective cholesterol lowering drug and that it is well tolerated. After stopping medication with probucol, serum cholesterol levels increased toward pretreatment values.

The decision to use probucol implies a long-term commitment, and this makes mandatory a careful selection of patients with primary hyperlipoproteinemias, taking into account family history, phenotype, age, sex, and response to diet.

REFERENCES

1. Armstrong, M. L. (1976): *Postgrad. Med. J.,* 52:456–461.
2. Barndt, R., Blankenhorn, D. H., Crawford, D. W., and Brooks, S. H. (1977): *Ann. Intern. Med.,* 86:139–146.
3. Connor, W. E. (1961): *Geriatrics,* 16:407–415.
4. Harris, R. S. (1974): *J. Am. Geriatr. Soc.,* 22:167–175.
5. Kannel, W. B., Castelli, W. P., Gordon, T., and McNamara, P. M. (1971): *Ann. Intern. Med.,* 74:1–12.
6. Keys, A. (1970): *Circulation [Suppl. 1],* 41:1–211.
7. LeLorier, J. (1977): *Arch. Intern. Med.,* 137:1429–1434.
8. Nash, D. T. (1974): *J. Clin. Pharmacol.,* 14:470–475.
9. Parsons, W. B. (1978): *Am. Heart J.,* 96:213–217.
10. Polachek, A. (1973): *Curr. Med. Res. Opin.,* 1:323–330.
11. The Pooling Project Research Group (1978): *J. Chronic Dis.,* 31:201–306.
12. Report from the Committee of Principal Investigators (1978): *Br. Heart J.,* 40:1069–1118.
13. Robertson, T. L. (1977): *Am. J. Cardiol.,* 39:244–249.
14. Salel, A. F. (1976): *Clin. Pharmacol. Ther.,* 20:690–694.
15. Tibblin, G., Wilhelmsen, L., and Werkö, L. (1975): *Am. J. Cardiol.,* 35:514–522.

Diet and Drugs in Atherosclerosis,
edited by G. Noseda, B. Lewis, and R. Paoletti.
Raven Press, New York © 1980.

Effect of Probucol on Human Bile Composition: Preliminary Observations

Z. Mareček, M. Jirsa, V. Kordač, and L. Kučerová

First Medical Department, Faculty of General Medicine, Charles University, Prague, Czechoslovakia

Triglyceride-lowering agents, such as clofibrate, increase biliary cholesterol saturation and gallstone incidence (3). The mechanism by which probucol lowers serum cholesterol is not yet well defined; it might increase fecal excretion of bile salts, fats, and cholesterol (4). We studied the effects of probucol on biliary bile acids and lipid composition in patients with type IIa hyperlipoproteinemia.

MATERIAL AND METHODS

We studied five outpatients with type IIa hyperlipoproteinemia (four males and one female), who had never been treated with probucol and who had discontinued other cholesterol-lowering agents for at least 1 month. The subjects, from 36 to 48 years of age, had serum cholesterol levels of 310 to 440 mg/dl.

An oral cholecystogram was performed in all subjects, and gallbladder disease was not found in any. All were examined initially and after ingestion of probucol (500 mg b.i.d.) for 8 weeks. Serum lipids were determined every 2 weeks during the study.

Bile was collected by duodenal drainage after intravenous injection of cholecystokinin (Pancreozymin®) before institution of therapy and again after 2 months of treatment.

Total bile acids were determined enzymatically with the 3-hydroxysteroid dehydrogenase method (Sterognost 3-alfa); cholesterol and phospholipids were measured colorimetrically. The degree of saturation of bile with cholesterol was calculated as the saturation (lithogenic) index (5).

Samples of gallbladder bile were hydrolyzed with 1 M KOH in closed steel tubes for 12 hr at 110°C. The bile acids were extracted with ethyl ether, methylated with diazomethane, converted to trimethylsilyl ether derivatives, and analyzed by gas-liquid chromatography on a 1% Hi-Eff BP8 column. This was carried out isothermally at 230°C using a Chrom 4 gas chromatograph and digital electronic integrator (1).

RESULTS

Body weight remained constant in all cases during treatment with probucol, and no side effects due to the drug were sought. There were no changes in diet. There was a significant decrease of serum cholesterol concentration, from 379 ± 32 mg/100 ml before treatment to 352 ± 28 after 1 month ($t = 3.105$, $p < 0.05$). After 2 months of treatment, the values were decreased to 310 ± 35 ($t = 7.418$, $p < 0.001$). Results were analyzed with Students' paired t-test. Serum triglyceride fell, but not significantly, from 2.9 ± 1.9 to 2.7 ± 1.6 mmoles/liter.

Changes in the Concentrations of Biliary Lipids

Bile composition is expressed as a percentage of total biliary lipids (mean $\pm$ SD). Changes in concentration of phospholipids were small and not significant: from $21.8\% \pm 5.5$ before treatment to $20.7\% \pm 3.9$. During probucol administration, the bile acid proportion of total lipids rose from $64.7\% \pm 9.3$ to $67.3\% \pm 7.1$; cholesterol concentration decreased from $13.4\% \pm 4.0$ to $11.9\% \pm 3.9$. None of these changes was statistically significant. The mean lithogenic index fell from 1.33 ± 0.29 before treatment to 1.28 ± 0.56 after 2 months of probucol (Fig. 1).

Bile Acid Composition (Molar Percent $\pm$ SD)

The percentage composition of cholic acid, chenodeoxycholic acid, and deoxycholic acid in the duodenal bile of the patients before treatment with probucol was (molar percent $\pm$ SD): cholic acid, $44.6 \pm 9.6\%$; chenodeoxycholic acid, $32.2 \pm 6.1\%$; deoxycholic acid, $23.2 \pm 12.6\%$. After 2 months of treatment

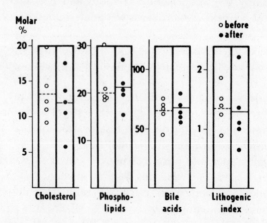

FIG. 1. Bile composition (relative molar composition) as percentage of total biliary lipids. Individual values before and after probucol.

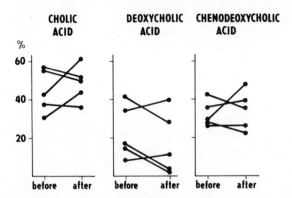

FIG. 2. Bile acids (cholic acid, deoxycholic acid, and chenodeoxycholic acid) as percentage of total bile acids. Individual values before and after probucol.

with probucol, the proportions of cholic acid and chenodeoxycholic acid rose from 44.6 ± 9.6% to 48.4 ± 7.9% and from 32.2% ± 6.1% to 34.2 ± 8.8%; the increase is not significant. The mean cholic acid/chenodeoxycholic acid ratio was 1.38 before and 1.41 after. Deoxycholic acid decreased from 23.2 ± 12.6% to 17.0 ± 15.0% (Fig. 2).

DISCUSSION

Changes in molar composition of biliary lipids are strikingly different from those commonly observed in bile composition after clofibrate treatment. Clofibrate increases the concentration of biliary cholesterol and reduces bile acid levels. These changes result in increased lithogenicity of bile, that is, supersaturation with cholesterol (2). After probucol administration, there were no significant changes; the trend was to decreased biliary cholesterol, increased bile acid, and thus decreased lithogenic index.

As mentioned above, changes in bile acid composition after probucol treatment were small and variable: the percentage composition of bile acids in our group of patients with type IIa hyperlipoproteinemia was similar to that reported by other authors (2). The decrease of deoxycholic acid after probucol treatment was greater than proportional changes of cholic acid and chenodeoxycholic acid but still statistically nonsignificant. One may hypothesize an action of the drug on microbial dehydroxylation of cholic acid in the intestine. It would be interesting to investigate the effect of probucol on the intestinal flora. Our results are preliminary and based on a small group of patients.

REFERENCES

1. Ahlberg, J., Angelin, B., Einarsson, K., Hellström, K., and Leijd, B. (1977): Influence of desoxycholic acid on biliary lipids in man. *Clin. Sci. Mol. Med.*, 53:249–256.
2. Ahlberg, J., Angelin, B., Einarsson, K., Hellström, K., and Leijd, B. (1977): Biliary lipid compo-

sition and gall-bladder disease in hyperlipoproteinemia. In: *Cholesterol and Bile Acid Metabolism in Norm- and Hyperlipoproteinemia,* edited by B. Angelin, pp. 11:1–12. Stockholm.

3. Coronary Drug Project (1975): Clofibrate and niacin in coronary heart disease. *JAMA,* 231:360–381.

4. Miettinen, T. A. (1972): Mode of action of a new hypocholesterolemic drug (DH-581) in familial hypercholesterolemia. *Atherosclerosis,* 15:163–176.

5. Thomas, P. J., and Hofmann, A. F. (1973): A simple calculation of the lithogenic index of bile expressing biliary lipid composition in rectangular coordinates. *Gastroenterology,* 65:698–700.

Diet and Drugs in Atherosclerosis,
edited by G. Noseda, B. Lewis, and R. Paoletti.
Raven Press, New York © 1980.

Effect of Probucol on Intestinal Absorption of Calcium and on Long-Term Anticoagulant Therapy in Patients With Hypercholesterolemia Associated With Cardiovascular Diseases

A. Rapado and M. Diaz Curiel

Unidad Metabolica, Fundacion Jiménez Díaz, Madrid-3, Spain

Modern therapy of primary hypercholesterolemia includes diet and various drugs, of which none is without serious side effects (3,10,18). Among these side effects, changes in intestinal absorption are worth mentioning. These changes may influence the metabolism of both calcium and vitamin K.

Probucol, a new drug agent which seems to selectively reduce levels of low-density lipoprotein cholesterol, is suitable for the long-term management of hypercholesterolemia (hyperlipoproteinemia type IIa) because of its good tolerance (1,5,12). The purpose of this chapter is to (a) evaluate, in a long-term follow-up, the effect of probucol in patients with severe cardiovascular disease associated with hypercholesterolemia, (b) assess the effect of this drug on calcium absorption; and (c) study its interaction with concurrent long-term anticoagulant therapy and, indirectly, with vitamin K metabolism.

MATERIAL AND METHODS

Twenty patients (11 males and nine females), ages 49–65, with a variety of cardiovascular diseases (seven with myocardial infarction, six with arterial hypertension, five with ischemic heart disease, and two with cerebrovascular lesions) associated with hypercholesterolemia (type IIa hyperlipoproteinemia) were treated with probucol. The dose was 500 mg every 12 hr for 6 to 24 months (mean, 14 months). The dosage was modified (decreased to 500 mg/day in two cases, and increased to 1,500 mg/day in three cases) in accordance with the response of serum cholesterol values. No significant side effects were observed. Drugs, such as digitalis, anticoumarins, or diuretics, were continued. Patients were advised to follow a low-cholesterol, low-saturated fat diet. Calcium and vitamin D supplements and other hypocholesterolemic drugs were not given.

During the trial, laboratory studies were carried out at 3-month intervals to rule out possible hematological, renal, hepatic, or bone abnormalities. Prothrombin time (Quick's) was assessed monthly in five patients who were receiving acenocoumarol. Calcium absorption tests were carried out in 16 cases both at baseline and during follow-up. Five microcuries ^{47}Ca were administered orally with a carrier of $CaCl_2 2H_2O$, the percentage of the administered dosage (α) being estimated per liter corrected in body weight and volume of the sample. The value of α was then estimated in blood samples obtained 1 hr after isotope administration following Marshall's method (11). Our normal range is 0.6 ± 0.15 but is adjusted for age. The biochemical methods employed have been described previously (14). Cholesterol was measured with the autoanalyzer SMAC. The Student's t-test for paired and unpaired samples was used.

RESULTS

Effect of Probucol on Serum Cholesterol and Triglyceride Levels

We found a statistically significant decrease ($p < 0.01$) in serum cholesterol with no significant changes in triglyceride values (Table 1).

Effect of Probucol on ^{47}Ca Absorption

In a group of five patients (not on other therapy), the ^{47}Ca absorption test did not show statistically significant differences in comparison with controls matched for age and sex after 6 months of continuous treatment with probucol (controls, 0.59 ± 0.08; trial patients, 0.54 ± 0.16; t, 0.34; NS). In four patients in whom the ^{47}Ca absorption test was carried out initially and after at least 6 months of treatment with probucol, no statistically significant changes were observed (Table 2). Statistical analysis was by the paired t-test. No differences were observed in the ^{47}Ca absorption test in patients also receiving other drugs (Table 3).

One 12-year old female patient had homozygous type IIa hyperlipoproteinemia with widespread xanthomas and a positive stress electrocardiogram (ECG). After treatment with diet plus 16 g/day cholestyramine for 3 months, she presented clinical and biochemical signs of rickets, corrected by 600,000 I.U./week i.m. vitamin D_3. After including probucol in her treatment (2,250 mg/day), the administration of cholestyramine and cholecalciferol was withdrawn without

TABLE 1. *Probucol in 20 patients with essential hypercholesterolemia*

	Cholesterol[a] (mg/dl)		Triglycerides[b] (mg/dl)	
	Basal	Probucol	Basal	Probucol
Mean	339	234	122.1	128.5
SD	44.6	54.1	45.2	43.9

[a] $t = 6.78$; $p < 0.01$.
[b] $t = 0.46$; NS.

TABLE 2. ^{47}Ca absorption test[a]

Case no.	Controls	Probucol
1	0.55	0.48
2	0.87	0.49
3	0.23	0.27
4	0.66	0.85

[a] $t = 0.455$; p NS.

TABLE 3. ^{47}Ca absorption test

Patients	No. of patients	Mean value	SEM
Controls[a]	8	0.45	0.07
Probucol[b]			
<6 months	12	0.47	0.07
>6 months	8	0.54	0.11

[a] $t = 0.31$; NS.
[b] $t = 0.52$; NS.

observing growth of xanthomas. The treadmill ECG became negative, and the mean values of cholesterol fell to 450 mg/dl from 660 mg/dl during 25 months of treatment with probucol (Fig. 1) (3).

The ^{47}Ca absorption test did not show changes in this patient during the treatment period. While she was on cholestyramine and vitamin D (i.m.), its value was 0.50; 18 months after the administration of probucol, it was 0.66.

Effect of Probucol on Prothrombin Time in Patients with Dicoumarins

Five patients entered the trial while they were on treatment with anticoagulants. During an average treatment period of 13.6 months with probucol, no changes were observed in prothrombin time (initially; 26.8% of normal control; on treatment, 25.4%). There was no need to modify the doses of acenocumarol (average, 2 mg/day) (Table 4).

DISCUSSION

Our study confirmed the beneficial effect of probucol with diet in controlling hypercholesterolemia; no significant changes in mean triglyceride levels were observed. The drug was well tolerated. These findings agree with those reported by LeLorier et al. (8), Heel et al. (5), Polachek et al. (15), Nash (13), and Taylor et al. (17), among others.

In our hands, an average dose of 1 g/day probucol has been effective in the control of hypercholesterolemia, although in some cases it could be reduced

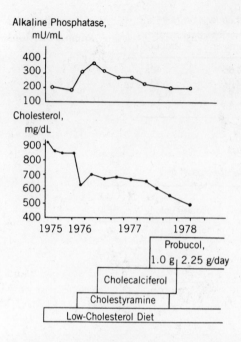

FIG. 1. A 12-year old female (E.C.L.) with homozygous hyperlipoproteinemia during treatment with probucol, who had developed clinical and biochemical signs of rickets following therapy with cholestyramine.

to 500 mg/day. When increased to 1,500 mg/day, no side effects were noted. The variable effect of the drug in homozygous hypercholesterolemia (8,12) may be related to pretreatment cholesterol values.

Some hypocholesterolemic drugs show side effects due to intestinal malabsorption, mainly of calcium, vitamin D, and vitamin K, or because they interfere with absorption of other drugs used in the treatment of cardiovascular diseases (2). High doses of cholestyramine modify the absorption of fat-soluble vitamins, necessitating supplementary vitamins in children (18). Cholestyramine also interferes with the absorption of digoxin, coumarins, thiazides, and antibiotics, which must be separately administered (4).

Clofibrate has a potential interaction with other drugs, especially anticoagulants. In fact, it is recommended to halve the dosage of anticoagulants when

TABLE 4. *Prothrombin time (% of normal control) in five patients under treatment with probucol*

Case no.	Basal[a]	Probucol[b]
1	25	23
2	27	30
3	22	26
4	28	30
5	25	25

Mean: [a] 25.4; [b] 26.8.
$t = 0.44$, NS.

starting treatment with clofibrate (9). Nicotinic acid therapy necessitates periodic assessment of hepatic function and increases vasodilation and hypotensive actions of ganglion-blocking agents (6).

D-Thyroxin is contraindicated in cardiovascular patients because of interaction with other drugs. It also seems to potentiate the effect of digitalis and anticoagulants (18). Neomycin, which is used in association with clofibrate in the treatment of hypercholesterolemia, has potential toxicity to the ear and kidney. Paraaminosalicylic acid (PAS), also used as a hypocholesterolemic agent, produces a malabsorption syndrome and is contraindicated in patients with impaired renal function (7).

Probucol is effective in the control of cholesterol levels due to type IIa hyperlipoproteinemia and does not interfere with either the intestinal absorption of calcium or vitamin D or the metabolism of vitamin K.

ACKNOWLEDGMENTS

Our thanks are due to Dr. Castro Mendoza, Dr. Gonzales Azpeitia, and Dr. J. Nuño who measured lipoprotein and to Dr. Castrillo and to Nieves Gandara, Beatriz Matesanz, Andrea de Blas, Rosario Palomino, and Mercedes del Valle in the Metabolic Unit.

We acknowledge the support of Laboratorios Lepetit, S.A., in providing us with probucol.

REFERENCES

1. Barnhart, J. W., Rytter, D. J., and Molello, J. A. (1977): An overview of the biochemical pharmacology of Probucol. *Lipids,* 12:29–34.
2. Davignon, J. (1977): Bases terapéuticas en las hiperlipoproteinemias. In: *Avances en el Control de la Hiperlipoproteinemias,* edited by J. M. Castrillo, M. Díaz-Curiel, and A. Rapado, pp. 83–107. Unidad Metabólica, Madrid.
3. Fredrickson, D. S., Goldstein, J. L., and Brown, M. S. (1978): The familial hyperlipoproteinemias. In: *The Metabolic Basis of Inherited Disease,* edited by J. B. Stanbury, J. B. Wyngaarden, and D. S. Fredrickson, pp. 604–680. McGraw-Hill, New York.
4. Gallo, D. G., Baily, K. R., and Shaffner, A. L. (1965): The interaction between cholestyramine and drugs. *Proc. Soc. Exp. Med. Biol.,* 120:60–62.
5. Heel, R. C., Bragden, R. W., Speight, T. M., and Avery, G. S. (1978): Probucol: A review of its pharmacological properties and therapeutic use in patients with hypercholesterolemia. *Drugs,* 15:409–428.
6. Holmes, W. L., Paoletti, R., and Kritchewsky, D. (1972): Nicotinic acid in the treatment of hypercholesterolemia. A long-term study. In: *Pharmacological Control of Lipid Metabolism,* pp. 27–34. Plenum Press, New York.
7. Kritchewsky, D. (1974): New drugs affecting lipid metabolism. *Lipids,* 9:97–102.
8. LeLorier, J., DuBreuil-Quidoz, S., Lussier-Cacan, S., Huang, Y. S., and Davignon, J. (1977): Diet and probucol in lowering cholesterol concentrations. *Arch. Int. Med.,* 137:1429–1434.
9. Levy, R. I., Morgauroth, J., and Rifkind, B. M. (1974): Treatment of hyperlipidemia. *N. Engl. J. Med.,* 293:1295–1298.
10. Lewis, B. (1976): *The Hyperlipidemias: Clinical and Laboratory Practice.* Blackwell, Oxford.
11. Marshall, D. H. (1976): Calcium and phosphate kinetics. In: *Calcium, Phosphate and Magnesium Metabolism,* edited by B. E. C. Nordin, pp. 257–261, Churchill Livingstone, Edinburgh.
12. Miettinen, T. A. (1972): Mode of action of a new hypocholesterinemic drug (DH-581) in familial hypercholesterolemia. *Atherosclerosis,* 15:163–176.

13. Nash, D. T. (1974): Safety and efficacy of probucol during one year of administration. *J. Clin. Pharmacol.,* 14:470–475.

14. Peces, R., González-Azpeitia, J. A., and Nuño, J. (1977): Incidencia de las hiperlipoproteinemias en la población española. In: *Avances en el Control de las Hiperlipoproteinemias,* edited by J. M. Castrillo, M. Díaz-Curiel, and A. Rapado. Unidad Metabólica, Madrid.

15. Polachek, A. A., Katz, H. M., Sack, J., Selig, J., and Littman, M. L. (1973): Probucol in the long-term treatment of hypercholesterolemia. *Curr. Med. Res. Opin.,* 1:323–330.

16. Rapado, A., Castrillo, J. M., and Díaz-Curiel, M. (1980): Use of diet and probucol. *Arch. Int. Med. (in press).*

17. Taylor, H. L., Nolan, R. B., Tedeschi, R. E., and Maurath, C. J. (1978): Combined results of the study of probucol at 1 g/day in eight centers. *Clin. Pharmacol. Ther.,* 23:131–136.

18. Yeshurun, D., and Gotto, A. M. (1976): Drug treatment of hyperlipidemia. *Am. J. Med.,* 60:379–388.

Diet and Drugs in Atherosclerosis,
edited by G. Noseda, B. Lewis, and R. Paoletti.
Raven Press, New York © 1980.

Probucol: An Evaluation of Effects on Plasma Lipids and Lipoproteins in 34 Cases of Primary Types IIa and IIb Hyperlipoproteinemia

J. Rouffy, R. Bakir, B. Chanu, J. Goy-Loeper, and J. P. Sauvanet

Departement de Lipoproteines Plasmatiques et Tissulaires, UER Médecine Paris VII, Villemin, and Service de Médecine Interne, Hôpital Saint-Louis, 75010 Paris, France

The need to treat atherogenic hyperlipoproteinemias (HLP) in the young subject is no longer a topic for debate. Primary treatment is dietary, using an isocaloric diet adapted to the type of HLP (1) or one modified to attain ideal body weight. Usually, modifications of diet will correct the endogenous hypertriglyceridemias (type IV) effectively and durably, and the hypertriglyceridemic component of mixed HLP (type IIb).

On the other hand, diet is, in general, less effective in the treatment of hypercholesterolemia caused by excess low density lipoprotein (LDL) in patients with the IIa or IIb pattern. Prospective studies have shown the atherogenic character of cholesterol LDL (C-LDL) and, to a lesser degree, of very low density lipoprotein (VLDL) and a strong negative correlation between the C-HDL level and atherosclerosis risk. Today, a lipid-active agent is expected to increase the cholesterol ratio: C-HDL/C-LDL + C-VLDL (2). The aim of this study was to specify the effects on these lipoproteins of probucol and to determine the clinical and biological tolerance of the drug.

PATIENTS AND METHODS

Patients

Distribution of Patients According to Duration of Treatment

Thirty-four patients participated in this study. Effectiveness and tolerance were observed for all patients between 1 and 3 months (t1), for 16 patients between 3 and 6 months (t2), for 12 patients between 6 and 12 months (t3), and for four patients for more than 12 months (t4).

HLP Type

The 34 patients in the study (18 men and 16 women; mean age, 47; age range, 19 to 72) had primary HLP, which did not reach satisfactory control with diet alone (HLP was characterized according to the criterion of WHO). Twenty-five had the IIa pattern, and nine IIb. All ambulant, long-term patients had stable weight close to their ideal weight and had accepted for several years an isocaloric, modified diet. Among them, 23 were previously treated with clofibrate, 22 with procetofen, and eight with cholestyramine without showing a sustained hypocholesterolemic effect or good tolerance of the treatment. Two patients had cerebral circulatory insufficiency, two arteriopathy of lower limbs, and 10 coronary insufficiency. Secondary HLP were carefully ruled out. No additional treatment having a known effect on lipids or lipoproteins was prescribed during the therapeutic trial. No patients showed obesity, severe hypertension, or diabetes, although some were smokers. Three patients were on long-term anticoagulant treatment (acenocoumarin in two and phenindione in one).

Treatment

All patients received 500 mg probucol twice daily.

Lipids and Lipoproteins

Before probucol treatment (t0), the subjects stopped all hypolipidic drugs for more than 6 months. In each therapeutic period (t1, t2, t3, t4), the levels of total lipids (TL), total cholesterol (TC), triglycerides (TG), C-HDL, C-LDL, C-VLDL, and triglyceride in HDL (TG-HDL), LDL (TG-LDL), and VLDL (TG-VLDL) were measured. Plasma was obtained by centrifugation of blood taken after a 12-hr fast. Triglyceride and cholesterol in plasma and in lipoproteins were determined by enzymatic methods (Boehringer). Lipoproteins were isolated by ultracentrifugation using the Beckman Airfuge at native plasma density and at a density of 1,063. Cholesterol and triglyceride in HDL and VLDL are measured directly, the C-LDL by difference.

The tolerance of the product and the possibility of unfavorable side effects were sought during each biological control by a complete medical examination. We also recorded a full blood count, urea, creatinine, bilirubin, SGOT and SGPT, alkaline phosphatase, total protein, urate, lactate dehydrogenase, creatine kinase, and γ-glutamyltranspeptidase (γ-GT).

The comparison between the values obtained at t0 and at the different therapeutic periods were made using Student's t-test.

RESULTS

Probucol Effects on Lipids and Lipoproteins

During the therapeutic periods, probucol reduced total lipids by 8 to 19%, total cholesterol by 8 to 12%, and C-LDL levels by 9 to 15% (Tables 1–4). Other lipid measurements (C-HDL, C-VLDL, total TG, TG-HDL, TG-LDL,

TABLE 1. Effects of probucol on lipids and lipoproteins (mg/100 ml) during therapeutic period t1.

Time	TL	TC	TG	C-HDL	C-LDL	C-VLDL	C-HDL C-LDL + C-VLDL	TG-HDL	TG-LDL	TG-VLDL
t0	1,148 ± 170	396 ± 80	118 ± 51	43.4 ± 11.5	293.7 ± 75.7	45.1 ± 18.8	0.13 ± 0.05	17.3 ± 5.8	37.6 ± 12.7	60.9 ± 60.04
t1	1,038 ± 170	350 ± 86	104 ± 50	43.2 ± 9.7	252.2 ± 82.3	45.4 ± 18.2	0.17 ± 0.07	15.8 ± 4.6	32.9 ± 10.8	54.2 ± 41.9
% Change	−10	−12	−12	0	−14	+1	+31	−9	−13	−11
p	<0.01	<0.01	>0.05	>0.05	<0.01	>0.05	<0.01	>0.05	<0.02	>0.05

N = 34.

TABLE 2. *Effects of probucol on lipids and lipoproteins (mg/100 ml) during therapeutic period t2.*

Time	TL	TC	TG	C-HDL	C-LDL	C-VLDL	C-HDL C-LDL + C-VLDL	TG-HDL	TG-LDL	TG-VLDL
t0	1,116 ± 186	377 ± 82	114 ± 58	42 ± 13	278 ± 81	47 ± 21	0.14 ± 0.05	17 ± 8	37 ± 13	51 ± 41
t2	991 ± 211	336 ± 93	99 ± 5	48 ± 9	249 ± 93	35 ± 14	0.17 ± 0.05	17 ± 5	30 ± 11	54 ± 40
% Change	−11	−11	−13	+14	−10	−26	+21	0	−19	+6
p	>0.05	>0.05	>0.05	>0.05	>0.05	>0.05	>0.05	>0.05	>0.05	>0.05

N = 16.

TABLE 3. *Effects of probucol on lipids and lipoproteins (mg/100 ml) during therapeutic period t3*

Time	TL	TC	TG	C-HDL	C-LDL	C-VLDL	C-LDL + C-VLDL / C-HDL	TG-HDL	TG-LDL	TG-VLDL
t0	1,058 ± 113	348 ± 48	122 ± 65	43 ± 13	250 ± 56	52 ± 22	0.15 ± 0.05	17 ± 8	39 ± 14	58 ± 16
t3	973 ± 175	320 ± 53	125 ± 87	50 ± 10	227 ± 47	44 ± 12	0.18 ± 0.04	19 ± 6	29 ± 12	76 ± 14
% Change	−8	−8	+12	+16	−9	−15	+20	+12	−26	−31
p	>0.05	>0.05	>0.05	>0.05	>0.05	>0.05	>0.05	>0.05	>0.05	>0.05

$N = 12$.

TABLE 4. Effects of probucol on lipids and lipoproteins (mg/100 ml) during therapeutic period t4[a]

Time	LT	CT	TG	C-HDL	C-LDL	C-VLDL	C-HDL C-LDL + C-VLDL	TG-HDL	TG-LDL	TG-VLDL
t0	995 ± 53	332 ± 17	99 ± 35	34 ± 5	239 ± 17	52 ± 14	0.12 ± 0.05	17 ± 8	31 ± 11	40 ± 10
t4	810 ± 36	284 ± 30	95 ± 31	38 ± 8	203 ± 22	39 ± 6	0.16 ± 0.03	19 ± 3	27 ± 9	52 ± 22
% Change	−19	−11	−4	+12	−15	−25	+32	+12	−13	+30
p	<0.01	<0.05	>0.05	>0.05	<0.05	>0.05	>0.05	>0.05	>0.05	>0.05

[a] N = 4.

TABLE 5. *Effect of probucol on biological parameters*

Mean values	No. of patients	Urea (0.10–0.45 g/liter)[a]	Creatinine (≤10 mg/liter)[a]	SGOT (≤25 μl)[a]	SGPT (≤25 μl)[a]	γ-GT (♂ <28 μm/ml)[a] (♀ <18 μm/ml)	Alkaline phosphatases (≤40 μl)[a]
t0	34	0.366 ($\sigma = 0.162$)	10.206 ($\sigma = 2.346$)	12.824 ($\sigma = 7.162$)	14.088 ($\sigma = 5.749$)	21.118 ($\sigma = 18.810$)	23.838 ($\sigma = 6.413$)
t1	34	0.370 ($\sigma = 0.091$)	10.529 ($\sigma = 2.164$)	13.029 ($\sigma = 9.675$)	15.353 ($\sigma = 11.190$)	17.941 ($\sigma = 12.378$)	21.956 ($\sigma = 6.919$)
t0	11	0.350 ($\sigma = 0.076$)	10.273 ($\sigma = 2.240$)	13.000 ($\sigma = 11.550$)	12.727 ($\sigma = 6.498$)	21.273 ($\sigma = 13.447$)	24.909 ($\sigma = 7.661$)
t2	11	0.359 ($\sigma = 0.090$)	10.364 ($\sigma = 2.461$)	17.091 ($\sigma = 10.193$)	16.545 ($\sigma = 5.989$)	23.091 ($\sigma = 16.991$)	24.545 ($\sigma = 10.434$)
t0	9	0.342 ($\sigma = 0.050$)	9.444 ($\sigma = 1.944$)	16.444 ($\sigma = 12.238$)	15.111 ($\sigma = 8.551$)	16.889 ($\sigma = 12.732$)	25.667 ($\sigma = 20.543$)
t3	9	0.356 ($\sigma = 0.099$)	10.000 ($\sigma = 2.550$)	15.667 ($\sigma = 8.559$)	17.667 ($\sigma = 12.913$)	40.111 ($\sigma = 64.982$)	28.000 ($\sigma = 10.461$)
t0	4	0.338 ($\sigma = 0.048$)	8.500 ($\sigma = 1.291$)	10.250 ($\sigma = 3.304$)	10.750 ($\sigma = 3.304$)	11.500 ($\sigma = 3.697$)	23.000 ($\sigma = 5.774$)
t4	4	0.375 ($\sigma = 0.050$)	9.500 ($\sigma = 2.217$)	8.750 ($\sigma = 2.217$)	9.500 ($\sigma = 4.509$)	15.750 ($\sigma = 6.801$)	22.825 ($\sigma = 6.570$)

[a] Range of normal values.

TG-VLDL) were not modified significantly. The ratio C-HDL/C-LDL + C-VLDL increased by 20 to 32%, mainly due to decreased C-LDL.

No significant drug-related symptoms or signs were observed, nor were abnormal trends noted in chemical or hematological measurements (urea, creatinine, alkaline phosphatase, SGOT, and SGPT, γ-GT levels), as shown in Table 5.

COMMENTS AND CONCLUSIONS

In this study, probucol appears as an effective agent to decrease lipidemia and total cholesterolemia as well as the cholesterol LDL level (therogenic cholesterol). The increase under probucol of HDL CH/LDL CH ratio with the consequent improvement on the atherogenic index is a favorable result. No interaction with anticoagulant has been observed.

REFERENCES

1. Beaumont, J. L., Carlson, L. A., Cooper, G. R., and Fejfar, Z. (1970): Classification of hyperlipidaemias and hyperlipoproteinemias. *Bull. WHO,* 43:891–915.
2. Paoletti, R., Ghiselli, G. C., Fumagalli, R., and Sirtori, C. R. (1978): New advances in atherosclerotic drugs. *International Conference on Atherosclerosis,* edited by L. A. Carlson, R. Paoletti, C. R. Sirtori, and G. Weber, pp. 29–34. Raven Press, New York.

Diet and Drugs in Atherosclerosis,
edited by G. Noseda, B. Lewis, and R. Paoletti.
Raven Press, New York © 1980.

Probucol Management of Hypercholesterolemia in Patients With Cardiovascular Disease

L. Scebat and J. Renais

Centre de Recherches Cardiologiques de L'Association Claude Bernard, Hôpital Boucicaut, 75015 Paris, France

The cholesterol-lowering effect of probucol in man is well documented (Colmore et al, 1969; Drake et al., 1969; Miettinen, 1972; Polachek et al., 1973; Davignon, 1974; McCaughan, 1974; Brown and De Wolfe, 1974; Harris et al., 1974; Nash, 1975; Salel et al., 1976; Lelorier et al. 1977). However, these studies were devoted to hyperlipemias as such, whatever the associated disease.

The purpose of the present work was to specify the cholesterol-lowering effect of probucol in patients with cardiovascular disease, and to investigate its possible interaction with drugs usually prescribed in this category of patients.

SUBJECTS AND METHODS

Thirty-three ambulatory outpatients (11 females, 22 males) were selected for this study. Their ages ranged from 43 to 78 years (mean, 60 years). None had received a lipid-lowering drug during the 3 preceding months. Eighteen had already been submitted to a low-fat, low-carbohydrate, low-alcohol diet. The same diet was prescribed to the 15 other patients.

In the 2-month placebo period, three blood samples were drawn for lipid determination; the mean was taken as the baseline value. The criterion for selection was a baseline serum cholesterol higher than 270 mg/dl independent of triglyceride levels.

All patients had cardiovascular disease; 15 had ischemic heart disease (eight associated with hypertension, two with ischemic disease of the legs), two with ischemic disease of the lower extremities, two with primary cardiomyopathy, 13 with hypertension, and one with extra systoles.

Thirteen were on antivitamin K therapy; 13 received a diuretic (bumetanide) for hypertension or edema. Probucol (500 mg twice/day) was administered for at least 12 months. Throughout the study, patients were examined every month during the first year, then every 3 months. All were evaluated for diet compliance and side effects, and all underwent physical examination, including electrocardiogram (ECG) at the beginning and at the end of the study. At each visit, routine chemistry, complete blood count, and urinalysis were performed. Plasma cholesterol (21) and triglyceride (20) levels were determined after an overnight fast, and paper electrophoresis was carried out (10). The results were statistically analyzed using the paired *t*-test, Student's *t*-test, and Fischer's *F*-test.

RESULTS

At the end of the placebo and diet period, cholesterol levels ranged from 271 to 408 mg/dl. The mean pretreatment level was 329 mg/dl ± 40. Triglyceride levels ranged from 65 to 195 mg/dl; the mean pretreatment level was 159 mg/dl ± 62.

Eleven patients had primary hyperbetalipoproteinemia (type IIa) with normal or slightly increased triglyceride levels; one was diabetic. Twenty-one had mixed hyperlipidemia (type IIb or type III). Three had diabetes. One had hypertriglyceridemia (type IV) (triglyceride 1,200 mg/dl). None exhibited xanthoma or xanthelasma. Fifteen had corneal arcus.

One patient dropped out in the second week because of diarrhea. The results obtained in the remaining 32 patients were used in this study. At the end of the first year, 12 patients were withdrawn from the trial because they were poor or nonresponders (cholesterol level lowered by less than 10%). On the whole, the mean duration of the treatment period was 18 months and exceeded

TABLE 1. *Mean cholesterol level (mg/dl) changes before and during 12 months of probucol administration in relation to the hyperlipidemia pattern*

Type	No. of patients	Serum cholesterol level		% Change
		Before	During	
Whole group	32	329.5 ± 40.1	281.1 ± 45.8	−14.5[a]
IIa	10	322.9 ± 44.6	264.1 ± 52.5	−18.2[a]
III (IIb + III)	21	329.5 ± 36.8	285.3 ± 38.8	−13.4[a]
IV	1	396	358.9	−9.4

[a] $p < 0.001$.

TABLE 2. *Mean triglyceride level (mg/dl) changes before and during 12 months of probucol administration in relation to the hyperlipidemia pattern*

Type	No. of patients	Serum triglyceride level		% Change
		Before	During	
Whole group	32	190 ± 79.9	158.7 ± 62.3	−16.5[a]
IIa	10	112.6 ± 31.2	112.9 ± 38.8	+0.3
III (IIb + III)	21	226.8 ± 68.6	180.5 ± 61.3	−20.4[b]
IV	1	1,206	1,255.3	+4.1

[a] $p < 0.05$; [b] $p < 0.02$.

24 months in nine patients (24 to 46 months). Serum cholesterol and serum triglyceride changes are summarized in Tables 1 and 2.

Interference With Drugs

Thirteen patients were already treated with antivitamin K when probucol was prescribed. There was no modification of the prothrombin time during the concomitant administration of these drugs. On the other hand, the anticoagulant drugs did not modify the cholesterol-lowering effect of probucol, as demonstrated in Table 3.

TABLE 3. *Comparison of mean cholesterol level changes during probucol administration in patients with and without antivitamin K therapy*

Therapy	No. of patients	Cholesterol level (mg/dl)			Responders	
		Before	During	Δ %	No.	%
With antivitamin K	13	314.3	267.2	−15	8	61.5
Without antivitamin K	19	338.8	290.6	−14.2	12	63.2

TABLE 4. *Comparison of mean serum cholesterol and triglyceride level changes during probucol administration in patients with and without diuretic therapy*

Therapy	No. of patients	Lipids (mg/100 ml)	Before	During	% Change
With diuretics	13	Cholesterol	338.2 ± 31.9	297.6 ± 40.3	−12.0[a]
		Triglyceride	206.5 ± 52.0	166.2 ± 46.7	−19.5[b]
Without diuretics	19	Cholesterol	323.6 ± 44.7	269.8 ± 47.0	−16.6[a]
		Triglyceride	179.5 ± 93.2	153.9 ± 71.2	−14.3

[a] $p < 0.001$; [b] $p < 0.05$.

Diuretics

Thirteen patients who received a diuretic (bumetanide) were compared with 19 patients without diuretics (Table 4). No appreciable difference was observed between the two groups.

DISCUSSION

Patients were instructed to adopt a modified diet and were questioned at each visit for diet compliance; but it is not certain that they all strictly adhered to the diet. There was a clear increase in serum cholesterol levels after holidays and feasts. This confirms the necessity to combine probucol therapy with dietary modification, although Harris et al. (7), and McCaughan (12) observed a strong decrease in serum cholesterol levels using probucol without changing the usual diet of their patients. In some patients who were previously poor diet responders, probucol caused a further fall in serum cholesterol level. The overall response to probucol was a 14.5% decrease in serum cholesterol, although some patients failed to respond. This is in accordance with previously published values (5,7, 11,14).

The cholesterol-lowering effect of probucol showed a 2-month lag period. In some patients, the favorable trend in cholesterol serum level occurred after the fourth month. The maximum effect occurred after 3 to 6 months of treatment.

Twelve patients were nonresponders (in seven patients, the serum cholesterol level decreased by 10% or less; in five others, it increased). Twenty patients were responders (62.5%). Their mean serum cholesterol level changed from 335 to 259 mg/dl (−22.5%). In relation to the classification of hyperlipoproteinemia, results are shown in Table 5 and Fig. 1. Although the cholesterol-lowering effect was more pronounced in type IIa patients, there were no statistically significant difference (Student's t-test) between the two groups.

Canosa (3) and Parsons (16) reported that probucol had lowered the serum cholesterol level by about the same extent in patients with hypercholesterolemia alone as in those with mixed hyperlipidemia. Conversely, Brown and de Wolfe (2) and Harris et al. (7) observed a lesser decrease in serum cholesterol level in type IIa patients. The reasons for these discrepancies are not clear. Nevertheless, probucol may be tried in the treatment of hypercholesterolemia, whatever the classification. The mean serum triglyceride levels were reduced by 16.5% ($p < 0.05$) for the whole group. However, the response was related to the typing (Table 6, Fig. 2). Probucol changed the serum triglyceride level only in the type III patients. In this type, the triglyceride reduction paralleled that of cholesterol. These results are in accordance with those reported by Harris et al. (7), who observed a statistically significant decrease in the triglyceride

TABLE 5. *Serum cholesterol level changes in probucol responders and poor or nonresponders in relation to the hyperlipidemia pattern*

Type	No. of patients	Cholesterol level (mg/100 ml)		% Change
		Before	During	
IIa	6 R	324.7 ± 47.4	239.9 ± 50.2	−26.1[a]
	4 N	320.2 ± 46.9	300.4 ± 38.2	−6.2
III (IIb + III)	14 R	340.2 ± 37.1	267.6 ± 33.9	−21.3[a]
	7 N	308.1 ± 27	320.5 ± 18.9	+4.0
IV	1 N	396.0	358.9	−9.4

[a] $p < 0.001$.
R, responders; N, nonresponders.

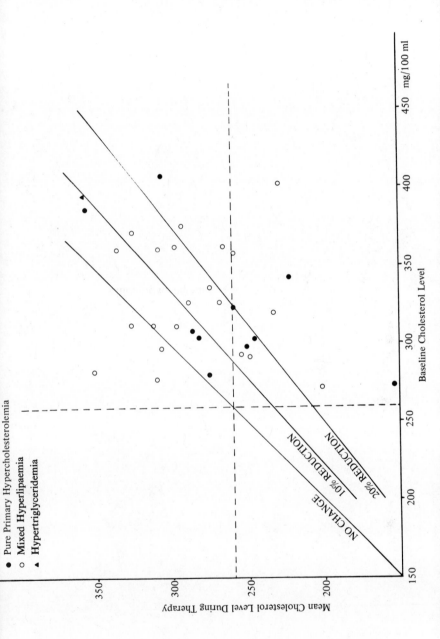

FIG. 1. Effect of probucol on serum cholesterol concentration during 12 months of therapy. Each symbol (corresponding to a hyperlipidemia pattern) is at the intersection of the serum cholesterol pretreatment value (abscissa) and of the treatment value (ordinate). The two dotted lines indicate the maximum serum cholesterol normal value in this laboratory.

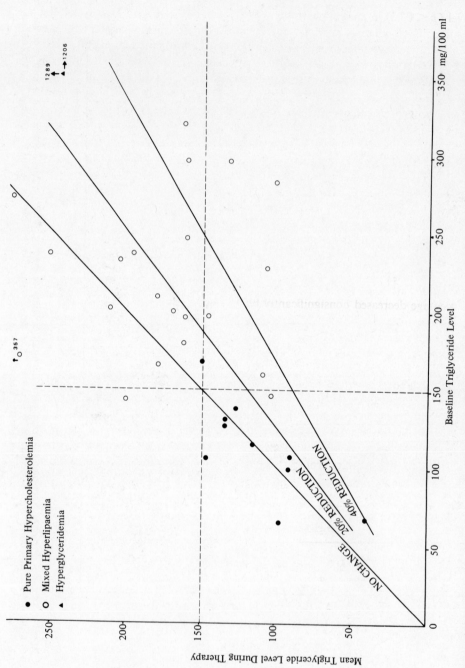

FIG. 2. Effect of probucol on serum triglyceride concentrations (see legend to Fig. 1). The two dotted lines indicate the maximum serum triglyceride normal value in this laboratory.

level ($p < 0.05$) in patients with types II, III, and IV patterns. However, these results differ from most previous studies, which did not show consistent changes in serum triglyceride concentration during probucol administration (8).

Fifteen patients were treated with probucol for 12 to 46 months. There was no further individual lipid reduction beyond that seen in the first year of therapy. In other long-term studies, the mean overall reduction in serum cholesterol level was greater after 4 years. This is probably the result of elimination of poor and nonresponders as these studies proceeded.

Among the 20 probucol responders, three disappeared from control toward the sixth month of therapy; despite continuing probucol administration, there was no further decrease in serum cholesterol concentration. Miettinen and Toivonen (14) have reported that the cholesterol-lowering effect of probucol could wane after 3 or 4 months of treatment. During the long-term administration of probucol, body weight was stable. There was neither modification of ECG nor evolution of cardiovascular disease. There was no significant change in blood glucose, urea, urate, bilirubin, creatinine, SGOT, SGPT, alkaline phosphatase, protein, or blood count. Harris et al. (7) and Polachek et al. (17) reported transient eosinophilia in some patients. In this study, the overall eosinophilia percentage decreased nonsignificantly by 15.2%.

No serious side effects were noted. Three patients complained of diarrhea, for which one patient discontinued treatment. The two others improved while continuing medication. These data are in keeping with those of previous reports (19). There was no interaction between probucol and antivitamin K. Harris et al. (7) had already observed the lack of effect on prothrombin time. Thus anticoagulant dosage did not need modification when probucol was prescribed, as is the case with some other lipid-lowering drugs (Table 3, Fig. 3).

The investigation of a possible interference between probucol and diuretics was justified by the observation of Ames and Hill (1) that there was a slight elevation of serum cholesterol level in some patients treated with chlorthalidone.

TABLE 6. *Probucol effect on triglyceride level in relation to the pattern of hyperlipidemia and to the cholesterol-lowering effect of the drug*

Type	No. of patients[a]	Triglyceride (mg/100 ml)		% Change
		Before	During	
IIa	10 WG	112.6 ± 31.2	112.9 ± 33.8	+0.3
	6 CR	119.0 ± 33.9	114.1 ± 42.9	−4.1
	4 CN	130.0 ± 28.1	111.2 ± 19.0	+8.0
III (IIb + III)	21 WG	226.8 ± 68.6	180.5 ± 61.3	−20.4[b]
	14 CR	231.0 ± 79.9	171.4 ± 41.8	−25.8[c]
	7 CN	218.3 ± 41.7	198.6 ± 90.4	−9.1

[a]WG, whole group; CR, cholesterol responders; CN, cholesterol nonresponders.
[b]$p < 0.05$; [c]$p < 0.01$.

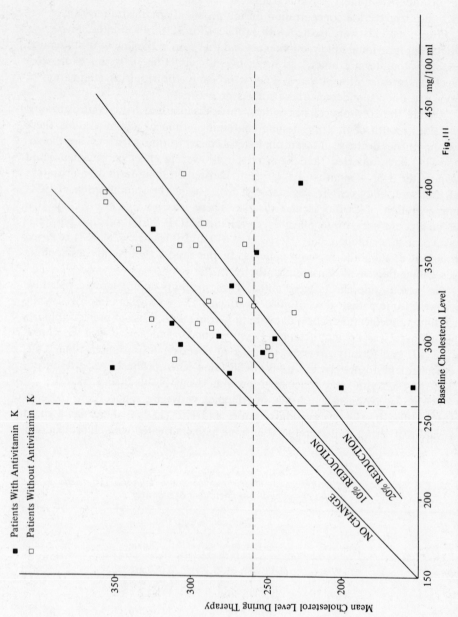

FIG. 3. Effect of probucol on serum cholesterol level in patients with and without antivitamin K therapy (see legend to Fig. 1).

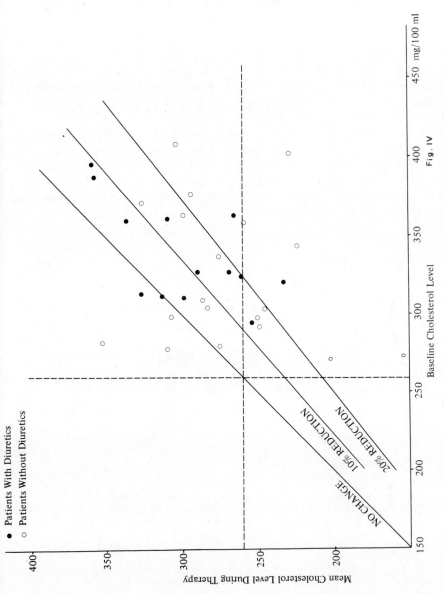

FIG. 4. Effect of probucol on serum cholesterol level in patients with and without diuretic therapy (see legend to Fig. 1).

Johnson et al. (9), however, did not confirm this assertion but noticed an increase in triglycerides. In an unpublished study of normolipidemic, hypertensive patients treated with bumetanide, we did not observe any significant change in cholesterol level. On the other hand, the triglyceride level increased from 73 to 98 mg/dl (+ 35%; $p < 0.02$). The present work shows that the decrease in serum cholesterol level was greater in patients without diuretics (−16.6%) than in those with (−12%) (Table 4, Fig. 4); this difference was not statistically significant. Conversely, the decrease in serum triglyceride level was greater in patients with diuretics (−19.5%) than in those without (−14.3%); again, the difference was not statistically significant.

Thus bumetanide does not modify the cholesterol-lowering effect of probucol. There was no interaction between probucol on the one hand and digoxin, beta-blocker drugs, amiodarone, and perhexiline on the other. Since cholesterol-lowering therapy often must be continued for decades in patients with cardiovascular disease and peculiarly ischemic heart disease, it is important to have established that probucol did not interact with these drugs, commonly prescribed in such patients, and that it had no serious adverse effects.

REFERENCES

1. Ames, R. P., and Hill, P. (1976): Increase in serum lipids during treatment of hypertension with chlorthalidone. *Lancet*, 1:721.
2. Brown, M. B., and de Wolfe, V. G. (1974): The additive effect of probucol on diet in hyperlipidemia. *Clin. Pharmacol. Ther.*, 16:44.
3. Canosa, F. L. (1975): Long-term hypocholesterolemic drug therapy with probucol (DH 581) in human subjects. *Clin. Pharmacol. Ther.*, 17:230.
4. Colmore, J., Norrby, A. S., and Vloedmand, D. (1969): DH 581: A new cholesterol lowering agent. *Int. Congress Pharmacol.*, 4:405.
5. Davignon, J. (1974): Clofibrate and DH 581 in the long term treatment of primary hyperlipoproteinemia. In: *Third International Symposium on Atherosclerosis*, pp. 794–797. Springer-Verlag, Berlin.
6. Drake, J. W., Bradford, R. H., McDearmon, M., and Furman, R. H. (1969): The effect of [4,4'(isopropylidenedithio)bis(2,6-di-t-butyl-phenol)] (DH581) on serum lipids and lipoproteins in human subjects. *Metabolism*, 18:916.
7. Harris, R. S., Gilmore, H. R., Bricker, L. A., Kiem, M., and Rubin, E. (1974): Long-term oral administration of probucol [4,4'(isopropyldenedithio)bis(2,6-di-t-butylphenol)] (DH 581) in the management of hypercholesterolemia. *J. Am. Geriatr. Soc.*, 22:167.
8. Heel, R. C., Brodgen, R. N., Speight, T. M., and Avery, G. S. (1978): Probucol: A review of its pharmacological properties and therapeutic use in patients with hypercholesterolemia. *Drugs*, 15:409.
9. Johnson, B. F., Munro-Faure, A. D., and Slack, J. (1976): Diuretic-induced hypertriglyceridemia. *Lancet*, i:1019.
10. Lees, R. S., and Hatch, P. T. (1963): Sharper separation of lipoprotein species by paper electrophoresis in albumin containing buffer. *J. Lab. Clin. Med.*, 6(1):518.
11. LeLorier, J., Dubreuil-Quidoz, S., Lussier-Cacan, S., Huang, Y. S., and Davignon, J. (1977): Diet and probucol in lowering cholesterol concentrations: Additive effects on plasma cholesterol concentration in patients with familial type II hyperlipoproteinemia. *Arch. Intern. Med.*, 137:1429.
12. McCaughan, D. (1974): Effect of probucol in lowering serum cholesterol. *Atherosclerosis*, 3:901.
13. Miettinen, T. A. (1972): Mode of action of a new hypercholesterolemic drug (DH 581) in familial hypercholesterolemia. *Atherosclerosis*, 15:163.

14. Miettinen, T. A., and Toivonen, I. (1975): Treatment of severe and mild hypercholesterolemia with probucol and neomycin. *Postgrad. Med. J. [Suppl. 8],* 51:71.
15. Nash, D. T. (1975): Probucol, a new cholesterol lowering drug. *J. Med.,* 6:305.
16. Parsons, W. B. (1978): Effect of probucol in hyperlipidemic patients during two years administration. *Am. Heart J.,* 96:213.
17. Polachek, A. A., Katz, H. M., Sack, J., Selig, J., and Littman, M. (1973): Probucol in the long term treatment of hypercholesterolemia. *Curr. Med. Res. Opin.,* 1:323.
18. Salel, A. F., Zelis, R., Sodhi, H. S., Price, J., and Mason, D. T. (1976): Probucol: A new cholesterol-lowering drug effective in patients with type II hyperlipoproteinemia. *Clin. Pharmacol. Ther.,* 20:690.
19. Taylor, H. L., Nolan, R. B., Tedeschi, R. E., and Maurath, C. J. (1978): Combined results of the study of probucol at 1gm/day in eight centers. *Clin. Pharmacol. Ther.,* 23:131.
20. Van Handel, E., and Zilversmith, D. B. (1957): Micromethod for the direct determination of serum triglycerides. *J. Lab. Clin. Med.,* 50:152.
21. Zlatkis, A., Zak, B., and Boyle, A. J. (1953): A new method for the direct determination of serum cholesterol. *J. Lab. Clin. Med.,* 41:486.

Diet and Drugs in Atherosclerosis,
edited by G. Noseda, B. Lewis, and R. Paoletti.
Raven Press, New York © 1980.

Effect of Probucol in Hypercholesterolemic Patients Resistant to Other Hypolipidemic Drugs

S. Stefanović and L. Vučić

Clinic A of Internal Medicine, University Medical Faculty, Belgrade, Yugoslavia

The cholesterol-lowering effect of the new agent probucol in familial types IIa and IIb hypercholesterolemia has been reported by several authors in different countries (1–8). We have sought to assess its efficacy in patients resistant to other hypolipidemic agents.

METHODS

We studied 15 ambulant patients with familial hypercholesterolemia, two of type IIa and four of type IIb. Their ages, sex, and duration of previous treatment are given in Table 1. All had been treated first with diet and then with clofibrate, with the addition of cholestyramine in three and polyunsaturated phosphatidyl-choline in five cases. None of these interventions had produced acceptable response in serum cholesterol. Baseline observations of cholesterol, triglyceride, and total lipid levels, hepatic and renal function, and hematology were made.

TABLE 1. *Pretreatment data*

Case no.	Age (years)	Sex	Previous therapy (years)
1	35	F	5
2	48	F	1
3	34	F	6
4	30	F	6
5	41	F	4
6	56	F	6
7	45	M	10
8	49	F	9
9	51	M	2
10	42	F	20
11	58	F	8
12	46	F	8
13	56	F	3
14	38	F	7
15	50	F	10

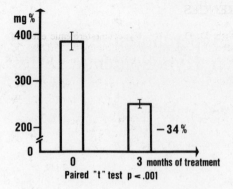

FIG. 1. Serum cholesterol levels before and 3 months after treatment with probucol, 1 g/day.

Thereafter, they were put on a hypocholesterolemic diet and treated with 1 g probucol/day in two divided doses. This was continued for 3 months. These observations were repeated monthly.

RESULTS

The mean fall in serum cholesterol levels at 3 months was 34% (Fig. 1). In all but one patient, cholesterol values were reduced to acceptable levels for the respective age groups, i.e., from 214 to 280 mg/dl (mean, 229 mg/dl). One patient was unaffected (baseline, 325 mg/dl; final level, 322 mg/dl).

Serum triglycerides increased from a mean of 122 to 156 mg/dl, still remaining within our normal range; this increase was possibly due to discontinuation of clofibrate (Fig. 2). During the treatment, we did not observe any clinical or laboratory abnormality. In one case, treatment was interrupted for reasons unrelated to the medication.

CONCLUSION

This study carried out in type IIa and type IIb familial hypercholesterolemic patients suggests that probucol is effective and well tolerated in patients selected for relative resistance to diet, clofibrate, and other drugs.

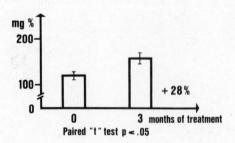

FIG. 2. Serum triglycerides (see Fig. 1).

REFERENCES

1. Barnhart, J. W., Sefranka, J. A., and McIntosh, D. D. (1970): Hypocholesterolemic effect of 4,4'-(isopropylidenedithio)-bis(2,6-di-t-butylphenol) (Probucol). *Am. J. Clin. Nutr.,* 23:1229.
2. Canosa, F. L. (1975): Long-term hypocholesterolemic drug therapy with probucol (DH-581) in human subjects. *Clin. Pharmacol. Ther.,* 17:230.
3. Davignon, J. (1974): Clofibrate and DH-581 in the long-term treatment of primary hyperlipoproteinemia. In: *Third International Symposium on Atherosclerosis,* pp. 794–797. Springer-Verlag, Berlin.
4. Harris, R. S., Gilmore, H. R., Bricker, L. A., Kiem, I. M., and Rubin, E. (1974): Long-term oral administration of probucol [4,4'(isopropylidenedithio)bis(2,6-di-t-butylphenol)] (DH-581) in the management of hypercholesterolemia. *J. Am. Geriatr. Soc.,* 22:167.
5. LeLorier, J., DuBreuil-Quidoz, S., Lussier-Cacan, S., Huang, Y. S., and Davignon, J. (1977): Diet and probucol in lowering cholesterol concentrations. *Arch. Intern. Med.,* 137:1429.
6. Parsons, W. B. (1978): Effect of probucol in hyperlipidemic patients during two years of administration. *Am. Heart J.,* 96:213.
7. Polachek, A. A., Katz, H. M., Sack, J., Selig, J., and Littman, M. (1973): Probucol in the long-term treatment of hypercholesterolerolaemia. *Curr. Med. Res. Opin.,* I:323.
8. Salel, A. F., Zelis, R., Sodhi, H. S., Price, J., and Mason, D. T. (1976): Probucol: a new cholesterol-lowering drug effective in patients with type II hyperlipoproteinemia. *Clin. Pharmacol. Ther.,* 20:690.

English Summaries

THE EFFECT OF PROBUCOL AND OTHER DRUGS ON STEROL SYNTHESIS IN HUMAN LYMPHOCYTES

A. Anastasi, D. J. Betteridge, and D. J. Galton

Current treatment of hypercholesterolemia is unsatisfactory and new hypo-cholesterolemic drugs are required. The human lymphocyte is a useful model in which to study the effects of potential hypocholesterolemic drugs on sterol synthesis.

In isolated lymphocytes, sterol synthesis is suppressed when cells are incubated with low-density lipoprotein (LDL). Removal of LDL from the medium leads to increased synthesis of sterols due to induction of HMG-CoA reductase, a rate-determining enzyme.

We have studied the effects of cycloheximide, a translational inhibitor of protein synthesis and cordycepin (3'-deoxyadenosine) a transcriptional inhibitor of mRNA synthesis on the induction of sterol synthesis in freshly isolated human lymphocytes incubated in a medium containing lipoprotein deficient serum (LPDS). We have studied other agents including compactin and probucol which may have a direct effect on the pathway.

Cycloheximide (20 μg/ml) inhibited the LPDS-mediated induction of sterol synthesis suggesting that the increase depends on *de novo* synthesis of enzymes.

Cordycepin (50 μg/ml) had no effect on the induction of sterol synthesis by LPDS, although reducing mRNA synthesis by 50%. Furthermore, in lymphocytes pre-incubated with LDL in the presence of cordycepin for 40 h (by which time the pool of mRNA with a short half-life should be greatly reduced), the subsequent rise in sterol synthesis after removal of LDL from the medium was the same as in cells pre-incubated in the absence of cordycepin. This suggests that the half-life of HMG-CoA reductase mRNA is relatively long and that now mRNA is not required for induction of sterol synthesis.

Compactin (0.2 μM) inhibited sterol synthesis by 65% without affecting the incorporation of ^{14}C-mevalonate into sterols, suggesting that the drug is specifically inhibiting the activity of HMG-CoA reductase.

Probucol, when emulsified in concentrations up to 1 mM with bovine serum albumin (in view of its poor solubility), produced about a 40% inhibition of sterol synthesis from ^{14}C-acetate. This possibly contributes to the hypocholesterolemic effect of the drug.

PHARMACOLOGY OF PROBUCOL

D. Kritchevsky

Probucol, 4,4' (isopropylidenedithio)*bis*(2,6-di-t-butylphenol) is an effective hypocholesterolemic agent in several species (mouse, rat, dog, monkey and man). The hypocholesterolemic response in mice is dose-related. In animals, the mechanism of action appears to be a combination of increased excretion of fecal bile acids, inhibition of cholesterol synthesis and decreased absorption. When tissue levels of cholesterol were compared in hypercholesterolemic control and drug-treated monkeys, there was a 52% drop in serum cholesterol.

The only other significant changes were a decrease in liver cholesterol and an increase in spleen cholesterol. No significant differences were seen in 17 other tissues. Thus, probucol treatment did not appear to cause any appreciable redistribution of cholesterol in the body. Based on studies in several hypercholesterolemic patients, Miettinen (*Atherosclerosis* 15, 163, 1972) concluded that probucol acted by inhibiting cholesterol synthesis and absorption and increasing bile acid excretion. When hypercholesterolemic monkeys are treated with probucol, they exhibit increased excretion of bile acids but not of neutral steroids.

Probucol induces ventricular fibrillation in dogs but is without side effects in all other species which have been tested. Administration of ^{14}C-labeled probucol resulted in excretion of 84% of radioactivity in the feces and 1–2% in the urine over 4 days. After giving isotopically labeled probucol, the half-lives of ^{14}C-labeled probucol are 0.8 and 12.8 days in the monkey, and 1 and 15.2 days in the dog. Probucol treatment does not affect activity of a number of liver enzymes: catylase, LDH, glutamic dehydrogenase nor does it cause changes in liver glycogen levels. When administered to hypercholesterolemic monkeys, probucol lowers aorta cholesterol by 25%. When fed to rabbits on an atherogenic regimen, probucol at 1% significantly inhibits atherosclerosis.

TOXICOLOGIC STUDIES ON PROBUCOL AND COMPARISON OF LIVER MORPHOLOGY IN RATS GIVEN PROBUCOL, FENOFIBRATE OR CLOFIBRATE

J. Molello, S. Barnard, and J. Lebeau

Probucol was given orally to 40 male and female rhesus monkeys at doses of 0, 60, 125, 250, or 500 mg/kg/day. Fourteen monkeys were killed at 18 and 24 months; 21 remained on test for 8 years. Observations included growth rate, hematology, clinical chemistry, urinalysis, organ weights and gross, histopathologic and electron-microscopic studies. Five unscheduled deaths occurred, none demonstrably related to treatment. No significant differences were observed between treated and control animals in respect of these observations.

Sprague-Dawley rats were given daily doses of approximately 500 mg/kg probucol, 250 mg/kg clofibrate or 100 mg/kg fenofibrate in their diets for periods of up to 91 days to assess their effects on liver cell ultrastructure. Control rats were given untreated basal rations. All compounds reduced serum cholesterol levels significantly. Liver tissues from probucol treated rats were comparable to those from untreated control animals.

Clofibrate and fenofibrate caused hepatocytomegaly, an increase in the number of peroxisomes and a mild alteration of the smooth and rough endoplasmic reticulum and mitochondria.

HYPOLIPIDEMIC EFFECT AND MECHANISM OF ACTION OF PROBUCOL IN MICE AND RABBITS

R. Infante and D. Petit

The effects of probucol on plasma and tissue lipids have been investigated in mice and rabbits receiving various diets (standard diet, fat-free diet, low-fat low-cholesterol diet, hypercholesterolemic diet).

In the first experiment, probucol induced a marked fall of serum cholesterol both in mice (− 33% and − 60% vs controls respectively, after 7 and 21 days of treatment with 0.6 g/kg food) and rabbits (− 37% and − 41% vs controls after 10 days with respectively 1 and 2.5 g/kg food). Hepatic lipids were unchanged.

When probucol was fed with synthetic diets containing 0, 1, 3, or 10% fat, the drug was ineffective at 0 and 1% fat levels. At 3% fat level, cholesterol was reduced and with the hyperlipidemic diet (10% fat and 1% cholesterol) it prevented the development of hypercholesterolemia. A rapid, marked and sustained decrease of plasma cholesterol and phospholipids was observed after a single i.v. injection in mice.

In rabbits, probucol prevented the hyperlipidemia induced by an i.v. injection of phospholipids.

In mice fed a normal standard diet for 7 to 21 days, probucol 0.6 g/kg food did not significantly affect ^{14}C-mevalonate incorporation into hepatic, intestinal and carcass cholesterol. Reduction of radioactivity incorporation into plasma cholesterol was observed.

Preliminary results in mice receiving probucol 0.6 g/kg diet during 4 weeks show a decrease in the very low density lipoprotein synthesis rate *in vivo*.

PROBUCOL IN THE LONG-TERM MANAGEMENT OF HYPERCHOLESTEROLEMIA

D. McCaughan

Probucol was studied in a double-blind, placebo controlled trial for one year in 118 male patients with primary hypercholesterolemia (pretreatment serum cholesterol levels 250 mg/dl or greater). The mean decrease in serum cholesterol in the probucol group (n = 88) from baseline for months 6 – 12 ranged from 16.2% to 20.9%. The mean decrease from baseline for the placebo-treated patients (n = 30) ranged from 5.2% to 12.7% (p < 0.001).

At the end of this one-year trial, 61 of the probucol-treated patients were continued on therapy in an open trial for up to nine years. After the second year of probucol treatment, the reduction in serum cholesterol ranged from 23.1% to 27.4% and was subsequently maintained.

Total mortality at the end of five years was 9%. The five-year incidence of coronary mortality and definite nonfatal myocardial infarction was 14%.

The drug was well tolerated. The most common side effect was transient loose stools or diarrhea. The present report suggests that probucol is safe and effective for the long-term lowering of serum cholesterol levels in patients with primary hypercholesterolemia.

EFFECT OF PROBUCOL AND DIET ON SERUM LIPIDS AND LIPOPROTEIN FRACTIONS IN PRIMARY HYPERCHOLESTEROLEMIA

R. Mordasini, M. Keller, and W. F. Riesen

The effect of probucol on serum lipoproteins was studied in 27 patients with primary hypercholesterolemia. The patients had received isocaloric, fat-reduced and fat-modified diet (NIH type II diet) for at least 3 months. This phase was followed by a pre-treatment period of 6 weeks, in which placebo was administered while the diet was continued. In the subsequent double-blind study, the patients received either diet and placebo (4 tablets per day) or diet and probucol (4 tablets of 250 mg in 2 administrations per day). Observations were made at monthly intervals. The following were analysed: cholesterol and triglyceride in serum and in LDL and HDL (isolated by ultracentrifugation) apo-B, apo-A-I (measured by radial immunodiffusion) and A-II (measured by radioimmunoassay).

Compared with the mean value during the placebo period, total cholesterol concentration fell in the probucol period by an average of 41 mg/100 ml (− 13%, p < 0.05). LDL cholesterol concentration was reduced in parallel to the total cholesterol, the average reduction being 42 mg/100 ml (− 16%, p < 0.025). A slight but statistically insignificant decrease was also noted in HDL cholesterol levels. In the placebo period no significant changes of total cholesterol, LDL or

HDL cholesterol concentration, were observed. Both during probucol and placebo periods serum triglyceride levels remained almost unchanged. The apo-B concentration was reduced by probucol by an average of 12%, but this change was not significant (p < 0.15). Under placebo treatment apo-B levels remained constant. The mean reduction of apo-A-I under probucol was 16% (p < 0.0005), that of apo-A-II 55% (p < 0.0005). In the placebo group a decrease of apo-A-I and apo-A-II levels was noted too; this decrease was only significant for apo-A-II (26%, p < 0.005).

In general, the probucol treatment was very well tolerated. In 4 patients, the study had to be discontinued, mainly due to subjective side-effects. Three of these were receiving placebo and 1 was taking probucol.

HIGH DENSITY LIPOPROTEIN LEVELS DURING A FIVE-YEAR MULTIFACTORIAL INTERVENTION AGAINST CORONARY HEART DISEASE RISK FACTORS

A. Miettinen, J. K. Huttunen, T. Kumlin
V. Naukkarinen, S. Mattila, and C. Enholm

Serum cholesterol (CH), triglycerides (TG), high density lipoprotein cholesterol (HDL-CH), HDL-A-I, HDL-A-II, and non-HDL-A-I were measured in 119 men who had participated for up to four years in a controlled trial to reduce the risk factors for coronary heart disease. The treatment included dietary advice, instructions for physical activity, and antihypertensive and antihyperlipidemic medication as needed. Total serum CH and TG were measured throughout the study, but HDL-CH and A-I and A-II only during the fourth year of the trial. Baseline values could not be used for HDL-CH, HDL-A-I and HDL-A-II because of a marked fall in the level when the sera were stored for up to four years at $-20\,°C$.

The levels of all serum lipids were similar in subjects treated with diet (n = 32) and with antihypertensive drugs (n = 19). As compared to these groups, subjects on clofibrate (n = 30) had similar levels of A-I, a 34% increase in A-II and a 13% decrease in HDL. Subjects treated with probucol (used for type IIa hyperlipoproteinemia (n = 25) showed a decrease in the level of total cholesterol (− 13%), HDL-CH (− 29%) and HDL-A-I (− 16%), but a similar level of HDL-A-II, as compared to the group treated with diet or antihypertensive medication. Non-HDL-A-I was also low. Subjects treated with the combination of clofibrate and probucol (mainly type IIb, n = 13) had inconsistent changes in serum lipids but exhibited a 55% decrease in HDL-CH, a 41% decrease in A-I, and a low non-HDL-A-I level, whereas the level of A-II was similar as compared to the diet group. The results suggest that though probucol and clofibrate reduce HDL-CH in long-term treatment, they decrease the cholesterol/apoliproprotein ratio of HDL, i.e. the mean cholesterol saturation of HDL fraction is lowered. The changes caused by clofibrate were partly associated with altered triglyceride concentration while those in the probucol group were correlated with the length of the treatment period.

EFFICACY AND TOLERANCE OF PROBUCOL AND CLOFIBRATE

J. L. De Gennes and J. Truffert

The hypocholesterolemic effect of probucol and clofibrate has been compared in a double-blind trial in 38 patients with primary hypercholesterolemia.

Nineteen patients received probucol (1 g/day) during 2 months and the other 19 received clofibrate (2 g/day) during the same period of time. All patients were on a low cholesterol, low saturated and high polyunsaturated fat diet started 2 months prior to the drug administration.

Addition of probucol to the dietary regimen induced a serum cholesterol fall of

13% (p < .05 versus placebo). In the group treated with clofibrate serum cholesterol decreased by 11% on average. This decrease was not statistically significant.

A serum cholesterol decrease exceeding 20% was observed in 31% of the patients in the probucol group and in 21% of the patients in the clofibrate group.

Serum triglycerides were not significantly modified by either drug. Both drugs were well tolerated.

Probucol can be usefully prescribed in hypercholesterolemic patients responding incompletely to clofibrate and its derivatives.

CLINICAL EXPERIENCE IN REGARD TO SAFETY AND CHOLESTEROL-LOWERING ACTION OF PROBUCOL

R. E. Tedeschi, H. L. Taylor, and B. L. Martz

Long-term, carefully monitored studies of probucol in the U.S. are reported, involving 1,133 patients treated for various periods. Eight hundred and eighty-one (881) patients were studied under a common protocol. By May 1979, 291 of these patients had been followed for five years; 139 had been followed for eight years. Sixty-eight percent of patients who received probucol 1 g/day for eight years exhibited a 15% or greater lowering of serum cholesterol concentration compared with the control level. Eighty-two percent of the probucol patients showed a 10% or greater lowering of serum cholesterol compared with controls. The mean decrease for the group was 19.9%. There was no evidence of escape from the cholesterol-lowering effect in these subjects.

The most frequent side effect was loose stools; others included flatulence, abdominal pain, nausea and vomiting. Blood counts, liver and renal function tests revealed no evidence of toxicity. An analysis of morbidity and mortality was made for all 1,133 patients who were treated with probucol, using life table analysis. Ninety-eight percent of these patients had a serum cholesterol ≥ 250 mg%. In addition, many of the patients had other coronary heart disease risk factors. The five-year cumulative mortality rate (all causes) was 6.5%. The five year cumulative event rate for nonfatal myocardial infarction in all probucol-treated patients with a history of myocardial infarction (n = 267) was 7.3%.

Differences in entry criteria, the size of the study group, and other variables have precluded a direct statistical comparison of the mortality and morbidity results during the probucol experience with other studies. However, using published data from the Coronary Drug Project as reference, the relatively low mortality and morbidity during probucol treatment suggest, but do not prove, a protective effect of probucol administration.

In view of the current interest in the possible deleterious effect of lipid-lowering agents on the biliary tract, we have analyzed the frequency of cholecystectomy and biliary disease in patients on long-term probucol. The six-year combined rate for biliary events (cholecystectomy, cholelithiasis, and cholecystitis) for males was 3.3% (n = 729) and 5.8% for females (n = 404), a combined rate of 4.1%. A life table six-year cumulative rate for cholecystectomy was ? 2% (n = 729) for males, and 2.7% for females (n = 404), with a combined six year cumulative rate of 2.3%. Because of differences in population characteristics, the frequently asymptomatic clinical course of cholelithiasis, and other variables, a direct statistical comparison with other study groups is not appropriate. However, the above rates certainly do not appear excessive.

PROBUCOL: SHORT- AND LONG-TERM TRIALS IN TYPE II HYPERLIPOPROTEINEMIA

V. Beaumont, J. C. Buxtorf, B. Jacotot, and J. L. Beaumont

A short term clinical trial of probucol versus placebo was carried out on 19 patients with type II hyperlipoproteinemia. Each patient received successively placebo and probucol 1 g/day each for 1 month, in random sequence. They continued to take their usual diet. Total cholesterol, phospholipids and triglyceride levels were compared at the end of each period, and evaluated with a paired "t" test. A decrease of 9% in mean total cholesterol was obtained with probucol (p < 0.001). No significant variation of phospholipid and triglyceride levels was observed. The persistence of probucol effects on serum lipids, its action on tissue lipids and its tolerance were investigated in an open trial in 20 patients with type II hyperlipoproteinemia. As in the short term trial, no special diet was prescribed. Serum lipid levels were determined initially and every 2 months for a 6 month period. Free and esterified cholesterol were measured in skin fragments before and at the end of the treatment and compared with observations on controls. Serum cholesterol levels showed a mean decrease of 9.9% (p < 0.001) similar to that in the short term trial. The decrease exceeded 10% in 60% of the patients. No significant change was noted in serum phospholipid and triglyceride levels.

A significant increase in the esterified cholesterol content of the skin after 6 months treatment was observed. No abnormalities in the routine laboratory tests were noted, though both SGOT and SGPT rose within the normal range. Hence the hypocholesterolemic effect of probucol is maintained during long term treatment, and appears to be safe. The significant increase of the esterified cholesterol fraction in the skin, in the absence of a significant change of total cholesterol needs further evaluation. It may be hypothesized that these qualitative changes may facilitate cholesterol removal and possibly correlate with the observed regression of xanthelasmas.

TREATMENT OF HYPERCHOLESTEROLEMIAS WITH PROBUCOL

R. Carmena and J. F. Ascaso

The hypolipidemic effect of probucol, given in addition to a low cholesterol, low saturated fat, high polyunsaturated fat diet, has been investigated in 20 patients with primary hyperlipoproteinemia (phenotype IIa in 7 cases and IIb in 13).

After 1 month on diet alone, the patients were given probucol 500 mg b.i.d. or placebo in a random fashion for 2 months. One month of diet preceded the second phase of the cross-over.

Diet alone reduced serum cholesterol from a mean value of 403.7 mg/dl to 375.1 mg/dl (− 7%, not statistically significant). The addition of probucol significantly enhanced the hypocholesterolemic effect of the diet (− 32%, p < .01), while it did not substantially alter serum triglycerides.

The tolerability of the drug was excellent.

EFFECT OF PROBUCOL ON
PRIMARY HYPERCHOLESTEROLEMIA

A. Gouveia, A. Noronha, I. Dionísio, S. Felix, B. Barros, and M. Carrageta

An open trial on probucol in patients with primary hypercholesterolemia was performed to determine effects of probucol on elevated serum levels of cholesterol, and to study the incidence and nature of adverse reactions. Patients were encouraged to follow a standard diet for one month and attended our clinic for physical examination and laboratory tests. The admission to the trial was limited to patients with an average of 3 measurements (by enzymatic methods) of baseline serum cholesterol level ⩾ 250 mg/100 ml (differences between the 3 values ⩽ 32 mg/100 ml) and with variations of weight ⩽ 5%.

From the 34 patients satisfying these criteria, 2 dropped out during the first week of medication owing to intestinal disturbances. There remained 15 men and 17 women, with average age 47 years (25 to 65 years) and 53 years (42 to 62 years) respectively. During 2 months of medication 32 patients took probucol 500 mg twice daily and continued to follow a standard diet.

Results confirmed that probucol is effective. At the end of the first month, lowering of serum cholesterol was already significant ($p < 0.001$), and cholesterol values dropped further on the second month. Variations of triglyceride levels were not significant.

No relevant findings were reported after physical examinations and laboratory tests. Probucol was well tolerated. Adverse reactions were limited to the 2 cases mentioned.

CLINICAL TRIAL OF A NEW CHOLESTEROL-LOWERING AGENT: PROBUCOL

A. Castro Ribeiro and A. Pereira Viana

In a double-blind design, probucol (500 mg twice daily) or placebo were randomly administered to 26 patients with primary hypercholesterolemia. For the one month preceding the medication period, all patients took placebo and were encouraged to follow a standard diet. Baseline values for serum cholesterol were established after three weekly measurements, using the enzymatic method.

In the probucol group, serum cholesterol dropped from an average value of 297 to 247 mg/100 ml after 3 months of medication. Analysis of covariance showed a significant difference ($p < 0.05$) in comparison with the placebo group. Serum cholesterol fell to less than 250 mg/100 ml in 7 patients on probucol and in 1 patient on placebo (Fisher test $p < 0.008$).

Triglyceride levels did not differ significantly between the two groups. Body weight remained practically unchanged. There were no withdrawals due to adverse reactions. Minor digestive disturbances were reported in 5 patients taking probucol and in 3 patients taking placebo.

Our trial confirms both that probucol is an effective cholesterol-lowering drug and that it is well tolerated.

EFFECT OF PROBUCOL ON BILE COMPOSITION IN MAN—PRELIMINARY OBSERVATIONS

Z. Mareček, M. Jirsa, V. Kordač, and L. Kučerová

We studied the effect of probucol on biliary bile acid and lipid composition in 5 patients with type IIa hyperlipidemia. None had previously received this drug. Other cholesterol-lowering agents were discontinued at least one month previously. Before treatment the serum cholesterol level ranged from 310 to 440 mg/dl.

After oral cholecystography to exclude gallstones and gallbladder disease, the patients were treated for two months with 1 g probucol daily. Serum lipids were determined every two weeks.

The bile was collected by duodenal drainage after i.v. injection of cholecystokinin, before and at the end of medication.

Total bile acids were measured enzymatically, cholesterol and phospholipids colorimetrically; the degree of bile saturation with cholesterol was calculated as the Thomas-Hoffman lithogenic index.

Bile acid composition was determined by gas-liquid chromatography; the methyl trimethylsilyl ethers were analyzed on a 1% Hi EFF 8 BP column.

On the basis of these preliminary findings, it appears that the changes in relative molar composition of biliary lipids after probucol are strikingly different from changes in bile composition after treatment with clofibrate.

Clofibrate increases the concentration of biliary cholesterol and reduces bile acid levels. These changes result in increased lithogenicity of bile, i.e., supersaturation with cholesterol. By contrast probucol reduces biliary cholesterol and increases bile acid content, thus the lithogenic index decreases. Changes in bile acid composition after probucol treatment were small and variable.

EFFECT OF PROBUCOL ON Ca INTESTINAL ABSORPTION AND ON LONG-TERM ANTICOAGULANT THERAPY IN PATIENTS WITH HYPERCHOLESTEROLEMIA ASSOCIATED WITH CARDIOVASCULAR DISEASE

A. Rapado and M. Diaz-Curiel

Probucol in doses varying from 0.5 to 1.5 g per day, together with a low cholesterol, low saturated fat diet, significantly decreased serum cholesterol (p < .01) in 20 type IIa patients. Treatment was for an average period of 14 months. Serum triglycerides were not modified by treatment.

The effect of the drug on calcium absorption was studied by measuring the ^{47}Ca intestinal absorption before and during probucol treatment. The effect on vitamin K activity was observed by monitoring prothrombin time in patients on chronic administration of anticoagulants. No drug interaction was evident.

Probucol was administered to a 12-year old homozygous type II hypercholesterolemic girl who had developed biochemical signs of rickets requiring therapy while taking cholestyramine. In this patient, probucol significantly decreased serum cholesterol concentration without changes in ^{47}Ca intestinal absorption and without biochemical signs of rickets.

PROBUCOL: EVALUATION OF EFFECTIVENESS ON LIPIDS AND LIPOPROTEINS

J. Rouffy, R. Bakir, B. Chanu, and J. Goy-Loeper

The effect of probucol 1 g/day on serum lipids and lipoproteins has been investigated in patients with primary hyperlipoproteinemia of types IIa and IIb, not responsive to diet. Some of them had previously failed to respond to clofibrate, procetofen and cholestyramine.

Treatment duration was 1 month in 34 patients (T_1), from 3 to 6 months in 16 (T_2), from 6 months to 1 year in 12 (T_3) and longer than 1 year in 4 (T_4).

A significant decrease of total serum lipids (from 8 to 19%) of total serum cholesterol (from 8 to 12%) and of LDL-cholesterol (from 9 to 15%) together with a significant increase of the ratio of HDL-CH to LDL-CH plus VLDL-CH were observed during all treatment periods with the exception of T_3, all potentially desirable results.

No interaction with anticoagulants has been observed.

This study demonstrated that probucol is an effective drug in lowering total serum lipids and cholesterol as well as LDL-cholesterol.

PROBUCOL MANAGEMENT OF HYPERCHOLESTEROLEMIA IN PATIENTS WITH CARDIOVASCULAR DISEASE

L. Scebat and J. Renais

Thirty-three patients with atherosclerotic cardiovascular disease and hypercholesterolemia type IIa (11 patients), type IIb or III (21 patients), and type IV (1 patient) were treated with probucol and a low-fat diet for 12 to 46 months. The mean serum cholesterol concentration decreased from 329.5 to 281.1 mg/dl (− 14.5%, p < 0.001).

Twelve patients were regarded as nonresponders (cholesterol decrease ≤ 10%), and 20 patients responded to diet with probucol (62.5% of the series). Three escaped from the cholesterol-lowering effect after the 6th month. The result obtained during the first year was maintained in 15 patients (47%).

Probucol lowered the plasma cholesterol level by about the same extent in primary hypercholesterolemia (type IIa) and in combined hyperlipidemia (types IIb and III).

No interaction was observed between probucol and other drugs prescribed for cardiovascular disease, particularly anticoagulants and diuretics.

No variations in liver and renal function tests, in glucose level or blood count were noted. Body weight remained stable. The ECG was not modified by treatment. Three patients complained of diarrhea which improved while on treatment in 2; in the 3rd therapy was withdrawn during the 2nd week.

EFFECT OF PROBUCOL IN HYPERCHOLESTEROLEMIC PATIENTS RESISTANT TO OTHER HYPOLIPIDEMIC DRUGS

S. Stefanović and L. Vučić

The effect of probucol on hypercholesterolemia has been studied in 15 patients: 11 with type IIa and 4 with type IIb hyperlipoproteinemia. Their hypercholesterolemia had been recognized for 1 to 20 years mean 7 years, and had never been satisfactorily controlled by diet, clofibrate, or, in some cases, cholestyramine or polyunsaturated phosphatidyl choline.

Baseline cholesterol levels ranged from 306 to 565 mg/dl, mean 385 mg/dl. All patients received 1 g of probucol daily for 90 days. Measurements were made at monthly intervals. At the end of treatment in all patients but one, cholesterol values were within normal range for the appropriate age group and ranged from 214 to 280 mg/dl (mean 229 mg/dl). Neither clinical nor laboratory side effects, nor subjective complaints were noted during probucol treatment.

Résumés en Français

EFFET DU PROBUCOL ET D'AUTRES MEDICAMENTS SUR LA SYNTHESE DES LYMPHOCYTES HUMAINS

A. Anastasi, D. J. Betteridge, and D. J. Galton

Les traitements actuels de l'hypercholestérolemie ne sont pas satisfaisants et ont a besoin de nouveaux médicaments hypocholestérolemiants. Le lymphocite humain est une cellule utîle dans l'étude de l'effet potentiel des medicaments sur la synthèse des stérols. Dans les lymphocytes isolées la synthèse des sterols est inhibée lorsque les cellules sont incubées avec les lipoproteines de basse densité (LDL). La suppression des LDL du milieu provoque une augmentation de la synthèse des stérols dependant de l'induction de la HMG-CoA réductase qui est l'enzyme limitante de cette voie métabolique.

Nous avons étudié les effets de la cycloheximide (un inhibiteur de la synthèse protéique au niveau de la traduction) et de la cordycepine (3'-desoxyadenosine) (un inhibiteur transcriptionel de la synthèse des mRNA) sur l'induction de la synthèse des sterols dans les lymphocytes humains fraîchement isolés et incubés dans un milieu contenant du serum de lipoproteinisé (LPDS).

Nous avons aussi étudié d'autres agents comme la compactine et le probucol qui pourraient avoir un effet sur ce métabolisme (synthèse des sterols).

La cycloheximide (20 μg/ml) inhibe l'induction de la synthèse des stérols LPDS—dépendante suggerant que l'augmentation dépends de la synthèse enzymatique *de novo*.

La cordycepine (50 µg/ml) n'a pas d'effet sur l'induction de la synthèse des sterols par le LPDS bien qu'elle réduise de 50% la synthèse des mRNA.

Par ailleurs, dans les lymphocytes preincubés avec des LDL en presence de cordycepine pendant 40 heures (un temps pendant lequel le pool de m RNA a demie vie courte doit être fortement réduit), l'augmentation de la synthèse des stérols après suppression des LDL du milieu était la même que dans les cellules preincubées en absence de cordycepine. Ceci suggère que la demi-vie du mRNA de la HMG-CoA réductase est relativement longue et qu'une nouvelle synthèse de mRNA n'est pas indispensable à l'induction de la synthèse des stérols.

La compactine (0.2 µg) inhibe la synthèse des stérols de 65% sans modifier l'incorporation de ^{14}C mevalonate dans les stérols suggerant que le produit inhibe specifiquement l'activité de la HMG-Coa réductase.

Le probucol en emulsion a des concentrations inferieures à 1 mM avec de la serum albumine bovine (à cause de sa faible solubilité) produit une inhibition d'environ 40% de la synthèse des sterols à partir du ^{14}C acetate. Ceci peut contribuer probablement à l'effet hypocholestérolemiant du médicament.

PHARMACOLOGIE DU PROBUCOL

D. Kritchevsky

Le probucol (4,4' (isopropylidène-dithio)*bis*(2,6-di-t-butylphenol) est un hypocholestérolémiant efficace chez différentes espèces animales (souris, rat, chien, singe) et chez l'homme.

Chez la souris, l'effet hypocholestérolémiant est lié à la dose administrée. Le mécanisme d'action a été étudié chez l'animal et l'effet hypocholestérolémiant semble étre dû à la fois à l'augmentation de l'excrétion fécale des acides biliaires, à l'inhibition de la synthèse du cholestérol et à la diminution de la résorption du cholestérol alimentaire.

Chez des singes hypercholestérolémiques, une diminution de 52% de la cholestérolémie a été observée dans le groupe traité par le probucol par rapport au groupe témoin. De même au niveau des tissus, le traitement par le probucol a entraîné une baisse significative du cholestérol hépatique et une augmentation également significative du cholestérol splénique; aucune différence significative n'a été mise en évidence dans les 17 autres tissus étudiés. Le traitement par le probucol ne semble donc pas provoquer de redistribution tissulaire du cholestérol dans l'organisme.

A partir d'études effectuées chez des malades hypercholestérolémiques Miettinin (*Atherosclerosis*, 15, 163, 1972) conclut que l'effet du probucol est dû à une inhibition de la synthèse du cholestérol et de sa résorption, et à une augmentation de l'excrétion des acides biliaires. Lorsque des singes hypercholestérolémiques sont traités par le probucol, l'excrétion des acides biliaires augmente mais celle des stéroîdes neutres n'est pas modifiée.

Le probucol provoque chez le chien une fibrillation ventriculaire mais aucun effet adverse n'a été constaté chez les autres animaux étudiés. Après administration de probucol marqué par le ^{14}C, 84% de la radioactivité se retrouve dans les fèces et 1 à 2% dans les urines, en 4 jours. Après administration de probucol marqué par le ^{14}C, les demi-vies du produit sont de 0,8 et 12,8 jours chez le singe et de 1 et 15, 2 jours chez le chien. Le traitement par le probucol n'exerce aucune influence sur l'activité de certaines catalases hépatiques (LDH déhydrogénase-lactique; déhydrogénase-glutamique) et ne modifie pas les taux de glycogène hépatique. Le probucol a réduit de 25% le taux de cholestérol aortique chez des singes hypercholestérolémiques.

Chez des lapins soumis à un régime athérogène, l'administration de probucol inhibe de maniere significative (p < 0,01) le processus athèroscléreux.

RESULTATS DES ETUDES TOXICOPATHOLOGIQUES SUR LE PROBUCOL ET ETUDE COMPARATIVE DE LA MORPHOLOGIE HEPATIQUE CHEZ DES RATS TRAITES PAR LE PROBUCOL, LE FENOFIBRATE ET LE CLOFIBRATE

J. Molello, S. Barnard, and J. Lebeau

Le probucol a été administré par voie orale à 40 singes Rhésus des deux sexes, à la dose de 0,60, 125, 250 ou 500 mg/kg/jour. Quatorze singes ont été sacrifiés après 18 et 24 mois de traitement; l'étude s'est prolongée pendant 8 ans chez 21 animaux. Les paramètres étudiés ont été le rythme de croissance, des données hématologiques et biochimiques, l'analyse des urines, le poids des organes. l'étude macroscopique, histologique et électromicroscopique des tissus. Cinq singes sont morts au cours de l'expérimentation, sans relation avec le traitement. Aucune différence significative n'a été constatée entre les animaux traités et témoins.

Les effets du probucol sur l'ultrastructure de la cellule hépatique ont été étudiés chez le rat Sprague-Dawley en les comparant à ceux du clofibrate et du fenofibrate. Les médicaments ont été mélangés aux rations alimentaires et administrés à des doses d'environ 500, 250, et 100 mg/kg/jour respectivement pour le probucol, le clofibrate et le fenofibrate pendant une période allant jusqu'à 91 jours. Les animaux témoins n'ont reçu que la ration alimentaire. Les trois médicaments ont réduit de façon significative le taux de cholestérol sérique.

La morphologie du tissu hépatique des rats traités par le probucol a été comparable à celle des animaux témoins. Le clofibrate et le fenofibrate ont provoqué une hépatocytomégalie, une augmentation du nombre des peroxysomes et de légères altérations du réticulum endoplasmique et des mitochondries. Les résultats de ces expériences, ainsi que celles d'autres études montrent que, à court terme comme à long terme, le probucol est bien toléré par la souris, le rat, le lapin, le singe et le cobaye soumis à des conditions expérimentales conventionnelles ou à un stress cardio-vasculaire sévère.

D'autre part, le chien est le seul chez lequel se développe une sensibilisation du myocarde à l'adrénaline et à la noradrénaline.

Contrairement à d'autres hypocholestérolémiants, le probucol n'altère pas la morphologie cellulaire du foie ni chez le rongeur ni chez le singe.

Les données fournies par ces études de toxicologie montrent que le probucol est un produit sûr.

EFFET HYPOCHOLESTEROLEMIANT ET MECANISME D'ACTION DU PROBUCOL CHEZ LA SOURIS ET LE LAPIN

R. Infante and D. Petit

L'effet du probucol sur le lipides plasmatiques et tissulaires a été étudié chez la souris et le lapin dans différentes conditions alimentaires (régime standard, régime sans lipide, régime à faible teneur en lipides et en cholestérol, régime hyper-cholestérolémiant).

Le probucol administré à des animaux soumis à un régime standard réduit de façon considérable le cholestérol sérique chez la souris (− 33% et − 60% par rapport aux témoins respectivement après 7 et 21 jours de traitement par 0,6 g/kg aliment, et chez le lapin) − 37% et − 41% par rapport aux témoins après 10 jours de traitement par des doses de 1 et 2,5 g/kg aliment respectivement) sans modifier les lipides hépatiques.

Chez les animaux soumis à régime comportant une teneur en lipides de 0%, 1%, 3% ou 10%, le probucol n'a manifesté aucune activité dans les 2 premières conditions (0% et 1%); en revanche, l'effet hypocholestérolémiant a été évident chez les animaux dont le régime contenait 3% de graisses; chez ceux qui avaient été soumis au régime hyperlipidémiant (10% de lipides, cholestérol à 1%), le probucol a empêché le développement de l'hyperlipidémie.

Chez la souris, l'administration intraveineuse d'une dose unique de probucol a provoqué une chute importante des taux sériques du cholestérol et des phospholipides.

Chez le lapin, le probucol a prévenu l'effet hyperlipidémiant d'une administration intraveineuse de phospholipides. Chez des souris soumises au régime standard, le traitement par le probucol (0,6 g/kg aliment) pendant 7 à 21 jours, n'a pas entraîné de modification significative de l'incorporation du mévalonate-^{14}C dans le cholestérol hépatique et intestinal ainsi que dans le cholestérol de la carcasse. En revanche, on a constaté une réduction de l'incorporation de la radioactivité dans le cholestérol plasmatique. Un effet spécifique du probucol sur les lipoprotéines a été envisagé. Les résultats préliminaires obtenus chez des souris traitées pendant 4 semaines par le probucol (0,6 g par kg aliment) ont mis en évidence une diminution de la synthèse des VLDL.

LE PROBUCOL DANS LE TRAITEMENT A LONG TERME DE L'HYPERCHOLESTEROLEMIE

D. McCaughan

Le probucol a été étudié dans un essai contrôlé en double aveugle versus placebo et d'une durée d'un an, chez 118 malades atteints d'hypercholestérolémie essentielle (cholestérolémie ⩾ 250 mg/dl avant traitement). Après 6 et 12 mois de traitement, la baisse moyenne du taux sérique du cholestérol était comprise entre 16,2% et 20,9% par rapport aux valeurs de base dans le groupe des 88 patients traités par le probucol et entre 5,2% et 12,7% chez les 30 patients traités par le placebo (p < 0,001). Le traitement par le probucol a été ensuite poursuivi en ouvert pendant des périodes allant jusqu'à 9 ans chez 61 sujets traités par ce médicament au cours de l'étude contrôlée.

Après la 2ème année de traitement par le probucol, la baisse du cholestérol sérique a été de 23,1% à 27,4%. Ces valeurs se sont conservées par la suite.

La mortalité totale à l'issue des 5 années de traitement a été de 9%. L'incidence sur 5 ans, de la mortalité par insuffisance coronarienne et des infarctus du myocarde traité avec succès a été de 14%.

Le médicament a été bien toléré. Les effets secondaires les plus fréquents ont été des épisodes de selles molles ou de diarrhées. Les résultats obtenus prouvent que le probucol est un médicament bien supporté par l'organisme, et efficace dans le traitement à long terme des hypercholestérolémies essentielles.

EFFET DU PROBUCOL ET DU REGIME DIETETIQUE SUR LES LIPIDES SERIQUES ET SUR LES FRACTIONS LIPOPROTEIQUES DANS L'HYPERCHOLESTEROLEMIE ESSENTIELLE

R. Mordasini, M. Keller, and W. F. Riesen

L'effet du probucol sur différentes fractions lipidiques a été étudié chez 27 patients souffrant d'hypercholestérolémie essentielle. Ces patients étaient soumis, pendant au moins 3 mois, à un régime diététique isocalorique à faible teneur en lipides avec modification du rapport acides gras saturés/acides gras non saturés (NIH régime de type II). Cette phase a été suivie d'un prétraitement d'une durée de 6 semaines comprenant régime plus placebo. Au cours de l'étude en double-aveugle qui a suivi, les patients ont été traités par le régime et le placebo (1 comprimé 4 fois par jour) ou par le régime et le probucol (1 comprimé de 250 mg 4 fois par jour). Les comprimés de placebo et de probucol avaient un aspect extérieur absolument identique. Les contrôles sur les patients externes ont été effectués à un mois d'intervalle. Il a été procédé à l'analyse des paramètres suivants: cholestérol et triglycérides sériques totaux et après ultracentrifugation cholestérol et triglycérides des lipoprotéines à faible densité (LDL) et à haute densité (HDL), apo B et apo AI (par RID) et apo AII (par RIA).

Comparée aux valeurs moyennes obtenues sous placebo, la concentration sérique du cholestérol total a été réduite par le probucol en moyenne de 41 mg/100 ml (− 13%, p < 0,05).

Le LDL-cholestérol a été considérablement réduit, parallèlement au cholestérol total (réduction moyenne 42 mg/100 ml, soit — 16%, p < 0,025). Une légère réduction, statistiquement non significative a également été constatée pour l'HDL-cholestérol.

L'administration de placebo n'a déterminé aucune variation significative du cholestérol total, du LDL-cholestérol et du HDL-cholestérol. La triglycéridemie s'est maintenue à peu prés constante, sous probucol comme sous placebo.

La concentration des apo B a été réduite en moyenne de 12% sous probucol; cette variation n'est cependant pas statistiquement significative (p < 0,15). Les taux d'apo B n'ont pas varié sous placebo. Dans le groupe traité par le probucol, on a constaté une baisse moyenne de 16% des apo AI (p < 0,0005) et de 55% des apo AII (p < 0,0005). Une réduction des concentrations d'apo AI et d'apo AII a également été observée dans le groupe traité par le placebo. Cette réduction cependant n'est statistiquement significative que pour les apo AII (− 26%, p < 0,005).

Le traitement par le probucol a été en général bien toléré. L'étude a été interrompue chez 4 patients, en raison d'effets secondaires, principalement subjectifs. Trois de ces patients étaient sous placebo, le quatrième sous probucol.

TAUX PLASMATIQUES DES LIPOPROTEINES DE HAUTE DENSITÉ AU COURS D'UN ESSAI CLINIQUE D'INTERVENTION SIMULTANÉE SUR PLUSIEURS FACTEURS DE RISQUE DE MALADIE CORONARIENNE

A. Miettinen, J. K. Huttunen, T. Kumlin
V. Naukkarinen, S. Mattila, and C. Enholm

Le cholestérol sérique (C), les triglycérides (TG), le cholestérol des lipoprotéines à haute densité (HDLC), les apoprotéines AI et AII des lipoprotéines à haute densité (HDL-AI, HDL-AII) et les apoprotéines AI des lipoprotéines à densité non élevée (AI non HDL) ont été déterminés chez 119 sujets de sexe masculin qui avaient participé pendant des périodes allant jusqu'à 4 ans à une enquête contrôlée ayant pour but de réduire les facteurs de risque des coronaropathies. Le traitement comprenait des conseils concernant la diététique et l'activité physique et, la prescription si nécessaire, d'antihypertensifs et d'hypolipidémiants. Les taux sériques du cholestérol total et des triglycérides ont été déterminés pendant toute la durée de l'étude, et le HDLC et les apolipoprotéines AI et AII n'ont été évalués qu'au cours de la quatrième année de l'essai. Il a été impossible d'utiliser les valeurs de base pour le HDLC et les HDL AI et AII, la conservation prolongée des sérums pendant 4 ans à − 20°C, déterminant une réduction considérable de leur concentration sérique.

Les taux sériques de tous les lipides se sont avérés semblables chez les sujets soumis au seul régime alimentaire (n = 32) et chez les sujets traités par les antihypertensifs (n = 19). Par rapport à ces groupes, les sujets traités par le clofibrate (n = 30) ont présenté des taux similaires des apolipoprotéines AI, une augmentation de 34% des apolipoprotéines AII et une diminution de 13% du HDLC.

Après traitement par le probucol (25 cas d'hyperlipoprotéinémie de type IIA) et comparativement au groupe des individus soumis au seul régime ou traités par des antihypertensifs, on a constaté une réduction du taux du cholestérol total (− 13%), du HDLC (− 29%) et des HDL AI (− 16%), mais des taux similaires des HDL AII. Le taux des apolipoprotéines AI non-HDL était également bas. Les sujets traités par le clofibrate et par le probucol en association (13 cas d'hyperlipoprotéinemie de type IIB principalement) n'ont accusé aucune modification importante des lipides sériques, mais ils ont présenté une réduction de 55% du HDLC, une réduction de 41% des AI et un faible taux d'AI non HDL; quant aux taux des apolipoprotéines AII, ils ont été semblables à ceux qui avaient été observés dans le groupe d'individus soumis au seul régime alimentaire. Ces résultats suggèrent que le probucol et le clofibrate réduisent le HDLC au cours de traitements prolongés, réduisent le rapport cholestérol/apolipoprotéine des HDL, c'est-à-dire que la saturation moyenne en cholestérol dans la fraction HDL est abaissée.

Les modifications produites par le clofibrate ont été en partie associées aux altérations de la concentration des triglycérides, tandis que les modifications constatées dans les groupes de patients traités par le probucol étaient en corrélation avec la durée du traitement.

EVALUATION DE L'EFFICACITE ET DE LA TOLERANCE DU PROBUCOL ET CLOFIBRATE

J. L. De Gennes and J. Truffert

L'effet hypocholestérolémiant du probucol et celui du clofibrate ont été comparés au cours d'une étude en double-aveugle, réalisée chez 38 patients atteints d'hypercholestérolémie essentielle.

La moitié de ces patients ont été traités pendant 2 mois par le probucol à la dose quotidienne d'un gramme; les 19 autres ont reçu du clofibrate (2 g/jour) pendant deux mois également. Tous ces patients suivaient un régime diététique à faible teneur en cholestérol et en acides gras saturés et à teneur élevée en acides gras polyinsaturés. Ce régime alimentaire avait débuté deux mois avant l'étude et pendant cette période les patients avaient reçu du placebo.

L'adjonction de probucol au régime alimentaire a réduit de 13% de taux de la cholestérolémie (p < 0,05) par rapport aux valeurs observées à la fin de la période régime diététique + placebo. Sous l'action du clofibrate, la baisse du taux de la cholestérolémie a été en moyenne de 11% (baisse non statistiquement significative).

La baisse du taux de la cholestérolémie a été supérieure à 20% chez 31% des patients traités par le probucol et chez 21% des cas traités par le clofibrate.

Les taux sériques des triglycérides n'a pas été modifié de façon significative par aucun des deux médicaments. Ces deux traitements ont été bien tolérés.

Le probucol peut être utilement employé dans le traitement des patients répondant peu au clofibrate et à ses dérivés. L'absence de pouvoir lithogène et de toute interaction avec les médicaments communément utilisés chez ces patients peut faire du probucol un médicament susceptible d'apporter un réel gain dans le traitement des hypercholestérolémies.

EXPERIENCE CLINIQUE SUR LE PROBUCOL: EFFET HYPOCHOLESTEROLEMIANT ET TOLERANCE

R. E. Tedeschi, H. L. Taylor, and B. L. Martz

L'effet à long terme du probucol a été évalué aux Etats-Unis sur un total de 1133 patients traités au cours d'une série d'études cliniques particulièrement contrôlées.

Sur ce total, 881 sujets ont été traités selon un protocole d'expérimentation identique et au mois de mai 1979, 291 de ces patients avaient été suivis pendant 5 ans et 139 pendant 8 ans; 68% des patients traités par le probucol pendant 8 ans à raison d'un gramme par jour présentaient une réduction supérieure ou égale à 15% de la cholestérolémie par rapport aux valeurs de base.

Quatre-vingt deux pourcent des patients traités par le probucol ont accusé une diminution de la cholestérolémie supérieure ou égale à 10% par rapport aux témoins. La réduction moyenne de la cholestérolémie dans ce groupe a atteint 19,9%. Aucun phénomène d'échappement n'a été observé chez ces malades.

L'effet secondaire le plus fréquent ont été de selles molles. On a constaté également des flatulences, des gastralgies, des nausées, des vomissements, des douleurs abdominales.

Les tests de laboratoire, qui comprenaient la numération sanguine et les tests fonctionnels hépatiques et rénaux, n'ont mis en évidence aucun signe de toxicité. L'analyse de la morbidité et de la mortalité a été effectuée pour les 1133 patients traités par le probucol, en appliquant la méthode des tables de mortalité. Chez 98% de ces patients, le taux de la cholestérolémie était supérieur ou égal à 250 mg% et plusieurs d'entre eux présentaient d'autres facteurs de risque des affections coronariennes.

L'incidence de la mortalité cumulative à la 5ème année (toutes causes confondues) s'est chiffrée à 6,5%. L'incidence cumulative à la 5ème année des cas non mortels d'infarctus du myocarde chez les patients ayant une histoire clinique d'infarctus myocardique (267 au total) et traités par le probucol, a été de 7,3%. Les différences constatées dans les critères d'admission et dans la dimension du groupe étudié, ainsi que d'autres variables, ont empêché toute comparaison statistique directe de la mortalité et de la morbidité entre cette étude sur le probucol et d'autres études. Si l'on se réfère toutefois, aux données publiées par le "Coronary Drug Project," les chiffres relativement peu élevés de morbidité en faveur d'un effet protecteur de ce médicament, même sans en donner la preuve proprement dite.

Compte tenu de l'intérêt reconnu de connaître l'effet potentiel des médicaments hypolipidémiants sur le tractus biliaire, nous avons analysé la survenue des cholécystectomies et des affections des voies biliaires chez les patients traités à long terme par le probucol. L'incidence cumulative à la 6ème année des affections des voies biliaires (cholécystectomie, lithiase biliaire, cholécystite) a été de 3,3% pour le sexe masculin (729 cas) et de 5,8% pour le sexe féminin (404 cas): d'où une incidence globale de 4,1%. L'incidence cumulative des cholécystectomies à la 6ème année a été de 2,2% pour le sexe masculin (729 cas) et de 2,7% pour le sexe féminin (404 cas), soit une incidence quel que soit le sexe de 2,3%. Les différences de caractéristiques des populations, l'évolution clinique fréquemment asymptomatique des lithiases biliaires et d'autres variables encore, n'ont pas permis d'effectuer de comparaison statistique avec les données provenant d'autres études. Néanmoins, les pourcentages cités plus haut ne semblent pas excessifs.

LE PROBUCOL DANS LE TRAITEMENT A COURT ET A LONG TERME DE L'HYPERLIPOPROTEINEMIE DU TYPE II

V. Beaumont, J. C. Buxtorf, B. Jacotot, and J. L. Beaumont

L'action du probucol a été évaluée dans une étude à court terme versus placebo chez 19 patients atteints d'hyperlipoprotéinémie du type II.

Chaque patient a été traité pendant un mois par le placebo et pendant 1 autre mois par le probucol (1 g/jour), l'ordre d'administration étant tiré au sort. Au cours de cette étude, les patients n'ont pas été soumis à un régime diététique particulier.

Il a été procédé à la comparaison des valeurs du cholestérol total, des phospholipides et des triglycérides, à la fin de chaque période de traitement. L'évaluation statistique a été effectuée à l'aide du test t de Student, cas des séries appariées. Le probucol a provoqué une diminution des taux sériques du cholestérol total de 9%

(p < 0,001) mais n'a pas modifié de façon statistiquement significative ni la phospholipidémie ni la triglycéridémie.

La persistance des effets du probucol sur les lipides sériques, son action sur les lipides tissulaires et sa tolérance clinique et biologique ont fait l'objet d'une étude en ouvert, effectuée chez 20 patients souffrant d'hyperlipoprotéinémie du type II. Au cours de cette étude, comme précédemment, les patients ont poursuivi leur régime alimentaire habituel.

Les lipides sériques ont été déterminés avant le début de l'étude et tous les deux mois, pendant une durée totale de 6 mois.

Avant et à la fin des 6 mois de traitement, des fragments de tissu cutané ont été prélevés afin de déterminer le cholestérol libre et estérifié. Les résultats obtenus ont été comparés aux valeurs correspondantes d'un groupe de sujets sains. A la fin de l'étude, on a constaté une diminution moyenne du taux sérique du cholestérol de 9,9% (p < 0,001) semblable à celle qui avait été observée après un mois de traitement lors de la première étude. La baisse du taux de la cholestérolémie a été supérieure à 10% chez 60% des patients. De même, les phospholipides et les triglycérides sériques n'ont pas varié de manière statistiquement significative. Le cholestérol estérifié dans les fragments de tissu cutané a augmenté de façon significative sous traitement. Les examens de laboratoires n'ont pas révélé de variation notable et l'augmentation observée du taux des SGPT et SGOT est resté dans les valeurs limites de la normale. Dans l'ensemble, la tolérance clinique du probucol a été satisfaisante.

Les auteurs concluent que le probucol est un médicament bien toléré, qui conserve son effet hypocholestérolémiant au cours des traitements prolongés.

L'augmentation significative du cholestérol estérifié cutané en l'absence d'une variation significative du cholestérol total nécessite des recherches ultérieures. A titre d'hypothèse de travail, on pourrait penser que ces variations qualitatives peuvent faciliter la mobilisation du cholestérol et être corrélées avec la régression constatée des xanthélasmas.

TRAITEMENT DES HYPERCHOLESTEROLEMIES PAR LE PROBUCOL

R. Carmena and J. F. Ascaso

L'effet hypolipidémiant d'un nouveau médicament, le probucol, a été étudié chez 20 patients atteints d'hyperlipoprotéinémie essentielle (phénotype IIa dans 7 cas et IIb dans 13 cas).

Tous ces malades ont été soumis à un régime à faible teneur en cholestérol et en acides gras saturés et à teneur élevée en acides gras poly-insaturés. Après un mois de régime alimentaire, sans médicament, les patients ont été répartis "par randomisation" en deux groupes: 10 patients ont d'abord reçu le probucol (500 mg deux fois par jour) pendant deux mois, puis lors de la deuxième phase, le placebo pendant deux autres mois; les 10 autres patients ont reçu les deux traitements dans l'ordre inverse. Les phases I et II ont été séparées par une période de 1 mois au cours de laquelle les patients n'ont été soumis qu'au régime alimentaire seul.

Le régime diététique a entraîné à lui seul une variation moyenne de la cholestérolémie de 403,7 mg/dl à 375,1 mg/dl (réduction de 7% non significative). L'addition de probucol a accru de manière manifeste l'effet hypocholestérolémiant du régime alimentaire (− 32%, p < 0,01). La triglycéridémie n'a pas été modifiée par le médicament.

La tolérance du probucol a été excellente.

EFFET DU PROBUCOL DANS
L'HYPERCHOLESTEROLEMIE ESSENTIELLE

A. Gouveia, A. Noronha, I. Dionisio, S. Felix,
B. Barros, and M. Carrageta

Cette étude, en ouvert, chez des patients atteints d'hypercholestérolémie essentielle, a eu pour but d'évaluer l'action hypocholestérolémiante du probucol et d'étudier la nature et l'incidence des effets adverses.

Les patients ont été encouragés à suivre un régime alimentaire standard pendant un mois et se sont soumis à une série d'examens cliniques et de recherches de laboratoire. Les patients rentrant dans l'étude avaient une cholestérolémie moyenne, effectuée sur 3 dosages, supérieure ou égale à 250 mg/100 ml (méthode enzymatique), et les valeurs individuelles ne différaient pas de plus de 32 mg/100 ml entre les 3 dosages. De plus, les variations du poids corporel ne dépassaient pas 5%.

Parmi les 34 patients satisfaisant aux critères d'admission, 2 ont interrompu le traitement au cours de la première semaine par suite de troubles intestinaux. L'étude a donc été effectuée sur 15 hommes et 17 femmes d'âge moyen de 47 ans (de 25 à 65 ans) et de 53 ans (de 42 à 62 ans) respectivement. Ces 32 patients ont reçu pendant 2 mois, du probucol à raison de 1 g/jour (2 comprimés de 250 mg au petit déjeuner, 2 autres au repas du soir, tout en poursuivant leur régime alimentaire standard.

Les résultats de cette étude confirment l'efficacité du probucol.

Les taux sériques du cholestérol, déjà réduits de façon significative à la fin du premier mois de traitement (p < 0,001), ont encore diminué au cours du second mois. Les taux sériques de triglycérides n'ont pas été modifiés de manière significative.

Aucune observation particulière n'a été signalée ni au cours des examens cliniques, ni en ce qui concerne les résultats des examens de laboratoire.

Le probucol a été bien toléré. On n'a relevé aucun effet secondaire, exceptés chez les deux patients déjà mentionnés.

ESSAI CLINIQUE D'UN NOUVEL
HYPOCHOLESTEROLEMIANT: LE PROBUCOL

A. Castro Ribeiro and A. Pereira Viana

Un essai en double-aveugle a été conduit chez 26 patients atteints d'hypercholestérolémie essentielle; les malades recevant selon la loi du hazard soit le probucol (500 mg deux fois par jour) soit le placebo.

Avant le début de l'étude, tous les malades ont été soumis pendant un mois à un régime alimentaire standard et traités simultanément par du placebo. Au cours de cette période, il a été procédé à trois déterminations, chacune à une semaine d'intervalle, de la cholestérolémie (méthode enzymatique) et la moyenne des données obtenues a été prise comme valeur de base. Après 3 mois de traitement par le probucol, le taux moyen de cholestérol sérique avait baissé de 297 à 247 mg/100 ml. L'analyse de la covariance a mis en évidence une différence significative (p < 0,05) entre ces patients et les sujets traités par le placebo.

On a constaté, en outre, un retour à la normale des taux sériques du cholestérol (< 250 mg/100 ml) chez 7 patients traités par le probucol et chez 1 patient sous placebo (test de Fisher p < 0,008). Les variations du taux des triglycérides n'ont pas été significatives d'un groupe à l'autre. Le poids corporel est demeuré pratiquement constant.

Aucun patient n'a dû interrompre le traitement par suite de quelque effet adverse. Cinq patients traités par le probucol et trois patients traités par le placebo ont accusé des troubles gastro-intestinaux d'importance modérée.

Les résultats obtenus chez ces malades du nord du Portugal confirment que le probucol est un hypocholestérolémiant efficace et bien toléré.

EFFET DU PROBUCOL SUR LA COMPOSITION BILIAIRE CHEZ L'HOMME. OBSERVATIONS PRELIMINAIRES

Z. Mareček, M. Jirsa, V. Kordač, and L. Kučerová

L'action du probucol sur les acides biliaires et sur les lipides de la bile a été étudiée chez 5 patients atteints d'hyperlipoprotéinémie du type IIa, présentant avant traitement des taux sériques de cholestérol entre 310 et 440 mg/dl. Ces sujets n'avaient jamais été traités précédemment par le probucol et n'avaient pas pris d'autres hypocholestérolémiants depuis au moins un mois. Après cholécystographie orale (en vue d'exclure toute présence de calculs biliaires et de cholécystopathie) les patients ont été traités pendant deux mois par le probucol à la dose d'un gramme par jour. Les lipides sériques ont été déterminés toutes les deux semaines au cours de l'étude. La bile a été collectée par tubage duodénal, après injection intraveineuse de cholécystoquinine, avant et à la fin du traitement.

Les acides biliaires ont été déterminés par la méthode enzymatique, le cholestérol et les phospholipides par la méthode colorimétrique; le degré de saturation de cholestérol dans la bile a été établi à l'aide de l'indice lithogénique de Thomas et Hoffman.

La composition en acides biliaires a été évaluée par chromatographie en phase gazeuse et les esters méthyl-triméthylsilyl ont été analysés sur colonne 1% Hi EFF 8 BP.

Les résultats obtenus semblent indiquer que les variations de la composition molaire relative des lipides biliaires provoquées par le probucol diffèrent considérablement de celles qui ont été observées après administration de clofibrate.

Le clofibrate provoque une augmentation de la concentration biliaire du cholestérol et une réduction des acides biliaires entraînant une augmentation du pouvoir lithogène de la bile par suite de la sursaturation de la bile en cholestérol.

Après administration de probucol, par contre, on constate une diminution du cholestérol biliaire et une augmentation des acides biliaires d'où une diminution de l'indice lithogénique. Les variations de la composition des acides biliaires après probucol sont d'importance modérée et ne s'avèrent pas constantes.

EFFETS DU PROBUCOL SUR L'ABSORPTION INTESTINAL DU CALCIUM ET SUR LA THERAPIE ANTICOAGULANTE PROLONGEE CHEZ LES PATIENTS SOUFFRANT D'HYPERCHOLESTEROLEMIE ASSOCIEE A DES AFFECTIONS CARDIO-VASCULAIRES

A. Rapado and M. Diaz-Curiel

Vingt patients atteints d'hypercholestérolémie de type IIa ont été traités pendant une période de 14 mois en moyenne par le probucol à des doses variant de 0,5 à 1,5 g/j et soumis à un régime diététique à faible teneur en cholestérol et en acides gras saturés. Ce traitement a déterminé une réduction significative du cholestérol sérique (-31%, $p < 0,01$) sans modifier le taux des triglycérides.

L'effet du probucol sur le métabolisme du calcium/vitamine D a été étudié en mesurant la résorption du Ca^{47} avant et après traitement. L'effet sur l'activité de la vitamine K a été déterminé en contrôlant le taux de prothrombine chez les malades en traitement chronique par les anticoagulants.

Aucune interaction n'a été constatée entre les médicaments utilisés. Il est particulièrement intéressant de signaler l'effet du probucol chez une jeune fille de 12 ans, homozygote, hyperlipoprotéinémique IIa, qui avait présenté au cours du traitement par la cholestyramine des signes biochimiques de rachitisme exigeant un traitement spécifique intensif. Le probucol a réduit de façon significative chez cette patiente le taux sérique du cholestérol, sans modifier aucunement la résorption intestinale du Ca^{47} et sans entraîner de symptômes biochimiques de rachitisme.

PROBUCOL: EVALUATION DE L'EFFET
SUR LES LIPIDES ET LES LIPOPROTEINES

J. Rouffy, R. Bakir, B. Chanu, and J. Goy-Loeper

L'effet du probucol (1 g / jour) sur les lipides et les lipoprotéines sériques a été étudié chez des patients atteints d'hyperlipoproteinémie essentielle IIa et IIb non réductibles per le régime diétique seul. Pour certain de ces malades, des traitements anterieur par la clofibrate, procétofén et cholestiramine s'étaient avéré d'efficacité non satisfaisante. La durée du traitement a été d'un mois chez 34 patients (T_1), de 3 à 6 mois chez 16 patients (T_2), de 6 mois à un an chez 12 patients (T_3) et de plus d'un an chez 4 patients (T_4).

A la fin des différentes périodes considérées, on a mis en évidence, sauf pour T_3, une réduction significative des lipides sériques totaux (de 8 à 19%), du cholestérol total (de 8 à 12%) et du LDL-cholestérol (de 9 à 15%), ainsi qu'une augmentation significative du rapport HDL-CH / LDL-CH + VLDL-CH.

Aucune interaction avec les anticoagulants n'a été observée. Cette étude a montré que le probucol est un médicament efficace pour réduire les lipides sériques totaux, le cholestérol total et le cholestérol des lipoprotéines à faible densité (LDL-CH) qui correspond à la fraction lipoprotéique la plus athèrogène.

Un autre résultat favorable du probucol est l'augmentation du rapport HDL-CH/LDL-CH − VLDL-CH améliorant ainsi l'indice athèrogène. La tolérance du produit a été excellente tant sur le plan clinique que biologique.

LE PROBUCOL DANS LE TRAITEMENT
DE L'HYPERCHOLESTEROLEMIE CHEZ DES PATIENTS
ATTEINTS DE TROUBLES CARDIO-VASCULAIRES

L. Scebat and J. Renais

Le probucol (500 mg 2 fois / jour), associé à un régime diététique à faible teneur en lipides, a été administré pendant une période de 12 à 46 mois, à 33 malades souffrant d'affections athéroscléreuses cardio-vasculaires et d'hypercholestérolémie de types IIa (n = 11), IIb + III (n = 21) et IV (n = 1). Globalement, ce traitement a provoqué une réduction des taux sériques moyens du cholestérol de 329,5 à 281 mg/dl (− 14,5%, p < 0,001). En fait, 12 malades n'ont pas répondu au traitement de manière suffisante (réduction du cholestérol ≤ 10%) et 20 malades (62,5%) ont favorablement réagi à ce traitement par le régime diététique + probucol.

Dans trois cas, on a constaté après le 6ème mois une réduction de l'effet hypocholestérolémiant du médicament.

Les résultats obtenus au cours de la première année se sont maintenus chez 15 malades (46,8%). L'effet du probucol sur le cholestérol sérique a été similaire chez les malades souffrant d'hypercholestérolémie de type IIa et chez ceux qui étaient atteints d'hyperlipémie mixte (types IIb + III).

Il n'a pas été observé d'interaction entre le probucol et les autres médicaments communément prescrits dans les affections cardiovasculaires, notamment avec les anti-vitamines K et les diurétiques.

Aucune variation des tests fonctionnels hépatiques et rénaux de la glycémie et de la formule sanguine n'a été observée. Le poids corporel n'a subi aucune modification particulière au cours de ce traitement de longue durée.

L'électrocardiogramme n'a pas été modifié par le traitement. Trois malades se sont plaint de diarrhée, celle-ci a regressé chez deux d'entre eux sous traitement mais a motivé chez le troisième l'arrêt du probucol après deux semaines de traitement.

EFFET DU PROBUCOL CHEZ DES HYPERCHOLESTEROLEMIQUES RESISTANT A D'AUTRES TRAITEMENTS HYPOLIPIDEMIQUES

S. Stefanović and L. Vučić

L'action du probucol sur l'hypercholestérolémie a été étudiée chez 15 patients, onze souffraient d'hyperlipoprotéinémie de type IIa et quatre d'hyperlipoprotéinémie de type IIb. Le diagnostic de l'affection avait été fait de 1 à 20 ans avant le début de cette étude (en moyenne 7 ans). Tous le patients avaient été précédemment traités, sans succès, d'abord par un régime diététique seul, puis associé au clofibrate et, dans certains cas, à la cholestyramine ou à la phosphatidylcholine.

Les concentrations sériques du cholestérol avant l'administration du probucol, étaient comprises entre 306 et 565 mg / dl ($\overline{X}$ = 385 mg / dl). Tous les patients ont reçu 1 g de probucol par jour pendant trois mois et les contrôles ont eu lieu à la fin de chaque mois. A la fin du traitement tous le patients, sauf un, présentaient des valeurs de la cholestérolémie dans les limites de la normale selon les groupes d'âge, c'est-à-dire entre 214 et 280 mg / dl ($\overline{X}$ = 229 mg / dl). Aucun effet adverse clinique objectif ou subjectif n'a été constaté pendant le traitement par le probucol; de même les résultats des examens de laboratoire n'ont pas relevé d'anomalie.

Deutsche Zusammenfassungen

WIRKUNG VON PROBUCOL UND VON ANDEREN ARZNEIMITTEL AUF DIE STEROLSYNTHESE IM LYMPHOZYTEN BEIM MENSCHEN

A. Anastasi, D. J. Betteridge, and D. J. Galton

Die gegenwärtig angewandten Behandlungsmethoden der Hypercholesterinämie sind unbefriedigend und erfordern deshalb den Einsatz neuer Wirkstoffe.

Menschliche Lymphozyten eignen sich vortrefflich zum Studium der Beeinflussung der Sterolsynthese durch potentiell die Serumcholesterasewerte senkende Präparate.

Sobald isolierte Lymphozyten in Gegenwart von LD-Lipoproteinen inkubiert werden, wird die Sterolsynthese unterbrochen. Nach Entfernung des LDL aus dem Inkubationsträger steigt die von der den Reaktionsablauf bestimmenden HMG-CoA-Reduktase induzierte Steroidsynthese an.

Wir untersuchten die Wirkung von Cycloheximid, eines Translationhemmers der Proteinsynthese, und von Cordycepin (3′-desoxyadenosin) eines Transkriptionhemmers der mRNA-Synthese, auf die Induktion der Sterolsynthese in frisch isoliertem und in lipoproteinarmem (LPDS) Serumnährboden inkubierter menschlicher Lymphozyten.

Wir untersuchten ferner auch andere Substanzen wie Compactin und Probucol, die gleichfalls unmittelbar die Synthesen beeinflussen könnten.

Cycloheximid (20 μg/ml) hemmt die Induktion der von LPDS bestimmten Sterolsynthese, so dass es naheliegend erscheint, dass der Anstieg durch eine *ex novo* ablaufende Enzymsynthese bedingt ist.

Cordycepin (50 μg/ml) übt keine Wirkung auf die Induktion der von LPDS bestimmten Sterolsynthese aus, wenngleich die mRNA-Synthese um 50% reduziert wird.

Bei mit LDL in Gegenwart von Cordycepin 40 Stunden lang vorinkubierten Lymphozyten (in dieser Zeitspanne dürfte der durch kurze Halbwertzeit gekennzeichnete mRNA-Pool stark reduziert worden sein) lag der nach Entzug des LDL aus dem Inkubationsmilieu feststellbare Anstieg der Sterolsynthese in der gleichen Grössenordnung wie bei ohne Cordycepinzugabe vorinkubierten Zellen. Daraus könnte geschlossen werden, dass die Halbwertzeit des HMG-CoA-Reduktase-mRNA relativ lang ist und sohin zur Induktion der Sterolsynthese kein mRNA mehr erforderlich ist.

Compactin (0,2 μg) hemmt die Steroidensynthese zu 65% ohne Modifizierung der

Einlagerung von ^{14}C-Mevalonat in die Steroiden, so dass anzunehmen ist, dass die Substanz die HMG-CoA-Reduktaseaktivität in spezifischer Weise hemmt.

Emulsionen von Probucol mit Rinderserumeiweiss in Konzentration bis 1 mM (die Substanz ist nur geringfügig löslich) hemmten zu rund 40% die Sterolsynthese aus ^{14}C-acetat.

Dieser Umstand könnte möglicherweise die hypocholesterolämische Wirkung der Substanz fördern.

ZUR PHARMAKOLOGIE VON PROBUCOL

D. Kritchevsky

Probucol, 4,4'(isopropyliden-dithio)bis(2,6-di-t-butylphenol), bewirkt bei verschiedenen Tiergattungen (Mäuse, Ratten, Hunde, Affen) sowie beim Menschen ausgeprägte Senkung des Blutcholesterinspiegels.

Bei der Maus steht die Senkung des Blutcholesterinspiegels in direktem Verhältnis zur applizierten Dosis.

Tierversuche zur Klärung des Wirkungsmechanismus scheinen für verstärkte Fäkalausscheidung der Gallensäuren sowie für Hemmung der Cholesterinsynthese und verringerte Absorption zu sprechen. Bei hypercholesterinämischen Affen liegt nach Behandlung mit Probucol der Serumcholesterolspiegel 52% unter den Werten der Kontrolltiere. Probucol bewirkt ferner signifikante Senkung des Leber-cholesterols und gleichfalls signifikante Erhöhung des Milzcholesterols, wogegen die Cholesterolgehalte weiterer 17 untersuchter Gewebe unbeeinflusst blieben. Die Behandlung mit Probucol scheint demnach keine merkliche Cholesterinverlagerung im Organismus auszulösen. Nach Miettinen (*Atherosclerosis,* 15, 163, 1972) manifestiert sich die Wirkung von Probucol durch Hemmung der Cholesterol-synthese und absorption sowie verstärkte Gallensäurenausscheidung.

Im Verlauf der Behandlung hypercholesterolämischer Affen mit Probucol kommt es zu verstärkter Exkretion der Gallensäuren, nicht aber Ausscheidung neutraler Steroide.

Beim Hund löst Probucol Herzkammerflattern aus. Bei den übrigen untersuchten Tiergattungen wurden keine Nebenwirkungen beobachtet. Nach Verabreichung von markiertem Probucol ^{14}C werden 84% der Radioaktivität mit den Fäces und 1–2% im Harn im Verlauf von 4 Tagen ausgeschieden. Die Halbwertzeit das mit ^{14}C markierten Probucol betrug 0,8 und 12,8 Tage beim Affen und 1 und 15,2 Tage beim Hund.

Die Darreichung von Probucol beeinflusst nicht die Aktivität bestimmter Leberenzyme wie Catalase, LDH (Milchsäuredehydrogenase), Glutaminsäure-dehydrogenase und verändert auch den Leberglykogenspiegel nicht.

Bei hypercholesterolämischen Affen bewirkt Probucol Senkung des Choles-terolspiegels der Aorta um 25%. Bei mit atherogener Diät ernährten Kanin-chen kommt es nach Verabreichung von Probucol in Konzentration von 1% zu signifikanter Atherosklerosehemmung.

ERGEBNISSE DER TOXIKOPATHOLOGISCHEN UNTERSUCHUNGEN MIT PROBUCOL UND VERGLEICH DER LEBERMORPHOLOGIE AN MIT PROBUCOL, PROCETOPHEN UND CLOFIBRAT BEHANDELTEN RATTEN

J. Molello, S. Barnard, and J. LeBeau

40 Affen beiderlei Geschlechts wurden mit Probucol per os (0, 60, 125, 250 und

500 mg/kg/die) behandelt. 14 Affen wurden nach 18 bzw. 24 Monaten Behandlungsdauer getötet. Bei 21 Tieren erstreckten sich die Beobachtungen auf einen Zeitraum von 8 Jahren. Als Vergleichsgrössen dienten Wachstumsrhythmus, hämatologische und hämatochemische Werte, Harnproben, Organgewicht sowie mikroskopischer, histologischer und elektromikroskopischer Gewebebefund. 5 Affen starben während der Beobachtungszeit, wobei der Tod nicht auf das varabreichte Präparat zurückzuführen war. Zwischen behandelten Versuchstieren und unbehandelten Kontrolltieren waren keine signifikanten Unterschiede feststellbar.

Die Wirkung von Probucol auf die Ultrastruktur der Leberzelle wurde an Sprague-Dawley-Ratten versus Clofibrat und Procetophen untersucht. Die Drogen wurden im Mengen von je ≈ 500, ≈ 250 und ≈ 100 mg/kg/die betreffends Probucol, Clofibrat und Procetophen, im Futter vermischt, bis zu 91 Tagen verabreicht. Die Kontrolltiere wurden lediglich mit Diätkost ernährt.

Alle drei Substanzen bewirkten signifikante Senkung des Serumcholesterinspiegels.

Die Lebermorphologie der mit Probucol behandelten Ratten unterschied sich nicht vom Befund bei unbehandelten Tieren. Clofibrat und Procetophen lösten Hepatozytomegalie, Anstieg der Peroxisomenzahl und leichte Veränderungen an Endoplasma retikulum und Mitochondrien aus.

Die Ergebnisse der hier und anderswo beschriebenen Untersuchungen geben an, dass Probucol bei den entweder unter normalen Bedingungen kurz-und langfristig behandelten oder einem schweren Kreislaufstress unterzogenen Mäusen, Ratten, Kaninchen, Affen und Meerschweinchen gut verträgt wird.

Dementgegen betragen sich die Hunde als Ausnahme, in dem sie eine Herzmuskelüberempfindlichkeit gegenüber Epinephrine und Nor-epinephrine entwickeln.

Probucol unterscheidet sich von den anderen lipidsenkenden Arzneimitteln, in dem es die Leberzellmorphologie in Nagetieren und submenschlichen Primaten nicht ändert.

Die Angaben dieser toxikologischen Untersuchungen geben an, dass Probucol ein sicheres Arzneimittel ist.

DIE BLUTCHOLESTEROLSENKENDE WIRKUNG VON PROBUCOL UND DESSEN WIRKUNGSMECHANISMUS BEI MAUS UND KANINCHEN

R. Infante and D. Petit

Die Wirkung von Probucol auf Blut- und Gewebefette wurde an der Maus und am Kaninchen unter verschiedenen Ernährungsmodalitäten (Standarddiät, fettlose Kost, fett- und cholesterolarme Kost, hypercholesterolämische Kost) untersucht.

Bei mit Standarddiät ernährten Tieren verminderte Probucol in auffälligem Mass den Serumcholesterolspiegel sowohl der Maus (− 33% und − 60% im Vergleich zu Kontrollgruppen nach 7 bzw. 21 Tagen Behandlung mit 0,6 g Probucol je kg Futter) als auch des Kaninchens (− 37% und − 41% im Vergleich zu Kontrollgruppen nach zehntägiger Behandlung mit 1 g bzw. 2,5 g Probucol je kg Futter) ohne die Leberlipide zu beeinflussen.

Bei Tieren, deren Kost einen Fettgehalt von 0%, 1%, 3% oder 10% aufwies, erbrachte Probucol bei der ersten zwei Versuchbedingungen keine Wirkung, wogegen die cholesterolsenkende Wirkung bei Verabreichung des Präparates mit der 3% fetthaltigen Diät augenfällig in Erscheinung trat und bei mit fettreichem Kost

(10% Fette, 1% Cholesterol), behandelten Tiere vorbengte Probucol die Hyperlipidämieentwicklung.

Bei Mäusen wurde nach einmaliger endovenöser Gabe von Probucol rascher, markanter und lang anhaltender Rückgang der Blutcholesterolwerte festgestellt. Beim Kaninchen hemmte die Substanz die durch endovenöse Verabreichung von Phospholipiden ausgelöste Hyperlipidämie.

Bei Mäusen mit Standarddiät bewirkte die 7 und 21 Tage dauernde Behandlung mit Probucol (0,6 g je kg Futter) keine signifikante Veränderung der Anlagerung von ^{14}C-Mevalonat im Cholesterolanteil der Leber, des Darmtrakts und des Skeletts. Es wurde verringerte Radioaktivitätsanreicherung im Plasmacholesterol beobachtet. Daraus dürfte auf eine spezifische Wirkung der Substanz auf die Eiweissfette zu schliessen sein.

Vorläufige Ergebnisse bei Mäusen, die 4 Wochen mit Probucol (0,6 g/kg Futter) behandelt wurden, bestätigten den retardierten Ablauf der VLDL-Synthese.

LANGZEITBEHANDLUNG DER HYPERCHOLESTEROLÄMIE MIT PROBUCOL

D. McCaughan

Probucol wurde im kontrollierten Doppelblindversuch versus Placebo ein Jahr lang an 118 Patienten mit essentieller Hypercholesterolämie (Serum-cholesterolspiegel vor Behandlungsbeginn ≥ 250 mg/dl) erprobt. Nach 6 und 12 Monaten Behandlung mit Probucol (n = 83) lag die durchschnittliche Serum-cholesterolsenkung im Vergleich zu den Ausgangswerten zwischen 16,2% und 20,9%. Bei den mit Placebo behandelten Patienten (n = 30) lagen die Senkungsraten zwischen 5,2% und 12,7% (p < 0,001).

Bei 61 der bereits in der Doppelblindstudie behandelten Patienten wurde die Probucoldarreichung anschliessend offen bis zu 9 Jahren weitergeführt.

Nach dem zweiten Jahr der Probucolbehandlung lag die Serum-cholesterolsenkung zwischen 23,1% und 27,4% und behielt diesen Wert weiter bei.

Die Gesamtsterblichkeitsrate betrug nach Ablauf von 5 Behandlungsjahren 9%. In dieser Zeitspanne belief sich die Frequenz der Todesfälle infolge Koronarinsuffizienz und nicht tödlich verlaufenen Myokardinfarkts auf 14%.

Das Präparat wurde gut vertragen. Zu den häufigsten Nebenerscheinungen zählten loser Stuhl oder Diarrhoe.

Die Ergebnisse beweisen, dass Probucol ein wirksames, gut verträgliches Präparat zur Langzeitbehandlung der essentiellen Hypercholesterolämie ist.

DIE WIRKUNG VON PROBUCOL UND DIÄT AUF SERUMLIPIDE UND LIPOPROTEINFRAKTIONEN BEI ESSENTIELLER HYPERCHOLESTEROLÄMIE

R. Mordasini, M. Keller, and W. F. Riesen

Die Wirkung von Probucol auf verschiedene Lipidfraktionen wurde bei 27 Patienten mit essentieller Hypercholesterolämie untersucht. Die Patienten wurden mindestens 3 Monate auf isokalorimetrische Diät mit niedrigem Lipidgehalt und modifiziertem Verhältnis zwischen gesättigten und ungesättigten Fettsäuren (NIH-Diät Type II) eingestellt. Auf diese erste Phase folgte eine Vorbehandlung über 6 Wochen, bei welcher zusammen mit der Diät auch Placebo gegeben wurde. Bei der anschliessenden Doppelblindstudie erhielten die Patienten Diät und Placebo (1 Tablette viermal täglich) oder Diät und Probucol (1 Tablette zu 250 mg viermal täglich). Die Probucol- und Placebotabletten hatten vollkommen identisches Aussehen.

Die ambulatorischen Patienten wurden monatlichen Kontrollen unterzogen.

Es wurden folgende Parameter bestimmt: Gesamtserumcholesterol und triglyceride; nach Ultrazentrifugation Cholesterol und Triglyceride der LD-Lipoproteine (LDL) und HD-Lipoproteine (HDL), Apo B und AI (mittels RID) sowie Apo AII (mittels RIA).

Im Vergleich zu den mit Placebo ermittelten Werten erwies sich unter Behandlung mit Probucol die Gesamtcholesterolkonzentration im Durchschnitt um 41 mg/100 ml (13%, p < 0,05) verringert. LDL-Cholesterol wurde parallel zum Gesamt-cholesterol gleichfalls im Durchschnitt um 42 mg/100 ml (− 16%, p < 0,025) merklich gesenkt. Eine leichte, statistisch nicht signifikante Senkung war bei HDL-Cholesterol zu verzeichnen.

Placebo löste keine signifikanten Veränderungen des Gesamtcholesterols, LDL-Cholesterols und HDL-Cholesterols aus. Die Triglyceridwerte blieben sowohl unter Probucol als auch unter Placebo nahezu unverändert.

Unter Behandlung mit Probucol nahm die Konzentration der Apo B im Mittel um 12% ab. Der Unterschied ist jedoch statistisch nicht signifikant (p < 0,15). Die Apo B-Spiegel blieben unter Placebo konstant. Bei den mit Probucol behandelten Patien-ten war eine durchschnittliche Senkung von 16% bei Apo AI (p < 0,0005) bzw. 55% bei Apo AII (p < 0,0005) feststellbar. Verringerte Konzentration von Apo I und Apo II wurde auch bei der mit Placebo behandelten Gruppe beobachtet.

Die Senkung war jedenfalls nur bei Apo II statistisch signifikant (− 26%, p < 0,005).

Probucol wurde allgemein gut vertragen. Bei 4 Patienten musste die Behandlung wegen meist subjektiver Nebenwirkungen vorzeitig abgebrochen werden. 3 dieser Patienten standen unter Placebo, einer unter Probucol.

HDL-SPIEGEL WÄHRENN EINER FÜNFJÄHRIGEN MULTIFACTORIELLEN INTERVENTION GEGEN RISIKOFAKTOREN KORONARER HERZKRANKHEITEN

T. A. Miettinen, J. K. Huttunen, T. Kumlin,
V. Naukkarinen, S. Mattila, and C. Enholm

Serumcholesterol (C), Triglyceride (TG), HD-Lipoproteincholesterol (HDLC), die HD-Apoproteine AI und AII der HD-Lipoproteine (HD-AI, HDL-AII) und die Apoproteine der nicht-HD-Lipoproteine (AII nicht-HDL) wurden bei 119 männlichen Probanden bestimmt, die sich bis zu 4 Jahre lang Versuchskontrollen unterzogen, die sich die Einschränkung de Risikofaktoren bei Koronarkrankheiten zum Ziel setzten. Die Behandlung umfasste Diätvorschriften, hygienische Massnahmen und - sofern erforderlich - Verabreichung blutdruck- und blutfettsenkender Präparate. Cholesterol- und Gesamttriglyceridspiegel wurden im Verlauf der Untersuchung in regelmässigen Abständen bestimmt, wogegen HDLC, HDL AI, HDL AII und AII nicht-HDL erst im 4. Jahr der Studie bestimmt wurden. Für die letzteren Werte lagen keine Vergleichsgrössen vor, da die Langzeitaufbewahrung bis zu 4 Jahren starken Verfall der Serumkonzentration nach sich zieht.

Die Gesamtserumfette waren bei nur auf Diät eingestellten Probanden (n = 32) und bei mit Antihypertonika behandelten Probanden (n = 19) ähnlich. Im Vergleich zu den vorgenannten Gruppen wiesen die mit Clofibrat behandelten Probanden (n = 30) vergleichbare AI-Spiegel, jedoch um 34% erhöhte AII-Werte und um 13% erhöhte HDLC-Werte auf. Nach Behandlung mit Probucol (Fälle mit Hyperlipo-proteinämie Type IIa; n = 25) waren verringerter Gesamtcholesterolspiegel (− 13%) sowie verringerte HDLC-Werte (− 29%) und HDL AI (− 16%) zu beobachten, doch traten keine Veränderungen bei HDL AII auf, deren Werte jenen der nur auf Diät gestellten oder mit Antihypertonika behandelten Probanden glichen. Nicht-HDL AI war gleichfalls gering. Die gleichzeitig mit Clofibrat und Probucol behandelten Probanden (grösstenteils Type IIb; n = 13) wiesen keine wesentlichen Serumfettspiegelveränderungen auf, doch stellte sich eine Verminderung von HDLC um 55% und von AI um 41% bei stets geringem nicht-HDL-AI ein, während die AII-Werte jenen der Diätgruppe glichen. Die Ergebnisse legen den Schluss nahe, dass - wenngleich Probucol und Clofibrat bei Langzeitbehandlung die HDLC-Werte senken - auch das Verhältnis Cholesterol/HDL-Apolipoprotein, also der mittlere Sättingungsstand des Cholesterols in der HDL-Fraktion, vermindert wird.

Die von Clofibrat ausgelösten Veränderungen gingen zum Teil mit modifizierten Triglyceridkonzentrationen einher, wogegen die in der Gruppe der mit Probucol behandelten Probanden zu beobachtenden Veränderungen mit der Behandlungsdauer korreliert waren.

PRÜFUNG DER WIRKSAMKEIT UND VERTRÄGLICHKEIT VON PROBUCOL UND VERGLEICH MIT CLOFIBRAT

J. L. De Gennes and J. Truffert

Probucol und Clofibrat wurden im Hinblick auf ihre hypocholesterolämische Wirkung in einer Doppelblindstudie an 38 Patienten mit essentieller Hypercholesterolämie verglichen.

Neunzehn Patienten wurden jeweils 2 Monate lang mit Probucol (1 g/die) und weitere 19 mit Clofibrat (2 g/die) behandelt.

Alle Patienten waren auf Spezialdiät mit geringem Gehalt an Cholesterol und gesättigten Fettsäuren sowie hohem Anteil an mehrfach ungesättigten Fettsäuren eingestellt, die 2 Monate vor Beginn der Vergleichsstudie einsetzte. Während der Vorbereitungszeit erhielten die Patienten Placebo.

Die Verabreichung von Probucol zusätzlich zur Diät bewirkte Senkung des Serumcholesterolspiegels um 13% (p < 0,05 im Vergleich zu den am Ende der Behandlung mit Diät + Placebo ermittelten Werten). Clofibrat bewirkte eine durchschnittliche Serumcholesterolsenkung von 11%. Dieser Wert liegt nicht im Bereich statistischer Signifikanz.

Die Cholesterolsenkung lag bei 31% der mit Probucol und bei 21% der mit Clofibrat behandelten Patienten über 20%.

Die Triglyceridwerte wurden von keinem der beiden Präparate signifikant verändert.

Beide Präparate wurden gut vertragen.

Probucol kann zur Behandlung von Patienten angezeigt sein, die auf Clofibrat und dessen Derivate nicht ansprechen.

Da Probucol nicht gallensteinbildend ist und auch keine Interaktion mit anderen Präparaten aufweist, die üblicherweise den vorgenannten Patienten verschrieben werden, könnte dieser Präparat einen ausschlaggebenden, zusätzlichen Beitrag zur Behandlung der Hypercholesterolämie leisten.

KLINISCHE PRÜFUNG DER UNBEDENKLICHKEIT UND DER CHOLESTEROLSENKENDEN WIRKUNG VON PROBUCOL

R. E. Tedeschi, H. L. Taylor, and B. L. Martz

Die Langzeitwirkung von Probucol wurde in den USA im Zuge klinischer Monitor-Studien an 1133 Patienten untersucht.

881 Patienten wurden nach einem allgemeinen Protokoll behandelt. Bis Mai 1979 wurden 291 dieser Patienten 5 Jahre, und weitere 139 acht Jahre lang beobachtet. 68% der mit Probucol (acht Jahre lang 1 g/die) behandelten Patienten liessen im

Vergleich zum Kontrollwert eine Verringerung von ≥ 15% des Serumcholesterolspiegels erkennen.

82% der mit Probucol behandelten Patienten wiesen im Vergleich zur Kontrollgruppe um ≥ 10% verringerte Cholesterolämie auf. Die durchschnittliche Cholesterolsenkung betrug in dieser Gruppe 19,9%. Resistenzerscheinungen wurden nicht beobachtet.

Als häufigste Begleiterscheinung trat loser Stuhl auf. Ferner traten Flatulenz, Gastralgie, Nausea, Erbrechen und Leibschmerzen auf.

Die Laborbefunde (Blutbild, Leber- und Nierenfunktion) liessen keine toxischen Anzeichen erkennen.

Aufgrund der Sterblichkeitstabellen wurde bei sämtlichen 1133 Patienten eine Morbiditäts- und Mortalitätsanalyse durchgeführt. 98% der Patienten wiesen Serumcholesterolspiegel ≥ 250 mg% auf, und zahlreiche Personen liessen zudem weitere Risikofaktoren von Koronarerkrankungen erkennen.

Die sämtliche Ursachen umfassende Gesamtsterblichkeit im fünften Jahr betrug 6,5%. Die Gesamtrate der nicht lätal verlaufenen Myokardinfarkte von Patienten mit Herzmuskelinfarktanamnese (n = 267) betrug im 5. Jahr 7,3% der mit Probucol behandelten Fälle. Verschiedene Zulassungskriterien und schwankende Gruppenzahlen sowie sonstige veränderliche Grössen erlaubten keinen statistischen Vergleich mit anderen Studien. Mit Bezug auf die im "Coronary Drug Project" veröffentlichten Angaben lässt die im Verlauf der Behandlung mit Probucol beobachtete, relativ geringe Morbiditäts- und Sterblichkeitsquote auf eine vermutliche vorbeugende Wirkung der Substanz schliessen, wenngleich diese Wirkung nicht nachgewiesen ist.

Im Hinblick auf die sich aufdrängende Befürchtung allfälliger Schädigung der Gallenwege seitens blutfettsenkender Substanzen, untersuchten wir die Häufigkeit der Cholezystektomien und aufgetretener Gallenwegeerkrankungen bei Patienten unter Dauertherapie mit Probucol. In sechs Jahren traten Erkrankungen der Gallenwege (Cholezystektomie, Cholelithiasis, Cholezystitis) bei 3,3% der Männer (n = 729) und 5,8% der Frauen (n = 404) auf. Die Gesamtquote beträgt 4,1%. Operative Entfernung der Gallenblase war gesamthaft im 6. Jahr bei 2,2% der Männer (n = 729) und 2,7% der Frauen (n = 404) erforderlich. Kombinationsquote 2,3%. Verschiedenartige individuelle Merkmale, der oft asymptomatische Verlauf und andere veränderliche Grössen liessen keinen unmittelbaren statistischen Vergleich mit den Angaben anderer Quellen zu. Die obenstehend angegebenen Prozentsätze sind jedenfalls bestimmt nicht zu hoch angesetzt.

PROBUCOL IN DER KURZ- UND LANGZEITBEHANDLUNG DER HYPERLIPOPROTEINÄMIE TYPE II

V. Beaumont, J. C. Buxtorf, B. Jacotot, and J. L. Beaumont

Die Wirkung von Probucol wurde im Vergleich zu Placebo in einer Kurzzeitstudie an 19 Patienten mit Hyperlipoproteinämie Type IIa erprobt.

Jeder Patient wurde im Verlauf eines Monats randomisiert mit Placebo und Probucol (1 g/die) behandelt. Die Patienten behielten dabei ihre gewohnte Diät bei.

Bei Abschluss der jeweiligen Behandlungsperioden wurden Gesamtcholesterol, Phospholipide und Triglyceride bestimmt. Die statistische Auswertung erfolgte mittels gekoppeltem t-Test nach Student.

Probucol bewirkte Senkung des Gesamtserumcholesterols um 9% (p < 0,001), während weder die Phospholipidämie noch die Triglyceridwerte statistisch signifikant verändert wurden. Die persistierende Wirkung von Probucol auf Serumlipide und Gewebelipide sowie die klinische und biologische Verträglichkeit wurden durch eine offene Studie an 20 Patienten mit Hyperlipoproteinämie Type II untersucht.

Auch in diesen Fällen hielten die Patienten ihre gewohnte Diät weiter ein.

Die Serumlipide wurden vor Beginn der Kontrolle sowie in Abständen von jeweils 2 Monaten während der gesamten Verabreichungsdauer von 6 Monaten bestimmt.

Zu Beginn und am Ende der 6 Monate wurden Hautteilchen zur Bestimmung des freien und veresterten Cholesterols entnommen. Die Resultate wurden mit den Ergebnissen einer Gruppe gesunder Probanden verglichen.

Abschliessend wurde im Schnitt eine Serumcholesterolsenkung von 9,9% (p < 0,001) beobachtet, was auf der gleichen Linie mit dem Befund nach einmonatiger Behandlung lag. Bei 60% der Patienten betrug die Cholesterolspiegelsenkung > 10%. Auch in diesem Fall bewirkte das Präparat keine signifikante Veränderung der Phospholipide und Triglyceride im Serum.

Der veresterte Cholesterolanteil der Haut wurde durch die Behandlung signifikant erhöht.

Die Laborbefunde ergaben keine Anomalien. SGOT und SGPT waren erhöht, lagen aber innerhalb der Norm.

Die klinische Verträglichkeit von Probucol war gesamthaft gut.

Die Autoren stellen abschliessend fest, dass Probucol bei Langzeitanwendung die Blutcholesterolwerte dauerhaft senkt und ein sicheres Präparat darstellt.

Der bemerkenswerte Anstieg der veresterten Cholesterolfraktion des Hautgewebes bei fehlender gleichzeitiger Veränderung des Gesamtcholesterolspiegels bedarf noch genauerer Untersuchung.

Als Arbeitshypothese könnte angenommen werden, dass diese qualitativen Veränderungen die Cholesterolmobilisierung fördern und mit der beobachteten Xanthelasmenrückbildung in Zusammenhang stehen könnten.

BEHANDLUNG DER HYPERCHOLESTEROLÄMIE MIT PROBUCOL

R. Carmena and J. F. Ascaso

Die hypolipidämische Wirkung des neuen Präparates Probucol wurde bei 20 Patienten mit essentieller Hyperlipoproteinämie (Phänotyp IIa in 7 Fällen, IIb in 13 Fällen) bestimmt.

Sämtliche Patienten waren auf cholesterol-und gesättigten fettsäuren-arme Diät sowie poly-ungesättigte fettsäuren-reiche Diät eingestellt.

Nach einem Monat ausschliesslicher Diätbehandlung wurden die Patienten zwei randomisierten Therapiemodalitäten unterzogen: 10 Patienten wurden zuerst zwei Monate lang mit Probucol (500 mg b.i.d.) und anschliessend weitere zwei Monate lang mit Placebo behandelt, bei den restlichen 10 Patienten wurde umgekehrt verfahren. Auch der zweiten Phase des cross-over ging ein Monat ausschliessliche Diätbehandlung voraus.

Alleinige Diätbehandlung bewirkte Rückgang der Cholesterinämie von durchschnittlich 403,7 mg/dl auf 375,1 mg/dl, was einer Reduzierung von 7% entspricht und sohin nicht signifikant ist. Die zusätzliche Verabreichung von Probucol verstärkte die hypocholesterinämische Wirkung dieser Diäte auf signifikante Weise (− 32%, p < 0,01). Die Triglyceridwerte wurden von dem Präparat nicht beeinflusst. Probucol wurde ausgezeichnet vertragen.

WIRKUNG VON PROBUCOL BEI ESSENTIELLER HYPERCHOLESTEROLÄMIE

A. Gouveia, A. Noronha, I. Dionisio, S. Felix, B. Barros, and M. Carrageta

Zweck dieser offenen Studie mit Patienten mit essentieller Hypercholesterolämie war die Bestimmung der durch Probucol ausgelösten Senkung des Blutcholesterolspiegels sowie die Erfassung von Art und Häufigkeit allfälliger Nebenwirkungen.

Die Patienten wurden zur Einhaltung einer Standarddiät für die Dauer eines Monats aufgefordert und unterzogen sich anschliessend klinischen und Laborkontrollen. Zugelassen wurden Patienten, die im Durchschnitt bei 3 Bestimmungen Serumcholesterolwerte $\geq$ 250 mg/100 ml (enzymatische Methodik) aufwiesen und deren Einzelwerte um nicht mehr als 32 mg/100 ml bei Körpergewichtsschwankung von $\leq$ 5% voneinander abwichen.

Zwei der insgesamt 34 erfassten Patienten brachen die Behandlung wegen Verdauungsstörungen in der ersten Woche ab. Die Bewertung bezieht sich demnach auf 15 Männer und 17 Frauen im Durchschnittsalter von 47 Jahren (von 25 bis 65 Jahren) bzw. 53 Jahren (von 42 bis 62 Jahren).

Die 32 Patienten wurden zwei Monate lang mit 1 g/die Probucol (2 Tabletten zu je 250 mg zum Frühstück, zwei weitere zum Mittagessen) behandelt, wobei die Standarddiät eingehalten wurde.

Die Ergebnisse der Untersuchung bestätigen die Wirksamkeit von Probucol.

Die bereits zu Ende des ersten Behandlungsmonats signifikant gefallenen Cholesterolwerte (p < 0,001) gingen im Verlauf des zweiten Monats weiter zurück. Die triglyceride erfuhren dabei keine nennenswerte Veränderung.

Die klinischen Untersuchungen wie auch die Laborbefunde lieferten keine erwähnenswerten Ergebnisse.

Probucol wurde gut vertragen. Abgesehen von den beiden eingangs erwähnten Fällen waren keine Nebenwirkungen feststellbar.

KLINISCHE ERFAHRUNGEN MIT EINEM NEUEN HYPOCHOLESTEROLÄMIKUM: PROBUCOL

A. Castro Ribeiro and A. Pereira Viana

Probucol (500 mg b.i.d.) und Placebo wurden randomisiert im Doppelblindverfahren an 26 Patienten mit essentieller Hypercholesterolämie erprobt. Ein Monat vor Beginn der Behandlung wurden die Patienten auf Standarddiät eingestellt und gleichzeitig mit Placebo behandelt. Im gleichen Zeitraum wurde dreimal der Cholesterolblutspiegel in wöchentlichen Abständen bestimmt. Der Mittelwert wurde als Ausgangswert angenommen.

Nach dreimonatiger Verabreichung von Probucol fielen die mittleren Serumcholesterolwerte von 297 auf 247 mg/100 ml.

Die Kovarianzanalyse ergab eine signifikante Differenz (p < 0,05) im Vergleich zu der mit Placebo behandelten Gruppe. Normalisierung der Serumcholesterolwerte (< 250 mg/100 ml) wurde ferner bei 7 mit Probucol und bei einem mit Placebo behandelten Patienten festgestellt (Fisher-test p < 0,008). Die Triglyceride Veränderungs-Werte zeigten bei beiden Gruppen keinen nennenswerten Unterschied. Das Körpergewicht blieb praktisch konstant.

Kein Patient war wegen Nebenerscheinungen zu vorzeitigem Therapieabbruch gezwungen. Fünf mit Probucol und 3 mit Placebo behandelte Patienten klagten über leichte gastrointestinale Störungen.

Die von uns erzielten Ergebnisse bestätigen, dass Probucol ein wirksames und gut verträgliches Hypocholesterolämikum ist.

WIRKUNG VON PROBUCOL AUF DIE ZUSAMMENSETZUNG DER GALLENFLÜSSIGKEIT BEIM MENSCHEN—VORLÄUFIGE BEOBACHTUNGEN

Z. Mareček, M. Jirsa, V. Kordač, L. Kučerová

Die Wirkung von Probucol auf die Gallensäure und den Fettanteil der Gallenflüssigkeit wurde bei 5 Patienten untersucht, die Hyperlipoproteinämie Type IIa und Serumcholesterolspiegel zwischen 310 und 440 mg/dl aufwiesen. Die Patienten waren zuvor noch nie mit Probucol behandelt worden und hatten die Einnahme sonstiger Hypocholesterolämika seit mindestens 1 Monat abgesetzt.

Nach oraler Cholezystographie zwecks Ausschluss des Vorhandenseins etwaiger Gallensteine und Gallenblasenleiden wurden die Patienten zwei Monate mit Probucol (1 g/die) behandelt. Die Blutfette wurden in Abständen von jeweils 2 Wochen bestimmt. Der Gallensaft wurde mittels Duodenaldrainage nach vorhergehender Injektion von Cholezystokinin vor sowie nach der Behandlung gesammelt.

Die Gallensäuren wurden enzymatisch, Cholesterol und Phospholipide kolorimetrisch bestimmt. Der Sättigungsgrad des Cholesterols im Gallensaft wurde nach dem lithogenen Index von Thomas und Hoffman bestimmt.

Die Zusammensetzung der Gallensäure wurde mittels Gas-Flüssig-Chromatographie ermittelt. Die Methyl-Trimethyl-silylester wurden in 1% Hi EFF 8 BP Säule analysiert.

Anhand der erhaltenen Ergebnisse scheint es, dass die von Probucol ausgelösten Veränderungen der Molarzusammensetzung der Gallenlipide sich weitgehend von den nach Verabreichung von Clofibrat zu beobachtenden Veränderungen unterscheiden.

Clofibrat erhöht die Gallencholesterolkonzentration und verringert die Gallensäurewerte. Das bedeutet erhöhte Gallensteinbildung infolge Cholesterolübersättigung der Galle.

Die Verabreichung von Probucol bewirkt dagegen verringerten Gallencholesterolspiegel und zunehmenden Gallensäurewerte, mit dementsprechender Senkung der für Gallensteinbildung.

Die Zusammensetzung der Gallensäuren erfährt unter Probucol nur geringfügige und unkonstante Veränderungen.

WECHSELWIRKUNG VON PROBUCOL MIT DER Ca-DARMRESORPTION UND DER LANGZEITBEHANDLUNG MIT ANTIKOAGULANTIEN BEI HYPERCHOLESTERINÄ-MISCHEN PATIENTEN MIT GLEICHZEITIGEN HERZ — UND KREISLAUFSTÖRUNGEN

A. Rapado and M. Diaz-Curiel

20 Hypercholesterolämiker (Type IIa) wurden durchschnittlich 14 Monate lang mit Probucol (0,5 bis 1,5 g / die) behandelt, bei gleichzeitiger cholesterol-und gesättigten fettsäuren-armer Diät. Die Behandlung bewirkte signifikante Serumcholesterolreduzierung (− 31%; p < 0,01) und liess den Triglyceridspiegel unverändert.

Die Wirkung von Probucol auf den Calcium/Vitamin D-Stoffwechsel wurde aufgrund der Wirkung auf die Intestinalabsorption von [47]Ca ermittelt. Die Wirkung auf Vitamin K wurde durch Bestimmung der Prothrombinzeit bei Patienten in Dauerbehandlung mit Antikoagulantien geprüft.

Es waren keine Interaktionen der Präparaten feststellbar. Besonders auffällig war die Wirkung von Probucol bei einem zwölfjährigen Mädchen mit homozigoter Hypercholesterolämie Type IIa, das im Verlauf der Cholestyraminbehandlung biochemische Anzeichen von Rachitis aufwies, die spezifische Intensivtherapie erforderten. Bei dieser Patientin löste Probucol ausgeprägten Abfall des Serumcholesterolspiegels ohne Beeinflussung der intestinalen [47]Ca-Absorption und ohne biochemische Rachitissymptome aus.

PROBUCOL: BEURTEILUNG DER WIRKSAMKEIT GEGEN LIPIDEN UND LIPOPROTEINEN

J. Rouffy, R. Bakir, B. Chanu, and J. Goy-Loeper

Die Wirkung von Probucol (1 g/die) auf Serumlipide und-lipoproteine wurde an Patienten untersucht, deren essentielle Lipoproteinämie Type IIa und IIb nicht auf Diät ansprach.

In einigen Patienten war nach worhergehenden Behandlungen mit Clofibrat, Prozetophen und Cholestyramin kein Erfolg eingetreten.

Die Behandlung erstreckte sich bei 34 Patienten (T_1) über 1 Monat, bei 16 (T_2) über 3 bis 6 Monate, bei 12 (T_3) über 6 bis 12 Monate und bei 4 Patienten (T_4) über mehr als ein Jahr.

Bei Abschluss der jeweiligen Behandlungsdauer wurde—mit Ausnahme von T_3— signifikanter Rückgang der Gesamtserumlipide (8 bis 19%), des Gesamtcholesterols (8 bis 12%) und des LDL-Cholesterols (9 bis 15%) sowie signifikanter Anstieg des Verhältnisses HDL-CH / LDL-CH + VLDL-CH festgestellt.

Interaktion mit Antikoagulantien wurde nicht beobachtet.

Die Untersuchung ergab, dass Probucol die Gesamtserumlipide, das Gesamt-serumcholesterol und das LDL-Cholesterol als die am stärksten atherogen wirkende Lipoproteinfraktion eindeutig reduziert.

Eine weitere günstige Wirkung des Probucol ist die Anhebung des Ver-hältnisses HDL-CH/LDL-CH +VLDL-CH unter gleichzeitiger Verbesserung des Atherogenindex.

Das Präparat wurde klinisch wie labortechnisch ausgezeichnet vertragen.

PROBUCOL IN DER BEHANDLUNG HYPERCHOLESTEROLÄMISCHER PATIENTEN MIT KARDIOVASKULÄREN STÖRUNGEN

L. Scebat and J. Renais

Probucol (500 mg b.i.d.) wurde zusammen mit fettarmer Diät 12 bis 46 Monate lang 33 Patienten mit atherosklerotisch bedingten kardiovaskulären Störungen und Hypercholesterolämie Type IIa (11 Patienten), IIb + III (21 Patienten), IV (1 Patient) verabreicht.

Gesamthaft bewirkte die Behandlung Cholesterolspiegelsenkung von anfänglicher Durchschnittskonzentration 329,5 auf 281,1 mg/dl (− 14,5%, p < 0,001).

12 Patienten sprachen auf die Behandlung nicht an (Cholesterolsenkung ⩽ 10%), bei 20 Patienten (62,5%) war die Behandlung Diät + Probucol erfolgreich. In 3 Fällen stellte sich Senkung des Blutcholesterolspiegels erst nach dem 6. Behandlungsmonat ein. Das im Ablauf des ersten Jahres erzielte Resultat blieb in 15 Fällen (46,8%) weiterhin beständig. Sowohl bei Patienten mit essentieller Hyper-cholesterolämie (Type IIa) als auch bei Patienten mit gemischter Hyperlipämie (Types IIB + III) war die Probucolwirkung auf Serumcholesterin vergleichbar.

Probucol geht keine Interaktion mit bei Herzgefässerkrankungen üblicherweise verschriebenen Präparaten ein und löst im besonderen keine Interaktion mit Antivitamin-K-Präparaten und Diuretika aus.

Leber- und Nierenfunktiontests sowie Blutzucker und Blutbild blieben unbeeinflusst.

Die Behandlung bewirkte keine Veränderung des EKG.

3 Patienten litten unter Diarrhoe. Bei 2 Patienten klang die Störung im Verlauf der Behandlung spontan ab, der dritte Patient musste die Therapie in der zweiten Woche abbrechen.

WIRKUNG VON PROBUCOL BEI GEGEN ANDERE BLUTFETTSENKENDE SUBSTANZEN REFRAKTÄREN HYPERCHOLESTEROLÄMIKERN

S. Stefanović and L. Vučić

Die Wirkung von Probucol auf die Hypercholesterolämie wurde bei 15 Patienten untersucht: 11 Patienten litten unter Hyperlipoproteinämie Type IIa und 4 Patienten Type IIb. Bei diesen Patienten war die Hypercholesterolämie bereits 1 bis 20 Jahre vor der hier beschriebenen Therapie diagnostiziert worden. Im Durchschnitt galt die

Diagnose seit 7 Jahren als gesichert. Sämtliche Patienten waren bereits vorher ohne Erfolg erst mit Diät allein, dann mit Diät und Clofibrat und zum Teil auch zusätzlich mit Cholestyramin oder Phosphatidilcholin behandelt worden. Vor der Verabreichung von Probucol lagen die Cholesterolspiegel zwischen 306 und 565 mg / dl ($\overline{X}$: 385 mg / dl). Alle Patienten erhielten drei Monate lang 1 g / die Probucol. Die Kontrollen wurden am Ende jedes Monats vorgenommen. Bei Abschluss lagen die Cholesterolwerte sämtlicher Patienten (mit einer einzigen Ausnahme) innerhalb der auf die Altersstufen bezogenen Norm, d.h. zwischen 214 und 280 mg / dl ($\overline{X}$: 229 mg / dl).

Während der Behandlung mit Probucol traten keine klinischen Nebenwirkungen oder abnorme Veränderungen der Laborbefunde auf. Es wurden auch keine subjektiven Beschwerden angegeben.

Riassunti in Italiano

EFFETTO DEL PROBUCOL E DI ALTRI FARMACI SULLA SINTESI DEGLI STEROLI NEI LINFOCITI UMANI

A. Anastasi, D. J. Betteridge, and D. J. Galton

Le misure terapeutiche attualmente impiegate per il trattamento dell'ipercolesterolemia sono insoddisfacenti e sono quindi necessari nuovi farmaci.

Il linfocito umano è una cellula che può essere utilmente impiegata nello studio degli effetti sulla sintesi sterolica delle sostanze potenzialmente ipocolesterolemizzanti.

In linfociti isolati, la sintesi sterolica viene soppressa quando le cellule sono incubate in presenza di lipoproteine a bassa densità (LDL).

Eliminando dal mezzo di incubazione le LDL, si osserva un incremento della sintesi degli steroidi dipendente dall'induzione della HMG-CoA reduttasi, che è l'enzima che determina l'andamento della reazione.

Abbiamo studiato gli effetti della cicloesimide, un inibitore della traduzione della sintesi proteica, e della cordicepina (3′ -desossiadenosina), un inibitore della trascrizione della sintesi dell'acido ribonucleico (mRNA), sull'induzione della sintesi sterolica in linfociti umani, isolati *ex vivo* ed incubati in un mezzo contenente siero delipoproteinizzato (LPDS).

Abbiamo anche studiato altre sostanze come il compactin e il probucol che possono avere un'azione diretta sull'andamento della sintesi.

La cicloesimide (20 μg/ml) ha inibito l'induzione della sintesi sterolica mediata da LPDS suggerendo che l'aumento sia dovuto ad una sintesi ex novo degli enzimi.

La cordicepina (50 μg/ml) non ha avuto alcun effetto sull'induzione della sintesi sterolica di LPDS, sebbene abbia ridotto la sintesi dell'mRNA del 50%.

Inoltre, in linfociti pre-incubati con LDL in presenza di cordicepina per 40 h (durante questo periodo il pool di mRNA con una breve emivita dovrebbe essere molto ridotto), l'incremento nella sintesi sterolica successiva alla rimozione delle LDL dal medium di incubazione è stato della stessa grandezza di quello riscontrato nelle cellule pre-incubate in assenza di cordicepina.

Ciò fa pensare che l'emivita della HMG-CoA-reduttasi mRNA sia relativamente lunga e che a questo punto l'mRNA non sia indispensabile per l'induzione della sintesi sterolica.

Il compactin (0,2 μg) ha inibito la sintesi degli steroidi del 65% senza modificare l'incorporazione del ^{14}C-mevalonato negli steroidi suggerendo che il farmaco abbia un effetto inibitore specifico dell'attività della HMG-CoA-reduttasi.

Emulsioni di probucol a concentrazioni fino a 1 mM in albumina sierica bovina (il farmaco è scarsamente solubile) hanno inibito di circa il 40% la sintesi sterolica da

[14]C-acetato. E' possibile che questo contribuisca all'azione ipocolesterolemizzante del farmaco.

FARMACOLOGIA DEL PROBUCOL
D. Kritchevsky

Il probucol, 4,4'(isopropilideneditio)*bis*(2,6-di-t-butilfenolo), ha dimostrato un'efficace azione ipocolesterolemizzante in diverse specie animali (topo, ratto, cane, scimmia) e nell'uomo.

Nel topo l'effetto ipocolesterolemizzante è direttamente correlato alla dose somministrata.

Studi sul meccanismo d'azione condotti nell'animale, sembrano deporre per un aumento dell'escrezione fecale degli acidi biliari, una inibizione della sintesi e una diminuzione dell'assorbimento del colesterolo. In scimmie, rese ipercolesterolemiche e trattate con probucol, il colesterolo sierico è risultato del 52% inferiore rispetto agli animali di controllo. Il probucol ha inoltre indotto una significativa diminuzione del colesterolo epatico ed un significativo aumento del colesterolo splenico mentre non ha modificato il tasso di colesterolo negli altri 17 tessuti esaminati. Il trattamento con probucol non sembra quindi provocare una apprezzabile ridistribuzione del colesterolo nell'organismo. Secondo Miettinen (*Atherosclerosis,* 15, 163, 1972), il probucol agisce mediante inibizione della sintesi e dell'assorbimento del colesterolo e aumento dell'escrezione degli acidi biliari.

Quando scimmie ipercolesterolemiche vengono trattate con probucol, si verifica un aumento nell'escrezione degli acidi biliari, ma non degli steroidi neutri.

Nel cane il probucol induce una fibrillazione ventricolare. In tutte le altre specie animali esaminate non si sono osservati effetti collaterali. Dopo somministrazione di probucol marcato con ^{14}C, l'84% della radioattività viene escreto nelle feci e l'1 - 2% nelle urine in 4 giorni. Dopo somministrazione di probucol marcato con [14]C l'emi vita del prodotto è risultata di 0,8 e 12,8 giorni nella scimmia e di 1 e 15,2 giorni nel cane.

Il trattamento con probucol non ha alcuna influenza sull'attività di alcuni enzimi epatici quali catalasi, LDH (lattico-deidrogenasi), glutammico deidrogenasi e non modifica i livelli di glicogeno epatico.

In scimmie rese ipercolesterolemiche, il probucol abbassa del 25% il tasso di colesterolo nell'aorta. In conigli mantenuti a dieta aterogenica, l'aggiunta di probucol ad una concentrazione dell'1% inibisce in modo statisticamente significativo il processo aterosclerotico.

RISULTATI DI STUDI TOSSICOPATOLOGICI SUL PROBUCOL E CONFRONTO DELLA MORFOLOGIA EPATICA IN RATTI TRATTATI CON PROBUCOL, FENOFIBRATO E CLOFIBRATO
J. Molello, S. Barnard, and J. Lebeau

Il probucol è stato somministrato per via orale a 40 scimmie d'ambo i sessi, in dosi di 0, 60, 125, 250 e 500 mg/kg/die.

14 scimmie sono state sacrificate dopo 18 e 24 mesi di trattamento; lo studio si è protratto per 8 anni in 21 animali. I parametri esaminati includevano: ritmo di crescita, dati ematologici ed ematochimici, analisi delle urine, peso degli organi, esame macroscopico, istologico ed elettromicroscopico dei tessuti. 5 scimmie sono morte durante la prova; nessun decesso era correlato alla somministrazione del farmaco. Non sono state messe in evidenza differenze significative fra gli animali trattati e i controlli.

L'effetto del probucol sull'ultrastruttura della cellula epatica è stato studiato nel ratto Sprague-Dawley in confronto al clofibrato e al fenofibrato. I farmaci sono stati somministrati, mescolati alla dieta, alle dosi di ≈ 500, ≈ 250 e ≈ 100 mg/kg/die rispettivamente per il probucol, clofibrato e fenofibrato per periodi di tempo fino a 91 giorni. Gli animali di controllo ricevevano la sola dieta.

I tre farmaci in esame hanno significativamente ridotto il tasso di colesterolo sierico.

La morfologia epatica nei ratti trattati con probucol non differiva da quella degli animali di controllo.

Il clofibrato e il fenofibrato hanno provocato epatocitomegalia, aumento del numero di peroxisomi e lievi alterazioni a carico del reticolo endoplasmatico e dei mitocondri. Il resultato di questi e di altri studi indicano che il probucol è ben tollerato in trattamenti a breve e a lungo termine in topi, ratti, conigli, scimmie e cavie sia in condizioni normali che sottoposti a gravi stress cardiovascolari. Il cane è l'unico animale che sviluppi una sensibilizzazione miocardica alla epinefrina e alla nor-epinefrina. Contrariamente ad altri farmaci ipocolesterolemizzanti, il probucol non altera la morfologia epatocellulare nei roditori e nelle scimmie.

I risultati di questi studi indicano che il probucol è un composto sicuro.

EFFETTO IPOCOLESTEROLEMIZZANTE E MECCANISMO D'AZIONE DEL PROBUCOL NEL TOPO E NEL CONIGLIO

R. Infante and D. Petit

L'effetto del probucol sui lipidi plasmatici e tissutali è stato studiato nel topo e nel coniglio alimentati con diete differenti (dieta standard, dieta priva di grassi, dieta a basso contenuto in grassi e colesterolo, dieta ipercolesterolemica).

Quando somministrato in animali mantenuti a dieta standard, il probucol riduce in maniera marcata il colesterolo sierico sia nel topo (− 33% e − 60% rispetto ai controlli rispettivamente dopo 7 e 21 giorni di trattamento con 0,6 g di probucol per kg di cibo) che nel coniglio (− 37% e − 41% verso i controlli dopo 10 giorni di trattamento con rispettivamente 1 g e 2,5 g di probucol per kg di cibo) senza modificare i lipidi epatici.

In animali mantenuti ad una dieta con contenuto lipidico dello 0%, 1%, 3% o 10%, il probucol non ha manifestato alcuna attività nelle prime 2 condizioni sperimentali. L'effetto ipocolesterolemizzante è stato evidente somministrando il prodotto con la dieta contenente grassi al 3%; negli animali sottoposti ad una dieta iperlipidemica (grassi al 10% e colesterolo all'1%) il probucol ha prevenuto lo sviluppo dell'iperlipemia.

Nel topo dopo una somministrazione endovenosa singola di probucol si è osservata una rapida, marcata e prolungata caduta del colesterolo epatico.

Nel coniglio il farmaco previene l'azione iperlipemizzante di una somministrazione endovenosa di fosfolipidi.

Nel topo a dieta standard il trattamento della durata di 7 e 21 giorni con probucol alla concentrazione di 0,6 g/kg di cibo non ha significativamente modificato l'incorporazione di ^{14}C-mevalonato nel colesterolo epatico, intestinale e della carcassa. Si è osservata una riduzione dell'incorporazione della radioattività nel colesterolo plasmatico. E' stato postulato un effetto specifico del farmaco sulle lipoproteine.

Risultati preliminari ottenuti in topi trattati per 4 settimane con probucol alla concentrazione di 0,6 g/kg di dieta, hanno dimostrato una diminuzione nella velocità di sintesi delle VLDL.

IL PROBUCOL NEL TRATTAMENTO A LUNGO TERMINE DELLA IPERCOLESTEROLEMIA

D. McCaughan

Il probucol è stato studiato secondo un disegno sperimentale doppio cieco, controllato verso placebo, della durata di un anno, in 118 pazienti con ipercolesterolemia essenziale (valori pre-trattamento di colesterolo sierico ⩾ 250 mg/dl). Dopo 6 e 12 mesi di trattamento, la riduzione media del colesterolo sierico, rispetto ai valori basali era compresa tra 16,2% e 20,9% nel gruppo di pazienti trattati con probucol (n. 88); tra 5,2% e 12,7% nei pazienti trattati con placebo (n. 30) (p < 0,001).

Il trattamento con probucol è quindi continuato in forma aperta per periodi di tempo fino a 9 anni in 61 dei pazienti già trattati con il farmaco nello studio controllato.

Dopo il secondo anno di trattamento con probucol, la riduzione del colesterolo sierico era compresa tra 23,1% e 27,4% e si è in seguito mantenuta sugli stessi valori.

La mortalità totale alla fine di 5 anni di trattamento è stata del 9%. L'incidenza a 5 anni della mortalità in seguito a insufficienza coronarica e a infarto del miocardio ad esito favorevole è stata del 14%.

Il farmaco è stato ben tollerato. Gli effetti collaterali più comunemente riscontrati sono stati: osservazione di feci non formate o episodi di diarrea.

I risultati ottenuti dimostrano che il probucol è un farmaco ben tollerato, efficace per il trattamento a lungo termine di pazienti con ipercolesterolemia essenziale.

EFFETTO DEL PROBUCOL E DELLA DIETA SUI LIPIDI SIERICI E SULLE FRAZIONI LIPOPROTEICHE NELL'IPERCOLESTEROLEMIA ESSENZIALE

R. Mordasini, M. Keller, and W. F. Riesen

L'effetto del probucol su varie frazioni lipidiche è stato studiato in 27 pazienti con ipercolesterolemia essenziale. I pazienti sono stati mantenuti a una dieta isocalorica a basso contenuto lipidico e rapporto acidi grassi saturi/insaturi modificato (dieta tipo II dell'NIH) per almeno 3 mesi. Questa fase era seguita da un periodo di pre-trattamento, della durata di 6 settimane, durante il quale insieme alla dieta veniva somministrato del placebo. Durante il successivo studio condotto in doppio cieco, i pazienti sono stati trattati con dieta e placebo (una compressa, 4 volte al giorno) o con dieta e probucol (una compressa da 250 mg 4 volte al giorno). Le compresse di placebo e di probucol erano tra loro indistinguibili. I controlli sui pazienti ambulatoriali sono stati eseguiti ad intervalli mensili.

Sono stati analizzati i seguenti parametri: colesterolo e trigliceridi sierici totali e, dopo ultracentrifugazione, colesterolo e trigliceridi delle lipoproteine a bassa densità (LDL) e ad alta densità (HDL), apoproteina B e AI (mediante RID) e apoproteina AII (mediante RIA).

In confronto ai valori medi ottenuti sotto placebo, durante probucol la concentrazione di colesterolo totale è stata in media ridotta di 41 mg/100 ml (−13%, p < 0.05). L'LDL-colesterolo è stato notevolmente ridotto parallelamente al colesterolo totale essendo la riduzione di 42 mg/100 ml in media (− 16%, p < 0.025). Una lieve riduzione, statisticamente non significativa, è stata anche osservata a carico dell'HDL-colesterolo.

La somministrazione di placebo non ha indotto variazioni significative del colesterolo totale, dell'LDL-colesterolo e dell'HDL-colesterolo. La trigliceridemia è rimasta pressoché inalterata sia sotto probucol che sotto placebo.

Sotto probucol la concentrazione delle apo B è stata in media ridotta del 12%, la variazione non è comunque statisticamente significativa (p < 0.15). I livelli di apo B sono rimasti costanti durante placebo. Nel gruppo trattato con probucol è stata osservata una riduzione media del 16% delle apo AI (p < 0.0005), e del 55% delle apo AII (p < 0.0005).

Una riduzione delle concentrazioni di apo AI ed apo AII è stata anche rilevata nel gruppo trattato con placebo.

Questa riduzione è comunque risultata statisticamente significativa solo per le apo

AII (− 26%, p < 0.005).

Il trattamento con probucol è stato in generale ben tollerato. Lo studio è stato interrotto in 4 pazienti per effetti collaterali per lo più soggettivi. Tre di questi pazienti erano sotto placebo e uno sotto probucol.

LIVELLI DI LIPOPROTEINE AD ALTA DENSITÀ RILEVATI IN 5 ANNI IN UNO STUDIO MULTIFACTORIALE SUI FATTORI DI RICHIO DELLE CARDIOPATIE CRONICHE

T. A. Miettinen, J. K. Huttunen, T. Kumlin, V. Naukkarinen, S. Mattila, and C. Enholm

Il colesterolo sierico (C), i trigliceridi (TG), il colesterolo delle lipoproteine ad alta densità (HDLC), le apoproteine AI e AII delle lipoproteine a non alta densità (AII non HDL), sono stati determinati in 119 soggetti di sesso maschile che avevano partecipato per periodi fino a 4 anni ad una indagine controllata avente lo scopo di ridurre i fattori di rischio delle coronaropatie. Il trattamento comprendeva consigli dietetici e igienici e, se necessario, la somministrazione di antiipertensivi e di ipolipidemizzanti. Il colesterolo ed i trigliceridi totali sono stati determinati a vari intervalli di tempo durante il corso della ricerca, l'HDLC, le HDL AI, le HDL AII e le AII non HDL sono state valutate soltanto durante il quarto anno dell'esperienza. Per questi parametri non si sono potuti utilizzare i valori basali in quanto la conservazione prolungata fino a 4 anni determina una notevole riduzione della loro concentrazione sierica.

I livelli dei lipidi sierici totali sono risultati simili nei soggetti sottoposti alla sola dieta (n. 32) e in quelli trattati con antiipertensivi (n. 19). Rispetto ai summenzionati gruppi, i soggetti trattati con clofibrato (n. 30) hanno presentato tassi simili di AI, un aumento del 34% di AII e un aumento del 13% di HDLC.

Dopo trattamento con probucol (impiegato nei 25 casi di iperlipoproteinemia di tipo IIa) è stata osservata una riduzione del tasso di colesterolo totale (− 13%), di HDLC (− 29%) e di HDL AI (− 16%) ma non di HDL AII il cui livello non differiva da quello rilevato negli individui sottoposti alla sola dieta o trattati con farmaci antiipertensivi. Il livello di AI non HDL era basso.

I soggetti trattati contemporaneamente con clofibrato e probucol (in massima parte individui di tipo IIb: n. 13) non hanno avuto sostanziali modifiche dei lipidi sierici ma hanno presentato una riduzione del 55% dell'HDLC, una riduzione del 41% delle AI e un basso livello di AI non HDL mentre i dati di AII erano simili a quelli osservati nel gruppo di individui sottoposti alla sola dieta. I resultati fanno supporre che sebbene il probucol e il clofibrato riducano l'HDLC durante il trattamento prolungato, essi riducano il rapporto colesterolo/apolipoproteina dell'HDL, ossia il livello medio di saturazione del colesterolo della frazione HDL.

Le modifiche indotte dal clofibrato erano in parte associate alle alterazioni della concentrazione dei trigliceridi, mentre le modifiche riscontrate nei gruppi di pazienti trattati con probucol erano correlate alla durata del trattamento.

EFFICACIA DEL TOLLERABILITA' DEL PROBUCOL E STUDIO COMPARATIVO VERSO CLOFIBRATO

J. L. De Gennes and J. Truffert

L'effetto ipocolesterolemizzante del probucol e del clofibrato sono stati valutati comparativamente in uno studio condotto in doppio cieco su 38 pazienti con ipercolesterolemia essenziale.

19 pazienti sono stati trattati per 2 mesi con probucol alla dose quotidiana di 1 g e gli altri 19 hanno ricevuto clofibrato — 2 g/die — durante lo stesso periodo di tempo. Tutti i pazienti erano mantenuti a una dieta a basso contenuto in colesterolo e

acidi grassi saturi e ad alto contenuto in acidi grassi polinsaturi iniziata 2 mesi prima dell'inizio dello studio. Durante questo periodo ai pazienti veniva somministrato del placebo.

L'aggiunta del probucol alla dieta, ha indotto una caduta del colesterolo sierico del 13% (p < 0.5 in confronto ai valori osservati alla fine del periodo dieta + placebo). Sotto l'azione del clofibrato, la diminuzione del colesterolo sierico è stata in media dell'11%. Tale valore non ha raggiunto i livelli di significatività.

La diminuzione del colesterolo è stata maggiore del 20% nel 31% dei pazienti trattati con probucol e nel 21% dei casi trattati con clofibrato.

Il livello dei trigliceridi non è stato significativamente modificato dai due farmaci.

Entrambi i trattamenti sono stati ben tollerati.

Il probucol può essere utilmente impiegato per il trattamento di pazienti resistenti al clofibrato ed ai suoi derivati.

La mancanza di potere litogenico unito all'assenza di interazioni con i farmaci comunemente impiegati in questo tipo di pazienti, possono fare del probucol un reale contributo additivo nel trattamento delle ipercolesterolemie.

EFFETTO IPOCOLESTEROLEMIZZANTE E TOLLERABILITA' DEL PROBUCOL

R. E. Tedeschi, H. L. Taylor, and B. L. Martz

L'effetto a lungo termine del probucol è stato valutato su 1133 pazienti trattati durante studi clinici attentamente seguiti negli U.S.A.

881 pazienti sono stati trattati, secondo un comune protocollo, fino al maggio 1979; 291 di questi pazienti sono stati seguiti per 5 anni e 139 per un periodo di 8 anni. Il 68% dei pazienti, trattati con probucol alla dose di 1 g/die per 8 anni, presentava una riduzione ≥ 15% della concentrazione sierica di colesterolo in confronto a valori basali.

L'82% dei pazienti trattati con probucol ha presentato una diminuzione della colesterolemia > 10% rispetto ai controlli. La riduzione media di colesterolo in questo gruppo è stata del 19.9%. Non è stata osservata resistenza.

L'effetto collaterale più frequentemente riportato è la presenza di feci non formate (loose stools). Sono stati inoltre osservati: flatulenza, gastralgie, nausea, vomito e dolori addominali.

I tests di laboratorio, comprendenti l'esame ematologico e le prove di funzionalità epatica e renale, non hanno messo in evidenza segni di tossicità.

L'analisi della morbilità e mortalità è stata eseguita per tutti i 1133 pazienti trattati con probucol, applicando il metodo delle tavole di mortalità. Il 98% di questi pazienti aveva un tasso di colesterolo sierico ≥ 250 mg e molti dei pazienti presentavano altri fattori di rischio per lo sviluppo di coronaropatie.

L'incidenza di mortalità cumulativa al 5° anno (comprendente tutte le cause) è stata del 6,5%. L'incidenza cumulativa al 5° anno di casi non mortali di infarto del miocardio in pazienti con storia di infarto miocardico (n. 267) e trattati con probucol, è stata del 7,3%. Differenze nei criteri di ammissione, nella dimensione del gruppo studiato ed altre variabili non hanno permesso un confronto statistico diretto di altri studi. Tuttavia, prendendo come riferimento i dati pubblicati dal "Coronary Drug Project," la relativamente bassa mortalità e morbilità osservata durante il trattamento con probucol, suggerisce, anche se non prova, un effetto protettivo del farmaco.

Considerando l'attuale interesse nel possibile effetto nocivo sul tratto biliare dei farmaci ipolipidemizzanti, abbiamo analizzato l'incidenza di colecistectomia e di affezioni delle vie biliari in pazienti trattati a lungo termine con probucol. L'incidenza cumulativa al 6° anno di affezioni delle vie biliari (colecistectomia, colelitiasi e colecistite) è risultata del 3,3% per i maschi (n. 729) e del 5,8% per le femmine (n.

404): una incidenza complessiva del 4,1%. L'incidenza cumulativa al 6° anno di colecistectomia è stata del 2,2% per i maschi (n. 729) e del 2,7% per le femmine (n. 404): una incidenza combinata del 2,3%.

Le differenze nelle caratteristiche delle popolazioni, il decorso clinico frequentemente asintomatico e altre variabili non hanno consentito un diretto confronto statistico con i dati provenienti da altri gruppi. Le percentuali sopra riportate non sono comunque eccessive.

IL PROBUCOL NEL TRATTAMENTO A BREVE E LUNGO TERMINE DELL'IPERLIPOPROTEINEMIA DI TIPO II

V. Beaumont, J. C. Buxtorf, B. Jacotot, and J. L. Beaumont

L'azione del probucol è stata valutata in confronto al placebo in uno studio a breve termine condotto in 19 pazienti con iperlipoproteinemia di tipo II.

Ciascun paziente è stato successivamente trattato, secondo uno schema randomizzato, con placebo e probucol (1 g / die) per un mese. I pazienti sono stati mantenuti alla loro dieta abituale.

Sono stati confrontati i valori di colesterolo totale, fosfolipidi e trigliceridi rilevati alla fine di ogni periodo di trattamento. La valutazione statistica è stata eseguita con il test "t" di Student per dati accoppiati.

Il probucol ha indotto una diminuzione del colesterolo sierico totale del 9% (p < 0.001) mentre non ha modificato in maniera statisticamente significativa sia la fosfolipidemia che la trigliceridemia. La persistenza degli effetti del probucol sui lipidi sierici, la sua azione sui lipidi tissutali e la sua tolleranza clinica e biologica, sono state l'oggetto di uno studio aperto condotto in 20 pazienti con iperlipoproteinemia di tipo II. Anche in questo studio i pazienti hanno mantenuto la loro dieta abituale.

I lipidi sierici sono stati determinati prima dell'inizio dello studio e ogni due mesi di trattamento per una durata totale di 6 mesi.

Prima e alla fine dei 6 mesi di trattamento sono stati prelevati frammenti di cute per la determinazione del colesterolo libero ed esterificato. I risultati ottenuti sono stati confrontati con i valori corrispondenti rilevati a un gruppo di soggetti sani.

Alla fine dello studio è stata osservata una diminuzione media di colesterolo sierico del 9,9% (p < 0.001) simile a quella rilevata dopo un mese di trattamento. La caduta del colesterolo è stata > 10% nel 60% dei pazienti.

Anche in questo caso i fosfolipidi e i trigliceridi sierici non sono stati significativamente modificati dal farmaco.

Il tasso di colesterolo esterificato della cute è stato significativamente aumentato dal trattamento.

Non si sono rilevate anomalie negli esami di laboratorio; i livelli di SGOT e di SGPT sono aumentati, mantenendosi però entro i limiti normali.

In complesso, la tolleranza clinica del probucol è stata buona. Gli Autori concludono che il probucol mantiene l'effetto ipocolesterolemizzante in trattamenti prolungati ed è un farmaco sicuro.

Il significativo aumento della frazione esterificata del colesterolo cutaneo in assenza di una significativa variazione del colesterolo totale necessita un'ulteriore valutazione.

Come ipotesi di lavoro si potrebbe pensare che tali variazioni qualitative possano facilitare la mobilizzazione del colesterolo e possano essere correlate con la osservata regressione degli xantelasmi.

TRATTAMENTO DELLE IPERCOLESTEROLEMIE CON PROBUCOL

R. Carmena and J. F. Ascaso

L'effetto ipolipidemizzante di un nuovo farmaco, il probucol, è stato studiato in 20 pazienti affetti da iperlipoproteinemia essenziale (fenotipo IIa in 7 casi e IIb in 13 casi). Tutti i pazienti ricevevano una dieta a basso contenuto di colesterolo e acidi grassi saturi e ad alto contenuto di acidi grassi polinsaturi.

Dopo un mese di sola dieta i pazienti sono stati assegnati mediante randomizzazione a due diverse sequenze di trattamento: 10 pazienti sono stati prima trattati con probucol (500 mg × 2/die) per due mesi e poi con placebo per altri due mesi; i rimanenti dieci hanno ricevuto i due trattamenti nell'ordine inverso. Un mese con sola dieta ha preceduto anche la seconda fase del cross-over.

La sola dieta ha indotto una variazione della colesterolemia da un valore medio di 403,7 mg/dl a 375,1 mg/dl con una riduzione del 7% che non ha raggiunto livelli di significatività. L'aggiunta di probucol ha significativamente incrementato l'effetto ipocolesterolemizzante della dieta (− 32%, p < 0.01). La trigliceridemia non è stata modificata dal farmaco.

La tollerabilità del probucol è stata eccellente.

EFFETTO DEL PROBUCOL
NELL'IPERCOLESTEROLEMIA ESSENZIALE

A. Gouveia, A Noronha, I. Dionisio, S. Felix, B. Barros, and M. Carrageta

Scopo di questo studio condotto in forma aperta in pazienti con ipercolesterolemia essenziale, è di valutare l'azione ipocolesterolemizzante del probucol e di studiare la natura e l'incidenza degli effetti collaterali.

I pazienti sono stati consigliati di seguire una dieta standard per un mese e sono stati quindi sottoposti ad esami clinici e di laboratorio.

Sono stati ammessi allo studio pazienti con una media di 3 determinazioni di colesterolo sierico ⩾ 250 mg/100 ml (metodo enzimatico) i cui valori singoli non differissero fra loro più di 32 mg/100 ml e con variazioni di peso corporeo ⩽ 5%.

Dei 34 pazienti ammessi, 2 hanno interrotto il trattamento durante la prima settimana per disturbi intestinali. Lo studio è stato quindi condotto su 15 uomini e 17 donne con età media rispettivamente di 47 anni (da 25 a 65 anni) e di 53 anni (da 42 a 62 anni).

I 32 pazienti sono stati trattati per 2 mesi con 1 g/die di probucol (2 compresse da 250 mg alla prima colazione e altre 2 compresse a pranzo) continuando a seguire una dieta standard. I risultati di questo studio confermano l'efficacia del probucol.

Il tasso di colesterolo già significativamente ridotto alla fine del primo mese di trattamento (p < 0.001), è diminuito ulteriormente durante il secondo mese. I trigliceridi non sono stati significativamente modificati.

Nessun reperto degno di nota è emerso dall'esame clinico e dalle analisi di laboratorio.

Il probucol è stato ben tollerato. Non si sono rilevati effetti secondari, ad eccezione che per i due pazienti sopra menzionati.

ESPERIENZA CLINICA SU UN NUOVO FARMACO
IPOCOLESTEROLEMIZZANTE: IL PROBUCOL

A. Castro Ribeiro and A. Pereira Viana

Il probucol (1 grammo/die) e il placebo sono stati somministrati secondo uno schema randomizzato con un disegno doppio cieco a 26 pazienti con ipercolesterolemia essenziale. Un mese prima dell'inizio dello studio i pazienti sono stati sottoposti ad una dieta standard e sono stati contemporaneamente trattati con placebo. Durante questo periodo sono state eseguite tre determinazioni della colesterolemia ad intervalli settimanali e la loro media è stata considerata come valore basale.

Dopo tre mesi di trattamento con probucol il livello medio del colesterolo sierico era passato da 297 a 247 mg/100 ml.

L'analisi della covarianza ha evidenziato una differenza significativa (p < 0.05) rispetto al gruppo di pazienti trattati con placebo. E' stata inoltre rilevata una normalizzazione dei livelli di colesterolo sierico (< 250 mg/100 ml) in 7 pazienti trattati con probucol e in 1 paziente sotto placebo (test di Fisher p < 0.008). Le variazioni dei livelli dei trigliceridi non sono state significativamente diverse nei due gruppi. Il peso corporeo è rimasto praticamente immodificato.

Nessun paziente ha dovuto interrompere lo studio a causa di effetti collaterali. 5 pazienti trattati con probucol e tre pazienti trattati con placebo hanno accusato disturbi gastro-enterici di modesta entità.

I risultati da noi ottenuti confermano che il probucol è un ipocolesterolemizzante efficace e ben tollerato.

EFFETTO DEL PROBUCOL SULLA COMPOSIZIONE BILIARE NELL'UOMO. OSSERVAZIONI PRELIMINARI

Z. Mareček, M. Jirsa, V. Kordač, and L. Kučerová

L'azione del probucol sugli acidi biliari e sulla componente lipidica della bile è stata studiata in 5 pazienti con iperlipoproteinemia di tipo IIa e con livelli sierici di colesterolo compresi tra 310 e 440 mg/dl. I soggetti non erano mai stati in precedenza trattati con probucol e avevano interrotto l'assunzione di qualsiasi farmaco ipocolesterolemizzante da almeno 1 mese.

Dopo una colecistografia orale, intesa ad escludere la presenza di calcoli biliari e di colecistopatie, i pazienti sono stati trattati per due mesi con probucol alla dose di 1 g/die. I lipidi sierici sono stati determinati ogni due settimane di trattamento. La bile è stata raccolta mediante drenaggio duodenale, previa iniezione di colescistochinina, prima e alla fine del trattamento.

Gli acidi biliari sono stati determinati con metodo enzimatico, il colesterolo ed i fosfolipidi con metodo colorimetrico; il grado di saturazione di colesterolo nella bile è stato determinato con l'indice litogenico di Thomas e Hoffmann.

La composizione degli acidi biliari è stata valutata mediante cromatografia gas-liquida e i metil-trimetilsilil esteri sono stati analizzati su colonna 1% Hi EFF 8 BP.

Dai risultati ottenuti sembra che le variazioni nella composizione molare relativa dei lipidi biliari indotte dal probucol siano notevolmente diverse da quelle osservate dopo somministrazione di clofibrato.

Il clofibrato provoca un aumento della concentrazione del colesterolo biliare e una riduzione degli acidi biliari con conseguente aumento della litogenicità della bile per supersaturazione della bile con colesterolo.

Dopo somministrazione di probucol si osserva invece una diminuzione del colesterolo biliare e un aumento degli acidi biliari con conseguente diminuzione dell'indice litogenico.

Le variazioni nella composizione degli acidi biliari rilevate dopo probucol sono di modesta entità e non costanti.

EFFETTI DEL PROBUCOL SULL'ASSORBIMENTO INTESTINALE NEL TRATTAMENTO CRONICO CON ANTICOAGULANTI IN PAZIENTI CON IPERCOLESTEROLEMIA ASSOCIATA AD AFFEZIONI CARDIOVASCOLARI

A. Rapado and M. Diaz-Curiel

20 pazienti affetti da ipercolesterolemia di tipo IIa sono stati trattati per un periodo medio di 14 mesi con probucol in dosi variabili da 0.5 a 1.5 g/die addizionato ad una dieta a basso contenuto di colesterolo e di acidi grassi saturi. Il trattamento ha significativamente ridotto il colesterolo sierico (− 31%, p < 0.01) e non ha modificato il livello dei trigliceridi.

L'effetto del probucol—1 g/die—sui lipidi e le lipoproteine sieriche è stato studi- alla sua azione sull'assorbimento intestinale di ^{47}Ca. L'attività della vitamina K è stata determinata mediante il controllo del tempo di protrombina in pazienti in trattamento cronico con anticoagulanti.

Non sono state evidenziate interazioni fra i farmaci.

Particolarmente interessante é stato l'effetto del probucol in una bambina di 12 anni, con iperlipoproteinemia di tipo IIa omozigote, che durante trattamento con colestiramina aveva presentato segni biochimici di rachitismo richiedenti una intensa terapia specifica. In questa paziente il probucol ha significativamente ridotto il tasso di colesterolo sierico senza modificazioni nell'assorbimento intestinale di ^{47}Ca e sen- za sintomi biochimici di rachitismo.

PROBUCOL: VALUTAZIONE DELL'EFFETTO SUI LIPIDI SIERICI E SULLE LIPOPROTEINE

J. Rouffy, R. Bakir, B. Chanu, J. Goy-Loeper

L'effetto del probucol — 1 g/die — sui lipidi e le lipoproteine sieriche è stato studiato in pazienti con iperlipoproteinemia essenziale di tipo IIa e IIb resistenti alla dieta.

Alcuni dei pazienti avevano in precedenza ricevuto colestiramina, clofibrato e procetofen con risultati insoddisfacenti.

La durata del trattamento è stata di 1 mese in 34 pazienti (T_1), da 3 a 6 mesi in 16 (T_2), da 6 mesi ad un anno in 12 (T_3) e di oltre 1 anno in 4 (T_4).

Alla fine dei vari periodi di trattamento considerati, ad eccezione del T_3, è stata osservata una riduzione significativa dei lipidi sierici totali (dall'8 al 19%), del colesterolo totale (dall'11 al 12%) e dell'LDL-colesterolo (dal 9 al 15%), e un significativo aumento del rapporto HDL-CH/LDL-CH + VLDL-CH.

Non si sono rilevate interazioni con anticoagulanti.

Questo studio ha dimostrato che il probucol è un farmaco efficace per la riduzione dei lipidi sierici totali, del colesterolo totale e del colesterolo delle lipoproteine a bassa densità che è la frazione lipoproteica più aterogenica.

Un altro favorevole risultato indotto dal probucol è l'aumento del rapporto HDL-CH/LDL-CH + VLDL-CH con conseguente miglioramento dell'indice aterogenico.

La tolleranza al prodotto è stata eccellente sia da un punto di vista clinico che di laboratorio.

IL PROBUCOL NEL TRATTAMENTO DELL'IPERCOLESTEROLEMIA IN PAZIENTI CON TURBE CARDIOVASCOLARI

L. Scebat and J. Renais

Il probucol (1 grammo/die) aggiunto ad una dieta a basso contenuto lipidico è stato somministrato durante un periodo variabile da 12 a 46 mesi a 33 pazienti con affezioni cardiovascolari su base aterosclerotica e con ipercolesterolemia di tipo IIa (11 pazienti), IIb e III (21 pazienti), IV (1 paziente).

In complesso il trattamento ha indotto una diminuzione del colesterolo da una concentrazione media di 329,5 a 281,1 mg/dl (− 14,5% p < 0.001). In particolare: 12 pazienti sono apparsi resistenti (riduzione del colesterolo ≤ 10%) e 20 pazienti (62,5%) hanno risposto al trattamento con dieta + probucol. In 3 casi si è osservata una diminuzione dell'effetto ipocolesterolemizzante del farmaco dopo il 6° mese. Il risultato ottenuto nel primo anno si è mantenuto in 15 pazienti con ipercolesterolemia essenziale (tipo IIa) e nei pazienti con iperlipemia mista (tipo IIb + III).

Il probucol non ha interagito con gli altri farmaci comunemente prescritti nelle affezioni cardiovascolari, in particolare con le sostanze antivitamina K e i diuretici.

Non sono state registrate variazioni di tests di funzionalità epatica e renale, della glicemia e dell'esame ematologico. Il peso corporeo è rimasto pressochè invariato.

L'elettrocardiogramma non è stato modificato dal trattamento.

3 pazienti hanno accusato episodi di diarrea, che si sono risolti durante il corso del trattamento in 2 soggetti e che nel terzo hanno richiesto la sospensione del probucol durante la seconda settimana.

EFFETTO DEL PROBUCOL IN PAZIENTI IPERCOLESTEROLEMICI RESISTENTI AD ALTRI TRATTAMENTI IPOLIPEMIZZANTI

S. Stefanović and L. Vučić

L'azione del probucol sull'ipercolesterolemia è stata studiata in 15 pazienti: undici con iperlipoproteinemia di tipo IIa e quattro di tipo IIb. In questi pazienti l'ipercolesterolemia era stata diagnosticata da 1 a 20 anni precedenti questa ricerca: in media durava 7 anni. Tutti i pazienti erano stati trattati senza successo prima con la dieta, poi con dieta e clofibrato con l'aggiunta in alcuni casi di colestiramina o fosfatidilcolina.

Le concentrazioni di colesterolo precedenti la somministrazione di probucol erano comprese fra 306 e 565 mg / dl ($\overline{X}$: 385 mg / dl). Tutti i pazienti sono stati trattati con 1 g di probucol al giorno per un periodo di tre mesi.

I controlli sono stati eseguiti alla fine di ogni mese. Alla fine del trattamento in tutti i pazienti, escluso uno, i valori di colesterolo erano compresi entro i limiti della norma per i rispettivi gruppi di età, ossia fra 214 e 280 mg/dl ($\overline{X}$: 229 mg/dl).

Durante la somministrazione di probucol non si sono rilevati effetti collaterali clinicamente evidenti o anomalie degli esami di laboratorio e non sono stati riportati disturbi soggettivi.

Resumos em Português

EFEITO DO PROBUCOL E OUTROS FÁRMACOS SOBRE A SÍNTESE DOS ESTERÓIDES NOS LINFÓCITOS HUMANOS

A. Anastasi, D. J. Betteridge, and D. J. Galton

Os meios terapêuticos empregados para o tratamento da hipercolesterolemia não são satisfatórios sendo, por isso, necessários novos fármacos. O linfócito humano é uma célula que pode ser utilmente empregada no estudo dos efeitos sobre a síntese dos esteróides por substâncias potencialmente hipocolesterolemizantes.

Nos linfócitos isolados, a síntese dos esteróides é suprimida quando as células são incubadas na presença de lipoproteínas de baixa densidade (LDL). Eliminadas as LDL do meio de incubação, observa-se um incremento da síntese dos esteróides dependentes da indução de HMG-CoA redutase, que é a enzima que determina o prosseguimento da reacção. Estudaram-se os efeitos da cicloeximida, um inibidor da descodificação da síntese proteica e da cordicepina (3' desoxiadenosina), um inibidor da transcrição da síntese do ácido ribonucleico mensageiro mRNA, sobre a indução da síntese dos esteróides nos linfócitos humanos, isolados extemporâneamente e incubados num meio contendo soro deslipoproteinizado (LPDS). Estudaram-se também outras substâncias tais como o compactin e o probucol, que podem ter uma ação directa na reação e síntese. A cicloeximida (20 μg/ml) inibe a indução da síntese de esteróides mediada por LPDS sugerindo que o aumento seja devido a uma síntese ex novo das enzimas.

A cordicepina (50 μg/ml) não mostrou efeito algum sobre a indução da síntese de esteróides pelo LPDS, apesar de reduzir a síntese do mRNA de 50%. Além disso, nos linfócitos pré-incubados com LDL na presença de cordicepina durante 40 h (neste tempo o pool do mRNA com semivida breve deveria ter-se reduzido muito), o incremento da síntese de esteróides após remoção do LDL do meio de incubação foi do mesmo valor que o encontrado nas células pré-incubadas, na ausência de cordicepina. Isto faz pensar que a semivida da HMG-CoA redutase mRNA é relativamente longa e que neste ponto o mRNA não é indispensável para a indução da síntese de esteróides.

O compactin (0.2 µg) inibe a síntese dos esteróides de 65% sem modificar a incorporação do ^{14}C mevalonato nos esteróides, sugerindo ter o fármaco um efeito inibidor específico da actividade da HMG-CoA redutase. Emulsões de probucol em concentrações até 1 mM, em albumina de boi (o fármaco é escassamente solúvel), inibe cerca de 40% a síntese de esteróides por ^{14}C-acetato.

É possível que isto possa contribuir para a ação hipocolesterolemizante do fármaco.

FARMACOLOGIA DO PROBUCOL
D. Kritchevsky

O probucol, 4,4' (isopropilideniditio)*bis*(2,6-di-t-butilfenol), demonstrou ter uma eficaz ação hipocolesterolemizante em diversas espécies animais (rato, ratazana, cão, macaco) e no homem.

No rato o efeito é diretamente proporcional à dose administrada. Estudos sobre o mecanismo de ação realizados em animais, parecem falar a favor de um aumento da excreção fecal dos ácidos biliares, uma inibição da síntese e uma diminuição da absorção do colesterol. Em macacos tornados hipercolesterolêmicos e tratados com probucol, verificou-se uma baixa do colesterol sérico (52% inferior ao dos animais de controle). O probucol, portanto, induziu de maneira significativa uma diminuição do colesterol hepático e um aumento do colesterol esplênico, não modificando a taxa de colesterol nos outros 17 tecidos examinados. O tratamento com probucol não parece, pois, provocar uma apreciável redistribuição do colesterol no organismo. Segundo Miettinen (*Atherosclerosis*, 15, 163, 1972), o probucol age mediante inibição da síntese e da absorção do colesterol e aumento da excreção dos ácidos biliares. Quando os macacos hipercolesterolêmicos são tratados com probucol, verifica-se um aumento da excreção dos ácidos biliares, mas não dos esteróides neutros. No cão o probucol induz uma fibrilação ventricular. Em todas as outras espécies animais examinadas não foram observados efeitos colaterais.

Após a administração de probucol marcado ^{14}C, 84% da radioactividade é eliminada pelas fezes e 1–2% pela urina, em 4 dias. Após administração de probucol marcado com ^{14}C a semivida do produto foi de 0,8 e 12,8 dias no macaco e de 1 e 15,2 dias no cão.

O tratamento com probucol não tem influência alguma sobre a actividade de algumas enzimas hepáticas tais como a catalase, LDH (desidrogenase láctica) desidrogenase glutâmica e não modifica os níveis do glicogênio hepático.

Nos macacos hipercolesterolêmicos o probucol baixa de 25% a taxa de colesterol na aorta. Nos coelhos mantidos em dieta aterogênica, a adição de probucol numa concentração de 1% inibe de modo significativo o processo aterosclerótico.

RESULTADOS DOS ESTUDOS TOXICOPATOLOGICOS COM PROBUCOL E UM ESTUDO COMPARATIVO DA MORFOLOGIA HEPÁTICA EM RATOS TRATADOS COM PROBUCOL FENOFIBRATE OU CLOFIBRATE
J. Molello, S. Barnard, and J. Lebeau

O probucol foi administrado por via oral em 40 macacos de ambos os sexos, nas doses de 0, 60, 125, 250 e 500 mg/kg/dia. 14 macacos foram sacrificados após 18 e 24 meses de tratamento; o estudo prolongou-se durante 8 anos em 21 animais. Os parâmetros examinados incluiam ritmo de crescimento, dados hematológicos e hematoquímicos, análises da urina, peso dos orgãos, exame macroscópico histológico e eletromicroscópico dos tecidos. Cinco macacos morreram durante as provas; nenhum óbito estava correlacionado com a administração do fármaco. Não foram postas em evidência diferenças significativas entre os animais tratados e os controles.

O efeito do probucol sobre a ultra-estrutura da célula hepática foi estudado no rato Sprague-Dowley em comparação com o clofibrate e o fenofibrate. Os fármacos foram administrados, misturados na dieta, nas doses aproximadas de 500, 250 e 100 mg/kg/dia respectivamente para o probucol, clofibrate e fenofibrate durante períodos de até 91 dias. Os animais de controle recebiam somente a dieta. Os 3 fármacos em exame reduziram significativamente a taxa de colesterol no soro. A morfologia hepática dos ratos tratados com probucol não se mostrou diferente da dos animais de controle. O clofibrate e o fenofibrate provocaram hepatocitomegalia, aumento do número de peroxisomas e leves alterações a cargo do retículo endoplasmático e das mitocôndrias.

Os resultados destas e de outras pesquisas indicam que o probucol é bem tolerado a curto e a longo prazo por camundongos, ratos, coelhos, macacos e cobaios mantidos em condições laboratoriais convencionais, ou quando submetidos a grave stress cardiovascular. Caes, por outro lado, são os únicos a desenvolver sensibilização miocárdica a epinefrina e nor epinefrina. Probucol não altera a morfologia hepatocellular de roedores e primatas como fazem outros agentes redutores do colesterol.

EFEITO HIPOCOLESTEROLEMIZANTE DO PROBUCOL E SEU MECANISMO DE AÇÃO NO RATO E NO COELHO

R. Infante and D. Petit

O efeito do probucol sobre os lípidos do plasma e dos tecidos foi estudado no rato e no coelho sob condições alimentares diversas (dieta padrão, dieta destituída de gorduras, dieta de baixo conteúdo em gorduras e colesterol, dieta hipercolesterolêmica).

Quando o probucol é administrado a animais sujeitos a dieta standard, reduz-se fortemente o colesterol sérico no rato (– 33% e – 60% em relação aos controles, após respectivamente 7 e 21 dias de tratamento com 0,6 g de probucol por kg de alimento) e no coelho (– 37% e – 41% de que o grupo de controle, após 10 dias de tratamento com respectivamente 1 g e 2,5 g de probucol por kg de alimento) sem modificação dos lípidos hepáticos. Nos animais sujeitos a uma dieta com um teor lipídico de 0%, 1%, 3% ou 10%, o probucol não manifestou atividade alguma nas primeiras 2 condições experimentais, mas o efeito hipocolesterolemizante foi já evidente nos casos com dieta contendo 3% de gorduras, e nos animais submetidos a uma dieta hiperlipídica (10% de gorduras e 1% de colesterol) o probucol preveniu o desenvolvimento da hiperlipidemia.

No rato, após uma única administração endovenosa de probucol, observouse uma rápida, marcada e prolongada descida do colesterol sérico. No coelho o fármaco preveniu o efeito hiperlipidêmico de uma administração endovenosa de fosfolípidos.

No rato, com dieta padrão, o tratamento durante 7 e 21 dias com probucol na concentração de 0,6 g/kg de alimento não modificou de maneira significativa a incorporação de ^{14}C-mevalonato no colesterol hepático, intestinal e ósseo.

Observou-se uma redução da incorporação da radiotividade no colesterol plasmático. Foi postulado um efeito específico do fármaco sobre as lipoproteínas.

Resultados preliminares obtidos em ratos tratados durante 4 semanas com probucol na concentração de 0,6 g/kg de dieta, demonstraram uma diminuição na velocidade de síntese das VLDL.

O PROBUCOL NO TRATAMENTO PROLONGADO DA HIPERCOLESTEROLEMIA

D. McCaughan

O probucol foi comparado com um placebo num ensaio duplo cego com a duração de um ano, em 118 doentes com hipercolesterolemia primária (valores de colesterol sérico, anteriores ao tratamento de: ⩾ 250 mg/dl). Após 6 a 12 meses de tratamento a redução média do colesterol sérico, em relação aos valores de base, foi entre 16.2% e 20.9% no grupo de doentes tratados com probucol (n = 88) e entre 5.2% - 12.7% nos doentes tratados com placebo (n = 30) (p < 0.001).

O tratamento com probucol foi depois continuado de forma aberta por períodos até 9 anos em 61 pacientes, já tratados com o fármaco no estudo controlado.

Após o segundo ano de tratamento com probucol, a redução do colesterol sérico estava compreendida entre 23.1% e 27.4% e manteve-se em seguida nestes valores.

A mortalidade ao fim de 5 anos de tratamento foi de 9%. Após 5 anos de tratamento , a incidência de mortalidade coronária ou de enfarte do miocárdio foi apenas de 14%.

O fármaco foi bem tolerado. Os efeitos colaterais mais usualmente observados foram casos de fezes não formadas ou diarréias. Os resultados obtidos demonstraram que o probucol é um fármaco bem tolerado, eficaz para o tratamento prolongado de pacientes com hipercolesterolemia primária.

EFEITO DO PROBUCOL E DA DIETA SOBRE OS LÍPIDES SÉRICOS E AS FRAÇÕES LIPOPROTEICAS NA HIPERCOLESTEROLÉMIA PRIMÁRIA

R. Mordasini, M. Keller, and W. F. Riesen

O efeito do probucol sobre as várias frações lipídicas foi estudado em 27 pacientes com hipercolesterolemia primária. Os doentes foram sujeitos a uma dieta isocalórica de baixo teor lipídico e com uma relação ácidos graxos saturados/ insaturados modificada (NIH dieta tipo II) pelo menos durante 3 meses. Esta fase foi seguida por um período de pré-tratamento, com a duração de 6 semanas, durante o qual juntamente à dieta era administrado o placebo. Seguiu-se depois o estudo em dupla ocultação; os pacientes foram tratados com dieta e placebo (1 comprimido 4 vezes ao dia) ou com dieta e probucol (1 comprimido de 250 mg 4 vezes ao dia). Os comprimidos de placebo e de probucol são indistinguíveis. Os controles dos doentes em regime ambulatórial foram feitos em intervalos mensais.

Foram analisados os seguintes parâmetros: colesterol e triglicérides totais e após ultracentrifugação, colesterol e triglicérides das lipoproteínas de baixa densidade (LDL) e de alta densidade (HDL), apo-B e apo AI (mediante RID) e apo-AII (mediante RIA).

Em comparação com os valores médios obtidos com o placebo a concentração de colesterol total durante a ação do probucol foi reduzida, em média, de 41 mg/100 ml (− 13%, p < 0.05). O LDL-colesterol foi notavelmente reduzido em comparação com o colesterol total, sendo a redução de 42 mg/100 ml, em média (− 16%, p < 0.025). Uma leve redução, estatisticamente não significativa, foi também obser- vada quanto ao colesterol das HDL.

A administração de placebo não induziu variações significativas do colesterol total, do colesterol das LDL e do colesterol das HDL. A trigliceridemia não foi praticamente alterada, quer com o tratamento com o probucol quer com o placebo. Com o uso do probucol a concentração das apo-B foi reduzida de 12%, a variação não é todavia estatisticamente significativa (p < 0.15). Os níveis de apo-B permaneceram constantes durante o uso do placebo.

No grupo com probucol foi observada uma redução média de 16% das apo-AI (p < 0.0005) e de apo-AII de 55% (p < 0.0005). Uma redução das concentrações de apo-AI e apo-AII foi também notada no grupo tratado com placebo.

Esta redução resultou, no entanto, estatisticamente significativa só para as apo-AII (− 26%, p < 0.005).

O tratamento com probucol foi em geral bem tolerado. O estudo foi interrompido em 4 pacientes devido a efeitos colaterais, geralmente de tipo subjetivo. Três destes 4 doentes estavam sendo tratados com placebo e só um com probucol.

NIVEIS DE LIPOPROTEINAS DE ALTA DENSIDADE UMA INTERVENÇÃO MULTIFACTORIAL DE CINCO ANOS CONTRA A DOENÇA CORONARIA

T. A. Miettinen, J. K. Huttunen, T. Kumlin,
V. Naukkarinen, S. Mattila, and C. Enholm

O colesterol sérico (COL) os triglicérides (TG), o colesterol das lipoproteínas de alta densidade (HDL-COL) as apoproteínas A-I e A-II das lipoproteínas de alta densidade (HDL-A-I, HDL-A-II) e as apoproteínas das lipoproteínas—não alta densidade (A-II não HDL) foram determinadas em 119 indivíduos do sexo masculino que haviam participado por períodos até 4 anos numa pesquisa controlada com o fim de reduzir os fatores de risco das coronaropatias. O tratamento compreendia conselhos dietéticos e higiénicos e, se necessário, a administração de anti-hipertensivos e de hipolipidemizantes. O colesterol e os triglicéridos totais foram determinados em vários intervalos de tempo durante o decorrer da pesquisa, o HDL-COL as HDL-A-I, as HDL-A-II e as A-II não HDL foram avaliadas somente durante o quarto ano da experiência. Com estes parâmetros não foi possível utilizarem-se os valores basais pois a conservação durante tempo tão prolongado (até 4 anos) determina uma notável redução das suas concentrações séricas.

Os níveis dos lípidos séricos totais resultaram semelhantes nos indivíduos submetidos somente à dieta (n = 32) e nos tratados com anti-hypertensivos (n = 19). Com respeito aos grupos acima citados, os indivíduos tratados com clofibrate (n = 30) apresentaram taxas semelhantes de A-I, um aumento de 34% de A-II e uma redução de 13% do HDL-COL.

Após tratamento com probucol (empregado em casos de hiperlipoproteinemia do tipo IIA; n = 25) há uma redução do colesterol total do soro (− 13%), HDL-COL − 29%) e de HDL-A-I (− 16%) mas não de HDL-A-II, cujo nível não se diferenciava daquele observado nos indivíduos submetidos somente à dieta ou tratados com fármacos anti-hipertensivos. O nível das A-I-não HDL era baixo.

Os indivíduos tratados simultâneamente com clofibrato e probucol (principalmente indivíduos de tipo IIb; n = 13) não tiveram substanciais modificações nos lípidos séricos, mas apresentaram uma redução de 55% no HDL-COL uma redução de 41% de A-I e um baixo nível de A-I-não HDL enquanto que os valores de A-II eram semelhantes aos observados nos indivíduos submetidos apenas a dieta. Os resultados fazem supor que, embora o probucol e o clofibrate reduzam o HDL-COL durante tratamentos prolongados, eles reduzem a relação colesterol/apolipoproteína das HDL, ou seja o nível médio de saturação do colesterol da fração HDL. As modificações induzidas pelo clofibrate vão em parte associadas às alterações da concentração dos triglicérides, enquanto que as modificações observadas nos grupos de pacientes tratados com probucol estão correlacionadas com a duração do tratamento.

AVALIAÇÃO DA EFICÁCIA E DA TOLERÂNCIA DO PROBUCOL E ESTUDO COMPARATIVO VERSUS CLOFIBRATE

J. L. De Gennes and J. Truffert

O efeito hipocolesterolemizante do probucol e do clofibrate foram avaliados comparativamente num estudo conduzido em duplo cego, em 36 doentes com hipercolesterolémia primária.

Dezenove doentes foram tratados durante 2 meses com probucol na dose diária de 1 g e os outros 19 receberam clofibrate—2 g/dia—durante o mesmo período.

Todos os doentes foram sujeitos a uma dieta de baixo teor em colesterol e ácidos graxos saturados e de alto teor em ácidos graxos polinsaturados iniciada 2 meses antes do começo do estudo. Durante este período os pacientes receberam placebo.

A junção do probucol à dieta induziu uma baixa do colesterol sérico de 13% (p < 0.05) em comparação com os valores observados no final do período do dieta + placebo. Sob a acção do clofibrate, a diminuição do colesterol sérico foi em média de 11%. Tal valor não alcançou níveis significativos.

A diminuição do colesterol foi maior do que 20% em 31% dos doentes tratados com probucol e em 21% dos casos tratados com clofibrate. O nível dos triglicérides não foi modificado de modo significativo pelos dois fármacos. Ambos os tratamentos foram bem tolerados. O probucol é de muita utilidade no tratamento de doentes resistentes ao clofibrate e seus derivados.

A falta de poder litogênico e a ausência de interações com os fármacos habitualmente empregados neste tipo de pacientes, podem fazer do probucol uma real contribuição no tratamento das hipercolesterolemias.

EXPERIÊNCIA CLÍNICA COM O PROBUCOL—EFICÁCIA HIPOCOLESTEROLEMIZANTE E TOLERANCIA

R. E. Tedeschi, B. L. Martz, and H. L. Taylor

O efeito do probucol, em tratamentos prolongados, foi avaliado em 1.133 pacientes tratados durante estudos clínicos dirigidos cuidadosamente nos E.U.A. 881 doentes foram tratados de acordo com um protocolo comum e, até Maio de 1979, 291 foram seguidos durante 5 anos, e 139 por um período de 8 anos. 68% destes pacientes tratados com probucol na dose de 1 g/dia durante 8 anos, apresentavam uma redução ≥ 15% da concentração sérica do colesterol em comparação com os valores basais. 82% dos pacientes tratados com probucol apresentavam uma diminuição da colesterolemia ≥ 10% com relação aos controles. A redução média do colesterol neste grupo foi de 19,9%. Não foi observado aparecimento de resistência.

O efeito colateral mais frequentemente referido foi a presença de fezes não formadas. Noutros foram observados flatulência, gastralgias, náuseas, vômitos e dores abdominais. Os testes de laboratório, compreendendo exames hematológicos e provas de função hepática e renal, não evidenciaram sinais de toxicidade.

A análise da morbilidade e mortalidade foi feita para todos os 1133 doentes tratados com probucol, aplicando o método dos índices de mortalidade. 98% dos doentes tinham uma taxa de colesterol sérico ≥ 250 mg% e muitos dos pacientes apresentavam outros fatores de risco para eventuais coronariopaties. A incidência de mortalidade cumulativa ao 5° ano (compreendendo todas as causas) foi de 6,5%. A incidência cumulativa ao 5° ano dos casos mortais de enfarte de miocárdio em pacientes com história de enfarte de miocárdio (n = 267) e tratados com probucol, foi de 7,3%. Diferenças nos critérios de admissão, na dimensão do grupo estudado e outras variaveis não permitiram uma comparação estatística direta de outros estudos. Todavia, tomando como referência os dados publicados pelo "Coronary Drug Project," a mortalidade e morbilidade relativamente baixas observadas durante o tratamento com probucol sugere também, mesmo que não prove, um efeito protetor do fármaco.

Considerando o atual interesse no possível efeito nocivo dos fármacos hipolipidemizantes sobre a árvore biliar, analisamos a incidência de colecistectomia e de afecções das vias biliares em doentes sujeitos a tratamento prolongado com probucol.

A incidência cumulativa ao 6° ano de afecções das vias biliares (colecistectomia, colelitíase e colecistite) foi de 3,3% para os homens (n = 729) e 5.8% para as mulheres (n = 404), resultando uma incidência combinada de 4,1%. O índice de mortalidade cumulativa ao 6° ano para a colecistectomia foi de 2,2% (n = 729) para homens e 2,7% para mulheres (n = 404), com uma incidência combinada de 2,3%. As diferenças nas características das populações não permitiram uma comparação estatística direta com os dados provenientes de outros grupos. Todavia, as percentagens acima relatadas, não são certamente excessivas.

O PROBUCOL NOS TRATAMENTOS CURTOS E PROLONGADOS DA HIPERLIPOPROTEINEMIA DE TIPO II

V. Beaumont, J. C. Buxtorf, B. Jacotot, and J. L. Beaumont

A ação do probucol foi avaliada em comparação com o placebo num estudo clínico de curta duração em 19 pacientes com hiperlipoproteinemia de tipo II.

Cada doente foi sucessivamente tratado, seguindo uma ordem randomizada, com placebo e probucol (1 g/dia) durante um mês. Os pacientes mantiveram a sua dieta habitual.

Foram comparados os valores de colesterol total, fosfolípides e triglicérides no fim de cada período de tratamento. A avaliação estatística foi feita com o teste de Student "t" em duplas.

O probucol induziu de modo estatisticamente significante uma diminuição média de 9% do colesterol total não interferindo nos níveis séricos de fosfolípidos e triglicéridos. A persistência dos efeitos do probucol sobre lípidos séricos, a sua ação sobre lípidos dos tecidos e a sua tolerância clínica e biológica, foram objecto de um estudo aberto conduzido em 20 doentes com hiperlipoproteinemia tipo II.

Também neste estudo os pacientes mantiveram a própria dieta habitual. Os lípidos séricos foram determinados antes do início do estudo e de cada dois meses de tratamento durante um total de 6 meses.

Antes e ao fim dos 6 meses de tratamento foram colhidos fragmentos de pele para a determinação do colesterol livre e esterificado. Os resultados obtidos foram comparados com os valores correspondentes revelados por um grupo de indivíduos sãos.

No fim do estudo foi observada uma diminuição média do colesterol sérico de 9.9% (p < 0.001) semelhante à revelada após um mês de tratamento. A diminuição do colesterol foi superior a 10% em 60% dos doentes. Também neste caso os fosfolípidos e os triglicérides séricos não foram modificados pelo fármaco de um modo significativo. A taxa de colesterol esterificado da pele foi evidentemente aumentada pelo tratamento.

Não se observaram anomalias nos exames de laboratório; os níveis de SGOT e de SGPT aumentaram, mantendo-se porém dentro dos limites normais.

No conjunto, a tolerância clínica do probucol foi boa. Os Autores concluem que o probucol mantém o efeito hipocolesterolemizante nos tratamentos prolongados e que o fármaco é seguro. O aumento significativo da fração esterificada do colesterol cutâneo na ausência de uma apreciável variação do colesterol total necessita de uma ulterior avaliação.

Como hipótese de trabalho poder-se-ia pensar que tais variações qualitativas possam facilitar a mobilização do colesterol e possam relacionar-se com a observada regressão dos xantelasmas.

TRATAMENTO DAS HIPERCOLESTEROLEMIAS COM PROBUCOL

R. Carmena and J. F. Ascaso

O efeito hipolipidemizante de um novo fármaco, o probucol, foi estudado em 20 pacientes portadores, de hiperlipoproteinemia primária (fenótipo IIa em 7 casos e IIb em 13).

Todos os pacientes receberam uma dieta de baixo conteúdo em colestero e ácidos graxos saturados, e de elevado conteúdo em ácidos graxos polinsaturados.

Após um mês somente de dieta, os doentes foram divididos mediante randomização em duas sequências de tratamento: 10 doentes tratados com probucol (500 mg, duas vezes ao dia) durante dois meses e depois com placebo por mais dois meses, e os restantes 10 receberam os dois tratamentos na ordem inversa. Um mês só de dieta precedeu também a segunda fase do cross-over.

A dieta só por si induziu uma variação da colesterolemia de um valor médio de 403.7 mg/dl para 375.1 mg/dl com uma redução de 7% o que não tem significado estatístico. A introdução de probucol incrementou de maneira evidente o efeito hipocolesterolemizante da dieta (− 32%, p < 0.01). A trigliceridemia não foi modificada pelo fármaco. A tolerância ao probucol foi excelente.

EFEITO DO PROBUCOL NA HIPERCOLESTEROLEMIA PRIMÁRIA

A. Gouveia, A. Noronha, I. Dionísio, S. Félix, B. Barros, and M. Carrageta

Realizámos este ensaio aberto do probucol em indivíduos com hipercolesterolémia primária, de acordo com os seguintes objetivos: (1) avaliar o efeito do probucol em níveis séricos elevados de colesterol e, também, na trigliceridemia; e (2) estudar a incidência e a natureza de reações adversas.

Nos 30 dias que precederam o início do período de medicação, todos os candidatos foram submetidos a exame clínico no nosso Serviço e a provas laboratoriais; durante as entrevistas com os médicos foram motivados a seguir hábitos regulares de alimentação. Foram admitidos ao ensaio os que (1) apresentavam média de 3 valores do colesterol total superior ou igual a 250 mg/dl (método enzimático), com diferenças entre os 3 valores não superiores a 32 mg/dl, e (2) mantinham peso corporal sem variações superiores a 5%.

Dos 34 indivíduos admitidos, dois abandonaram o ensaio na primeira semana de medicação, devido a alterações do trânsito intestinal (1 caso de diarréia e 1 caso de obstipação). Assim, foram estudados 15 homens e 17 mulheres, com idades médias de 47 anos (25 – 65) e de 53 anos (42 – 62), respectivamente.

O período de medicação foi de 2 meses com a posologia diária de 1 g de probucol (2 comprimidos de 250 mg ao café da manhã e outros 2 comprimidos ao jantar); todos os indivíduos continuaram a seguir hábitos regulares de alimentação.

Os resultados demonstram a eficácia do probucol. Ao fim do primeiro mês de medicação, a descida da colesterolemia já era significativa (p < 0.001); o valor médio do colesterol sérico passou de 295 para 245 mg/dl. Ao fim do segundo mês, baixou ainda mais para 228 mg/dl. Portanto, durante o período de medicação de 2 meses a descida foi de 22.7%. Os triglicérides não variaram de modo significativo, não se registaram alterações nas provas laboratoriais e, além dos 2 casos já mencionados, não houve reações adversas.

ENSAIO CLÍNICO DE UM NOVO AGENTE HIPOCOLESTEROLEMIZANTE (PROBUCOL)

A. Castro Ribeiro and A. Pereira Viana

Seguindo um esquema de duplo cego, distribuímos ao acaso 26 indivíduos com hipercolesterolemia primária por dois grupos de tratamento; probucol (500 mg duas vezes por dia) e placebo.

Nos 30 dias que antecederam o ensaio, todos os indivíduos tomaram placebo e foram encorajados a seguir hábitos regulares de dieta. Os valores basais da colesterolemia foram estabelecidos nesse período, pela média aritmética de 3 determinações espaçadas pelo menos de 1 semana; usou-se o método enzimático, aferido por controle de qualidade interno e externo.

Nos 13 indivíduos que tomaram 1 g diário de probucol, durante 3 meses, o valor médio da colesterolemia baixou de 297 para 247 mg/100 ml (16,8%). A análise da covariância mostrou diferença significativa em comparação com o resultado obtido nos 13 indivíduos que tomaram placebo (p < 0,05); a colesterolemia "normalizou" (< 250 mg/100 ml) em 7 indivíduos medicados com probucol, e apenas em 1 indivíduo dos que tomaram placebo (Fisher p = 0,008).

De salientar a subida da colesterolemia após a parada da medicação, pelo que consideramos que a terapêutica com probucol deverá ser mantida.

As variações da trigliceridemia não permitiram estabelecer diferenças significativas entre os grupos de tratamento. O peso corporal não variou de modo importante. Nenhum dos indivíduos abandonou o ensaio por motivo de reações adversas; alterações digestivas ligeiras foram registadas em 5 indivíduos do grupo probucol e em 3 indivíduos do grupo placebo.

Concluímos que o probucol é um hipocolesterolemizante eficaz e bem tolerado nesta amostra da população do Norte de Portugal.

EFEITO DO PROBUCOL SOBRE A COMPOSIÇÃO DA BILE, NO HOMEM—OBSERVAÇÕES PRELIMINARES

Z. Mareček, M. Jirsa, V. Kordač, and L. Kucerova

A ação do probucol sobre os ácidos biliares e sobre a componente lipídica da bile foi estudada em 5 pacientes com hiperlipoproteinemia de tipo IIa e com níveis séricos de colesterol compreendidos entre 310 e 440 mg/dl.

Os indivíduos não haviam sido nunca tratados com probucol e haviam interrompido o uso de todo e qualquer fármaco hipocolesterolemizante pelo menos há um mês.

Após uma colecistografia oral, feita para excluir a presença de cálculos biliares e de colecistopatias, os pacientes foram tratados durante dois meses com probucol na dose de 1 g/dia. Os lípides séricos foram determinados no final de cada duas semanas de tratamento. A bile foi recolhida mediante drenagem duodenal, após injeção de colecistoquinina, antes de iniciar o tratamento e no final do mesmo.

Os ácidos bibliares foram determinados por método enzimático, o colesterol e os fosfolípides por método colorimétrico; o grau de saturação da bile em colesterol pelo índice litogênico de Thomas e Hoffmann.

A composição dos ácidos bibliares foi avaliada mediante cromatografia (gás-líquide) e os ésteres de metil-trimetilsilil foram analisados sobre coluna Hi EFF 8 BP, a 1%.

Pelos resultados obtidos parece que as variações na composição molar relativa dos lípidos biliares induzidas pelo probucol são notavelmente diferentes daquelas observadas após administração de clofibrate.

O clofibrate provoca um aumento da concentração do colesterol biliar e uma redução dos ácidos biliares com consequente aumento da litogênese da bile, e supersaturação da bile com colesterol.

Após administração de probucol observa-se, ao contrário, uma diminuição do colesterol biliar e um aumento dos ácidos biliares com consequente diminuição do indice litogênico.

As variações na composição dos ácidos biliares observadas após o uso de probucol são de modesta intensidade e não são constantes.

EFEITOS DO PROBUCOL NA ABSORÇÃO INTESTINAL DE CÁLCIO E NO TRATAMENTO ANTICOAGULANTE PROLONGADO EM PACIENTES COM HIPERCOLESTEROLEMIA ASSOCIADA A AFECÇÕES CARDIOVASCULARES

A. Rapado and M. Diaz-Curiel

Vinte pacientes hipercolesterolemicos do tipo IIa foram tratados por um período médio de 14 meses, com probucol em doses variáveis de 0,5 a 1,5 g / dia adicionado a uma dieta de baixo teor em colesterol e em ácidos graxos saturados. O tratamento realmente reduziu o colesterol sérico (− 31%, p < 0.01) e não modificou o nível dos triglicérides. O efeito do probucol sobre o metabolismo do cálcio / vitamina D foi estudado, mediante medições da absorção intestinal do ^{47}Ca, antes e durante o tratamento com probucol. A atividade sobre a vitamina K foi determinada mediante o controle do tempo de protrombina em doentes em tratamento crônico com anticoagulantes.

Não foram evidenciadas interações entre os fármacos. Particularmente interessante foi o efeito do probucol numa menina de 12 anos homozigota para a hiperlipoproteinemia de tipo IIa, que durante o tratamento com colestiramina havia apresentado sinais bioquímicos de raquitismo exigindo uma intensa terapia específica. Nesta paciente o probucol reduziu de modo significativo a taxa de colesterol sérico sem modificações na absorção intestinal do ^{47}Ca e sem sinais bioquímicos de raquitismo.

PROBUCOL: AVALIAÇÃO DA EFICÁCIA SOBRE OS LÍPIDES E LIPOPROTEINAS

J. Rouffy, B. Chanu, R. Bakir, and J. Goy-Loeper

O efeito do probucol—1 g / dia—nos lípides e lipoproteínas séricas foi estudado em pacientes com hiperlipoproteinemia primária de tipo IIa e IIb resistentes à dieta; alguns destes doentes não tinham, previamente, dado resposta satisfatoria ao clofibrate, procetofen e à colestiramina.

A duração do tratamento foi de 1 mês em 34 pacientes (T_1), de 3 a 6 meses em 16 (T_2), de 6 meses a um ano em 12 (T_3) e superior a 1 ano em 4 (T_4).

No fim dos vários períodos de tratamento, com excepção de T_3, foi observada uma redução significativa dos lípides séricos totais (de 8 a 19%) do colesterol total (de 8 a 12%) e de LDL-colesterol (de 9 a 15%) e um evidente aumento da relação HDL-COL / LDL-COL + VLDL-COL.

Não foram notadas interações com os anticoagulantes. Este estudo tem demonstrado que o probucol é um fármaco eficaz para a redução dos lípides séricos totais, do colesterol total e do colesterol das lipoproteínas de baixa densidade que é fracção lipoproteica mais aterogênica.

Um outro resultado favorável induzido pelo probucol é o aumento da relação HDL-COL / LDL-COL + VLDL-COL com consequente melhora do índex aterogênico.

A tolerância ao produto foi excelente tanto do ponto de vista clínico como laboratorial.

O PROBUCOL NO TRATAMENTO DA HIPERCOLESTEROLEMIA EM PACIENTES COM DISTÚRBIOS CARDIOVASCULARES

L. Scebat and J. Renais

O probucol (500 mg duas vezes / dia) e uma dieta de baixo teor lipídico foram prescritos, durante um período variável de 12 a 46 meses, a 33 pacientes com afecções cardiovasculares de base aterosclerótica e com hipercolesterolemia de tipo IIa ((11 doentes), IIb + III (21 doentes), tipo IV (1 doente).

No conjunto o tratamento induziu uma diminuição do colesterol de uma concentração média de 329.5 para 281.1 mg / dl (− 14.5% p < 0.001). 12 pacientes não tiveram resposta satisfatória (redução do colesterol ≤ 10%), e 20 pacientes (62.5%) responderam ao tratamento com a dieta + probucol.

Em 3 casos observou-se uma diminuição do efeito hipocolesterolemizante do fármaco após o 6°-mês. O resultado obtido no primeiro ano mantevese em 15 pacientes (46.8%). O efeito do probucol sobre o colesterol sérico foi semelhante nos pacientes com hipercolesterolemia primária (tipo IIa) e nos com hiperlipemia mista (tipo IIb + III).

O probucol não interagiu com os outros fármacos usualmente prescritos nas afecções cardiovasculares, em particular com as substâncias antivitamina K e os diuréticos.

Não foram registradas alterações das provas de função hepática e renal, da glicemia e do exame hematológico. O peso corporal permaneceu quase invariável. O eletrocardiograma não foi modificado pelo tratamento. Três pacientes tiveram diarréia, que se resolveu durante o curso do tratamento em 2 indivíduos, e que causou a suspensão do probucol durante a segunda semana, no terceiro indivíduo.

EFECTO DEL PROBUCOL Y DE OTROS MEDICAMENTOS EN LA SINTESIS DE LOS ESTEROLES TRATAMENTOS HIPOLIPIDÊMICOS

S. Stefanović and L. Vucić

A ação do probucol sobre a hipercolesterolemia foi estudada em 15 pacientes: 11 com hiperlipoproteinemia de tipo IIa e quatro de tipo IIb. Nestes pacientes a hipercolesterolemia foi diagnosticada entre 1 e 20 anos antes deste estudo: em média durava há 7 anos.

Todos os pacientes haviam sido tratados sem sucesso, num primeiro tempo, com a dieta, e num segundo com a dieta e clofibrate, ou com a junção, em alguns casos, de colestiramina ou fosfatidilcolina. As concentrações de colesterol anteriores à administração do probucol estavam compreendidas entre 306 e 565 mg/dl ($\overline{X}$: 385 mg/dl). Todos os pacientes foram tratados com 1 g de probucol por dia, durante um período de três meses. Os controles foram feitos no fim de cada mês. No final do tratamento em todos os pacientes, com exceção de um, os valores de colesterol estavam compreendidos dentro dos limites normais para as respectivas idades, ou seja entre 214 e 280 mg/dl (X: 229 mg/dl).

Durante a administração do probucol não foram observados efeitos colaterais clinicamente evidentes ou anomalias nos exames de laboratorio e não foram notados distúrbios subjetivos.

Resúmenes en Español

EFECTO DEL PROBUCOL Y DE OTROS MEDICAMENTOS EN LA SINTESI DE LOS ESTEROLES EN LOS LINFOCITOS HUMANOS

A. Anastasi, D. J. Betteridge, and D. J. Galton

Los recursos terapéuticos empleados en la actualidad para el tratamiento de la hipercolesterolemia no son satisfactorios y por lo tanto existe la necesidad de hallar nuevos medicamentos.

El linfocito humano es una célula que puede ser empleada con utilidad en el estudio de los efectos que sobre la síntesis esteroide pueden ejercer las substancias potencialmente hipocolesterolemiantes.

En linfocitos aislados, la síntesis esteroide es suprimida cuando las células son incubadas en presencia del lipoproteínas de baja densidad (LDL). Cuando del medio de incubación son eliminadas las LDL, se observa un aumento de la síntesis de los esteroides debido a la inducción de la HMG-CoA reductasa, la enzima que determina el progreso de la reacción.

Hemos estudiado los efectos del cicloheximide, un inhibidor de la traslación de la síntesis proteica, y de la cordicepina (3'-desoxiadenosina), un inhibidor de la transcripción de la síntesis de ácido ribonucleico (mRNA) en la inducción de la síntesis esteroide en linfocitos humanos, recién aislados e incubados en un medio conteniente suero con bajo contenido de lipoproteínas (LPDS). También hemos estudiado otras substancias tales como el Compactin y el Probucol que pueden ejercer una acción directa sobre el progreso de la síntesis. El cicloheximide (20 µg/ml) ha inhibido la inducción de la syntesis esteroide mediata por LPDS surgiriendo que el aumento se debe a una síntesis *ex novo* de las enzimas.

La cordicepina (50 µg/ml) no posee efecto alguno en la inducción de la síntesis esteroide de LPDS, no obstante haya reducido de un 50% la síntesis del mRNA. Además, en linfocitos preincubados con LDL en presencia de cordicepina durante 40 h (en este período el "pool" de mRNA con una breve semivida debería resultar muy reducido), el aumento de la síntesis esteroide sucesiva a la remoción del LDL del medio de incubación ha resultado ser de la misma importancia que el observado en las células preincubadas sin cordicepina. Esto sugiere que la semivida de la HMG-CoA-reductasa mRNA sea relativamente larga y que el mRNA no sea indispensable para la inducción de la síntesis esteroide.

El compactin (0.2 µg) ha inhibido en un 65% la síntesis de los esteroides sin modificar la incorporación del ^{14}C mevalonato en los esteroles sugiriendo que el medicamento ejerce un efecto inhibidor específico de la actividad de la HMG-CoA-reductasa.

Emulsiones de probucol en concentraciones hasta 1 mM en albúmina sérica bovina (medio en el cual el medicamento es poco soluble) han inhibido en un 40% aproximadamente la síntesis esteroide a partir del ^{14}C-acetato. Es posible que esto contribuya a la acción hipocolesterolemiante del medicamento.

FARMACOLOGIA DEL PROBUCOL

D. Kritchevsky

El Probucol, 4,4'(isopropilideneditio)*bis*(2,6-di-t-butilfenol), demostró una eficaz acción hipocolesterolemiante en distintas especies animales (ratón, rata, perro, mono) y en el hombre.

En el ratón el efecto hipocolesterolemiante resulta directamente relacionado a la dosis administrada. Estudios conducidos en el animal sobre el mecanismo de acción, parecen indicar un aumento de la excreción fecal de los ácidos biliares, una inhibición de la síntesis y una disminución de la absorción del colesterol. En monos hipercolesterolémicos tratados con probucol, el colesterol sérico resultó ser inferior al 52% respecto al de los animales de control. Además, el probucol provocó una significativa disminución del colesterol hepático y un significativo aumento del colesterol esplénico mientras no modificó la tasa de colesterol en los demás 17 tejidos examinados. Por lo tanto el tratamiento con probucol no parece provocar una apreciable redistribución del colesterol en el organismo. De acuerdo con Miettinen (*Atherosclerosis,* 15, 163, 1972), el probucol actúa por medio de la inhibición de la síntesis y de la absorción del colesterol, aumentando la excreción de los ácidos biliares.

Cuando monos hipercolesterolémicos son tratados con probucol, se observa un aumento de la excreción de los ácidos biliares y no de los esteroides neutros.

En el perro el probucol induce fibrilación ventricular, aunque en las demás especies animales examinadas no se han observado estos efectos colaterales. Después de la administración de probucol marcado con ^{14}C, durante 4 días el 84% de la radiactividad es excretado con las heces y el 1 – 2% con la orina. Después de la administración de probucol marcado con ^{14}C, la semivida del medicamento ha resultado de 0,8 y 12,8 días en el mono, siendo de 1 y 15,2 días en el perro.

El tratamiento con probucol no influye sobre la actividad de las enzimas hepáticas tales como catalasas, LDH (lactato-deshidrogenasa) y glutamato-deshidrogenasa, y no modifica los niveles de glucógeno hepático.

Cuando se administra a monos hipercolesterolémicos, el probucol disminuye del

25% la tasa de colesterol de la aorta. En conejos sometidos a dieta aterogénica, adicionando probucol en una concentración del 1%, hay una significativa inhibición del proceso aterosclerótico.

RESULTADOS DE ESTUDIOS TOXICOPATOLOGICOS CON PROBUCOL Y ESTUDIO COMPARATIVO SOBRE LA MORFOLOGIA HEPATICA DE RATAS TRATADAS CON PROBUCOL, FENOFIBRATO Y CLOFIBRATO

J. Molello, S. Barnard, and J. Lebeau

El probucol fue administrado por vía oral a 40 monos de ambos sexos a la dosis de 0, 60, 125, 250 y 500 mg/kg/día. Se han sacrificado 14 monos después de 18 y 24 meses de tratamiento; en 21 animales el ensayo se ha alargado durante 8 años. Los parámetros examinados incluían el ritmo de crecimiento, datos hematológicos y hematoquímicos, análisis de las orinas, peso de los órganos, examen macroscópico, histológico y electromicroscópico de los tejidos. Cinco monos murieron durante el ensayo, no siendo nigún fallecimiento debido a la administración del medicamento. No se han observado diferencias significativas entre los animales tratados y los controles.

Se ha ensayado el efecto del probucol, comparado con el clofibrato y el fenofibrato, sobre la ultraestructura de la célula hepática de ratas Sprague-Dawley. Los medicamentos se administraron mezclados con la dieta, a las dosis de aproximadamente 500, 250, 100 mg/kg/día respectivamente de probucol, clofibrato y fenofibrato durante un período de tiempo que alcanzaba hasta los 91 días. Los animales de control recibieron solamente la dieta. Los 3 medicamentos examinados han reducido significativamente la tasa de colesterol sérico.

La morfología hepática de las ratas tratadas con probucol no se diferenció respecto a los animales de control.

El clofibrato y el fenofibrato han provocado hepatocitomegalia, aumento del número de peroxisomas y ligeras alteraciones del retículo endoplasmático y de las mitocondrias. Los resultados de estos y otros experimentos demuestran que el probucol, en tratamientos a corto y largo plazo, es bien tolerado por ratones, ratas, conejos, monos y cobayos mantenidos en condiciones normales de laboratorio, o sometidos a un fuerte stress cardiovascular. En cambio los perros no siguen esta regla y desarrollan una sensibilización miocárdica a la epinefrina e a la norepinefrina.

Contrariamente a lo que ocurre con algunos agentes anticolesterolémicos, el probucol no altera la morfología hepatocelular de los roedores y de los primates subhumanos. Los datos obtenidos en estos estudios toxicológicos indican que el probucol es un compuesto seguro.

EFECTO HIPOCOLESTEROLEMIANTE DEL PROBUCOL Y SU MECANISMO DE ACCION EN EL RATON Y EN EL CONEJO

R. Infante and D. Petit

El efecto del probucol en los lípidos plasmáticos y tisulares ha sido ensayado en el ratón y en el conejo bajo distintas condiciones alimenticias (dieta standard, dietas sin grasas, dieta con un reducido contenido de grasas y colesterol, dieta hipercolesterolémica).

Cuando es administrado a animales sometidos a dieta standard, el probucol reduce marcadamente el colesterol sérico en el ratón (− 33% y − 60% en comparación con los controles respectivamente después de 7 y 21 días de tratamiento con 0.6 g de probucol por cada kg de comida) y en el conejo (− 37% y − 41% en comparación con los controles después de 10 días de tratamiento con 1 g y 2.5 g de probucol por cada kg de comida, respectivamente) sin modificar los lípidos hepáticos.

En animales sometidos a una dieta con contenido lipídico igual al 0%, 1%, 3% ó 10%, el probucol no ha determinado ninguna actividad en las dos primeras condiciones experimentales mencionadas. El efecto hipocolesterolemiante ha resultado evidente cuando el medicamento fue administrado con la dieta con contenido de grasas del 3% y en aquellos animales sometidos a una dieta hiperlipídica (grasas al 10% y colesterol al 1%) el probucol además previno el desarrollo de la hiperlipemia.

En el ratón, después de una única administración intravenosa de probucol, se ha observado una rápida, marcada y prolongada disminución de la tasa de colesterol hemático. En el conejo el medicamento ha prevenido el efecto hiperlipídico de una administración intravenosa de fosfolípidos. En el ratón sometido a dieta standard el tratamiento durante 7 y 21 días con probucol a la concentración de 0.6 g/kg con la comida no ha modificado significativamente la incorporación de ^{14}C-mevalonato en el colesterol hepático, intestinal y en el esqueleto.

Se ha observado una disminución de la incorporación de la radiactividad en el colesterol plasmático. Se ha postulado un efecto específico del medicamento a nivel de las lipoproteínas.

Resultados preliminares obtenidos en ratones tratados durante 4 semanas con probucol a la concentración de 0.6 g/kg con la dieta, han demostrado una disminución de la velocidad de síntesis de las VLDL.

EL PROBUCOL EN EL TRATAMIENTO CRONICO DE LA HIPERCOLESTEROLEMIA

D. McCaughan

Se ha estudiado el probucol, de acuerdo con un diseño experimental en doble ciego, controlado vs placebo, durante un año, en 118 pacientes afectados de hipercolesterolemia esencial (valores pre-tratamiento de colesterol sérico $\geqslant$ 250 mg/dl). Después de 6 y 12 meses de tratamiento, la disminución media de colesterol sérico respecto a los valores basales, oscilaba entre 16.2 y 20.9% en el grupo de pacientes tratados con probucol (n. 88), y entre 5.2% – 12.7% en los pacientes tratados con placebo (n. 30) (p < 0.001).

Se ha continuado el tratamiento de probucol en forma no controlada durante períodos de tiempo de hasta 9 años en 61 de los enfermos ya tratados con el medicamento durante el estudio controlado.

Después del segundo año de tratamiento con probucol, la disminución de colesterol sérico variaba entre 23.1 y 27.4%, continuando posteriormente alrededor de los mismos valores. La mortalidad total al término de los 5 años de tratamiento fue del 9%. La incidencia de la mortalidad por causas coronarias y aquella de infartos miocárdicos no fatales durante cinco años, fue del 14%.

El medicamento fue bien tolerado. Los efectos colaterales observados más frecuentemente fueron ablandamiento de las heces y diarrea.

Los resultados obtenidos demuestran que el probucol es un medicamento bien tolerado, eficaz para el tratamiento crónico de pacientes afectados de hipercolesterolemia esencial.

EFECTO DEL PROBUCOL Y DE LA DIETA SOBRE LOS LIPIDOS SERICOS Y LAS FRACCIONES LIPOPROTEICAS EN LA HIPERCOLESTEROLEMIA ESENCIAL

R. Mordasini, M. Keller, and W. F. Riesen

El efecto del probucol sobre varias fracciones lipídicas se ha estudiado en 27 pacientes con hipercolesterolemia esencial.

Los pacientes recibieron durante por lo menos tres meses una dieta isocalórica de bajo contenido lipídico y con una relación modificada de ácidos grasos saturados/insaturados (NIH dieta tipo II). A esta fase seguió un período de pretratamiento, de 6 semanas, durante el cual, asociado a la dieta se administraba el placebo. Durante el subsiguiente estudio llevado a cabo en doble ciego, se han tratado los pacientes con dieta y placebo (1 comprimido 4 veces al día) o con dieta y probucol (1 comprimido de 250 mg 4 veces al día). Los comprimidos de placebo y de probucol eran iguales entre sí. Los controles de los pacientes ambulatorios se efectuaron con intervalos mensuales. Se han analizado los parámetros indicados a continuación: colesterol y triglicéridos séricos totales y, después de ultracentrifugación, colesterol y triglicéridos de las lipoproteínas de baja densidad (LDL) y alta densidad (HDL), apo B y AI (por medio de RID) y apo AII (por medio de RIA). Comparado con los valores medios obtenidos con placebo, durante el tratamiento con probucol la concentración de colesterol total ha resultado reducida en un promedio del 41 mg/100 ml (− 13%, p < 0.05). El LDL-colesterol se ha reducido notablemente asociado al colesterol total, siendo la disminución en promedio del 42 mg/100 ml (− 16%, p < 0.025).

También se ha observado una ligera disminución, estadísticamente no significativa, del nivel del HDL-colesterol. La administración de placebo no provocó modificaciones significativas del colesterol total, del LDL-colesterol y del HDL-colesterol. La trigliceridemia no se modificó tanto con el tratamiento con probucol como con placebo.

Bajo tratamiento con probucol la concentración de las apo B resultó reducida en un promedio del 12%, siendo esta variación no estadísticamente significativa (p < 0.15). Los niveles de apo B han quedado constantes durante el tratamiento con placebo. En el grupo tratado con probucol se ha observado una disminución media del 16% de las apo AI (p < 0.0005), y del 55% de las apo AII (p < 0.0005). Se observó también una disminución de las concentraciones de apo AI y apo AII en el grupo tratado con placebo.

De cualquier manera esta disminución ha resultado estadísticamente significativa solamente para las apo AII (− 26%, p < 0.005).

El tratamiento con probucol ha resultado habitualmente bien tolerado. El estudio fue interrumpido en 4 pacientes debido a efectos colaterales principalmente subjetivos. Tres de estos pacientes estaban sometidos a tratamiento con placebo y uno bajo tratamiento con probucol.

NIVELES DE LIPOPROTEINAS DE ALTA DENSIDAD DURANTE UN PERIODO DE CINCO AÑOS DE INTERVENCION MULTFACTORIAL CONTRA LOS FACTORES DE RIESGO DE LA ENFERMEDAD CORONARIA

T. A. Miettinen, J. K. Huttunen, T. Kumlin,
V. Naukkarinen, S. Mattila, and C. Enholm

El colesterol sérico (C), los triglicéridos (TG), el colesterol de las lipoproteínas de alta densidad (HDLC), las apoproteínas AI y AII de las lipoproteínas con alta densidad (HDL-AI, HDL-AII) y las apoproteínas AII de las lipoproteínas de no alta densidad (AII no HDL), han sido determinados en 119 sujetos de sexo masculino que habían participado durante períodos de hasta 4 años en una investigación controlada conducida con la finalidad de reducir los factores de riesgo de las coronariopatías. El tratamiento implicaba también una orientación dietética e higiénica y, cuando se considerase necesario, la administración de medicamentos antihipertensivos e hipolipidemiantes.

El colesterol y los triglicéridos totales se han determinado a varios intervalos durante el desarrollo de la investigación mientras el HDLC, las HDL-AI, las HDL-AII y las AII no HDL se han valorado solamente durante el cuarto año del ensayo.

Por estos parãmetros no ha resultado posible valerse de los valores basales ya que la conservación prolongada hasta los cuatro años determina una destacada disminución de su concentración sérica. Los niveles de lípidos séricos totales han resultado parecidos en los sujetos sometidos a dieta solamente (n. 32) y en los tratados con medicamentos antihipertensivos (n. 19). Respecto a los grupos mencionados, los sujetos tratados con clofibrato (n. 305 han presentado tasas parecidas de AI, un aumento de AII igual al 34% y un aumento de HDLC equivalente al 13%.

Después de tratamiento con probucol, empleado en casos de hiperlipoproteinemia de tipo IIA (n. 25), se ha observado una disminución de la tasa de colesterol total (− 13%), de HDLC (− 29%) y de HDL AI (− 16%), mientras no se hallaba diferencias de HDL-AII cuyo nivel no se diferenciaba respecto al encontrado en sujetos sometidos solamente a dieta o tratados con medicamentos antihipertensivos. El nivel de los n-HDL-AI era reducido.

Los sujetos tratados al mismo tiempo con clofibrato y probucol (en mayoría individuos de tipo IIB: n. 13) no han sufrido substanciales modificaciones de los lípidos séricos presentando sin embrago una disminución del 55% en el HDLC, una disminución del 41% en las AI y un reducido nivel de no-HDL-AI mientras los datos de AII resultaban parecidos a los observados en el grupo de sujetos sometidos solamente a la dieta. Los resultados hacen suponer que, no obstante el probucol y el clofibrato disminuyen el HDLC durante tratamiento prolongado, al mismo tiempo reducen la relación colesterol/apoliporoteína de las HDL, esto es el nivel medio de saturación del colesterol de la fracción HDL.

Las modificaciones producidas por el clofibrato resultaban en parte asociadas a las alteraciones de la concentración de los triglicéridos, mientras las modificaciones observadas en los grupos de pacientes tratados con probucol fueron relacionadas con la duración del tratamiento.

EFICACIA Y TOLERANCIA DEL PROBUCOL VERSUS CLOFIBRATO

J. L. De Gennes and J. Truffert

El efecto hipocolesterolemiante del probucol y del clofibrato se han comparado en un estudio llevado a cabo en doble ciego en 38 pacientes afectados de hiper-colesterolemia esencial.

19 pacientes han sido tratados durante dos meses con probucol a la dosis diaria de 1 g y los demás 19 con clofibrato—2 g/día—durante el mismo período.

Todos los pacientes habían observado una dieta con bajo contenido de colesterol y ãcidos grasos saturados y con alto contenido de ácidos grasos polinsaturados iniciada dos meses antes del comienzo del estudio. Durante este período se administraba placebo a los enfermos. La adición de probucol a la dieta provocó una disminución del colesterol sérico del 13% (p < 0.05 en comparación con los valores observados al final del período dieta + placebo). Con el tratamiento con clofibrato, la disminución del colesterol sérico ha resultado del 11%. Este valor no ha alcanzado niveles significativos. La disminución del colesterol ha resultado superior al 20% en el 31% de los pacientes tratados con probucol y en el 21% de los casos tratados con clofibrato.

El nivel de los triglicéridos no ha resultado significativamente modificado por el empleo de los dos medicamentos.

Ambos tratamientos han sido bien tolerados.

El probucol puede ser eficazmente empleado para el tratamiento de los pacientes resistentes al clofibrato y sus derivados.

La ausencia de poder litógeno y de interacciones con los medicamentos normalmente empleados en este tipo de pacientes, hace que probucol sea una efectiva contribución adicional para el tratamiento de las hipercolesterolemia.

EXPERIENCIA CLINICA CON EL PROBUCOL: EFECTO HIPOCOLESTEROLEMIANTE Y TOLERANCIA

R. E. Tedeschi, H. L. Taylor, and B. L. Martz

El efecto a largo plazo del probucol ha sido valorado en 1,133 enfermos tratados en el curso de estudios clínicos cuidadosamente controlados en U.S.A.

Se han tratado 881 enfermos de acuerdo con un protocolo común y, a finales de mayo de 1979, 291 de éstos habían sido controlados durante un período de cinco años y 139 durante un período de 8 años. El 68% de los enfermos tratados con probucol a la dosis de 1 g/día durante 8 años, presentaba una disminución ≥ 15% de la concentración sérica de colesterol respecto a los valores basales. El 82% de los enfermos tratados con probucol ha presentado una disminución de la colesterolemia ≥ 10% respecto a los controles. La disminución media de colesterol en este grupo ha resultado del 19.9%. No hubo evidencias de fenómeno de "escape" en estos pacientes.

El efecto colateral más frecuentemente citado ha resultado la presencia de heces blandas. Se ha observado, además, flatulencia, gastralgias, náusea, vómito y dolores abdominales.

Las pruebas de laboratorio correspondientes al examen hematológico y las pruebas de funcionalidad hepática y renal, no han evidenciado signos de toxicidad.

El análisis de la morbilidad y de la mortalidad ha sido efectuado en todos los 1,133 enfermos tratados con probucol, aplicando el método de las tablas de mortalidad. El 98% de estos enfermos tenía una tasa de colesterol sérico ≥ 250 mg% y muchos presentaban otros factores de riesgo para el desarrollo de coronariopatías.

El porcentaje de mortalidad acumulativa al 5° año (considerando todas las causas) ha resultado el 6.5%. El porcentaje acumulativo al 5° año de casos no mortales de infarto miocárdico en enfermos con historia de infarto de miocardio (n. 267) tratados con probucol, ha resultado igual al 7.3%. Diferencias en los criterios de admisión y en la importancia del grupo estudiado, así como otras variables, no han permitido una comparación estadística directa con otros ensayos. Sin embargo, tomando como referencia los datos publicados por el "Coronary Drug Project," la relativamente reducida mortalidad y morbilidad observada durante el tratamiento con probucol, indica, aunque no demuestra, un efecto protector del medicamento.

Teniendo en cuenta el actual interés en el posible efecto dañino de los medicamentos hipolipidemiantes sobre el tracto biliar hemos examinado la importancia de las colecistectomías y de las afecciones de las vías biliares en enfermos tratados durante largo plazo con probucol. El valor acumulativo de las afecciones de las vías biliares al 6° año (colecistectomía, colelitiasis y colecistitis) ha resultado igual al 3.3% para los varones (n. 729) y al 5.8% para las hembras (n. 404): con un porcentaje total del 4.1%. La importancia acumulativa de colecistectomías al 6° año ha resultado igual al 2.2% en los varones (n. 729) y al 2.7% en las hembras (N. 404) con un valor global del 2.3%.

Las diferentes características de las poblaciones, el decurso clínico a menudo asintomático y otras variables no han permitido una directa comparación estadística con los datos obtenidos por otros grupos. De cualquier manera, los valores porcentuales anteriormente indicados ciertamente no son excesivos.

EL PROBUCOL EN EL TRATAMIENTO A CORTO Y LARGO PLAZO DE LA HIPERLIPOPROTEINEMIA DE TIPO II

V. Beaumont, J. C. Buxtorf, B. Jacotot, and J. L. Beaumont

La acción del probucol ha sido valorada en comparación con placebo en un estudio a corto plazo llevado a cabo en 19 pacientes afectados de hiperlipoproteinemia de tipo II. Cada paciente fue sometido sucesivamente a un tratamiento randomizado con placebo y probucol (1 g/día) durante un mes.

Los pacientes seguían su dieta habitual. Se han comparado los valores de colesterol total, fosfolípidos y triglicéridos determinados al término de cada período de tratamiento. La valoración estadística se ha efectuado con la prueba de Student "t" pareada.

El probucol produjo una disminución del colesterol sérico total del 9% (p < 0.001) mientras no modificó en modo estadísticamente significativo la fosfolipidemia y la trigliceridemia. La persistencia de los efectos del probucol sobre los lípidos séricos, su acción sobre los lípidos tisulares y su tolerancia clínica y biológica, han sido objeto de un estudio abierto en 20 pacientes con hiperlipoproteinemia de tipo II.

También en este estudio los pacientes han seguido su dieta habitual. La determinación de los lípidos séricos se ha efectuado antes del inicio del estudio y cada dos meses de tratamiento durante seis meses en conjunto.

Antes de empezar el tratamiento y al final de los seis meses se analizaron fragmentos cutáneos para determinar el colesterol libre y esterificado. Los resultados han sido comparados con los valores correspondientes obtenidos de un grupo de sujetos sanos.

Al final del estudio se ha observado una disminución media de colesterol sérico igual al 9.9% (p < 0.001) parecida al valor encontrado después de un mes de tratamiento. La caida del colesterol resultó > 10% en el 60% de los pacientes. También en este caso el medicamento no ha modificado significativamente los fosfolípidos y los triglicéridos séricos. El tratamiento ha aumentado significativamente la tasa de colesterol esterificado cutáneo.

No se han encontrado anomalías en los exámenes de laboratorio; los niveles de SGOT y de SGPT han aumentado, quedando sin embargo posteriormente en valores normales. En conjunto la tolerancia clínica del probucol ha resultado buena.

Los Autores concluyen que el probucol sigue manteniendo el efecto hipocolesterolemiante durante tratamientos prolongados y que es un medicamento seguro. El aumento significativo de la fracción esterificada del colesterol cutáneo sin una significativa modificación del colesterol total necesita una ulterior valoración. Como hipótesis de trabajo es posible opinar que estas modificaciones cualitativas pueden favorecer la movilización del colesterol pudiendo ser relacionadas con la regresión observada de los xantelasmas.

TRATAMIENTO DE LAS HIPERCOLESTEROLEMIAS CON PROBUCOL

R. Carmena and J. F. Ascaso

El efecto hipolipidemiante de un nuevo medicamento, el probucol, ha sido ensayado en 20 pacientes afectados por hiperlipoproteinemia esencial (fenotipo IIa en 7 casos y IIb en 13 casos).

Todos los pacientes seguían una dieta de bajo contenido de colesterol y ácidos grasos saturados y con alto contenido de ácidos grasos polinsaturados. Después de un mes solamente de dieta se han asignado por medio de randomización los pacientes a dos distintos esquemas de tratamiento: 10 pacientes han sido sometidos durante dos meses al tratamiento con probucol (500 mg b.i.d.) y luego durante los dos meses sucesivos al tratamiento con placebo mientras los demás 10 pacientes has recibido los dos tratamientos en orden inverso. Un mes con dieta sola ha precedido también la segunda fase del cross-over. La dieta sola ha producido una disminución de la colesterolemia desde un valor medio de 403.7 mg/dl hasta 375.1 mg/dl con una reducción del 7% que no ha alcanzado niveles significativos.

La adición de probucol ha aumentado significativamente el efecto hipocolesterol-

emiante de la dieta (− 32%, p < 0.01). El medicamento no ha modificado la tasa de triglicéridos.
La tolerancia del probucol ha resultado excelente.

EFECTO DEL PROBUCOL EN LA HIPERCOLESTEROLEMIA ESENCIAL

A Gouveia, A. Noronha, I. Dionisio, S. Felix, B. Barros, and M. Carrageta

La finalidad de este estudio conducido en forma no controlada en pacientes afectados de hipercolesterolemia esencial, era valorar la acción hipocolesterolemiante del probucol y estudiar la naturaleza y la frecuencia de los efectos colaterales.

A los pacientes se les recomendó seguir una dieta standard durante un mes, siendo sometidos seguidamente a exámenes clínicos y de laboratorio. Se han admitido en el estudio pacientes con una media de tres determinaciones de colesterol sérico ⩾ 250 mg/100 ml (método enzimático) cuyos valores no debían diferenciarse entre ellos más de 32 mg/100 ml y con variaciones de peso corporal ⩾ 5%. De los 34 pacientes incluidos en el ensayo, 2 han interrumpido el tratamiento durante la primera semana debido a trastornos intestinales. Por lo tanto el ensayo se ha llevado a cabo en 15 varones y 17 hembras con edad media respectivamente de 47 años (desde los 25 hasta los 65 años) y de 53 años (desde los 42 hasta los 62 años). Los 32 pacientes han sido sometidos durante dos meses al tratamiento de 1 g/día de probucol (2 comprimidos de 250 mg con el desayuno y otros dos con la cena) continuando la dieta standard.

Los resultados de este estudio confirman la eficacia del probucol.

La tasa de colesterol, ya significativamente disminuida al final del primer mes de tratamiento (p < 0.001), se ha reducido ulteriormente durante el segundo mes. Los triglicéridos no resultaron significativamente modificados.

No había ningún dato de importancia en los exámenes clínicos y en los análisis de laboratorio.

El probucol ha resultado bien tolerado. No se han observado efectos colaterales con la excepción de los dos pacientes anteriormente mencionados.

ENSAYO CLINICO CON UN NUEVO MEDICAMENTO HIPOCOLESTEROLEMIANTE: EL PROBUCOL

A. Castro Ribeiro and A. Pereira Viana

Se ha administrado el probucol (500 mg b.i.d.) y el placebo a 26 pacientes afectados por hipercolesterolemia esencial, de acuerdo con un esquema randomizado a doble ciego. Un mes antes de empezar el ensayo los pacientes han sido sometidos a una dieta standard, siendo al mismo tiempo tratados con placebo. Durante este período se han efectuado tres determinaciones de la colesterolemia a intervalos semanales, siendo la media de estos valores considerada dato basal. Después de tres meses de tratamiento con probucol el nivel medio del colesteral sérico había disminuido desde 297 hasta 247 mg/100 ml. El análisis de la covarianza ha evidenciado una diferencia significativa (p < 0.05) respecto al grupo de pacientes tratados con placebo. Además se ha observado una normalización de los niveles de colesterol sérico (< 250 mg/100 ml) en 7 pacientes tratados con probucol y un paciente bajo placebo (prueba de Fisher p < 0.008).

Las variaciones de los niveles de triglicéridos no han resultado significativamente distintas en los dos grupos. El peso corporal ha quedado prácticamente sin modificaciones. Ningún enfermo ha tenido que interrumpir el ensayo debido a los efectos colaterales. 5 pacientes tratados con probucol y tres pacientes tratados con placebo tuvieron trastornos gastrointestinales de modesta entidad.

Los resultados que hemos observado confirman que el probucol es un hipocolesterolemiante eficaz y bien tolerado.

EFECTO DEL PROBUCOL SOBRE LA COMPOSICION BILIAR EN EL HOMBRE. OBSERVACIONES PRELIMINARES

Z. Mareček, M. Jirsa, V. Kordač, and L. Kucěrová

La acción del probucol sobre los ácidos biliares y sobre la componente lipídica de la bilis ha sido ensayada en 5 pacientes con hiperlipoproteinemia de tipo IIa y con niveles séricos de colesterol incluidos entre 310 y 440 mg/dl. Los sujetos no habían sido nunca tratados con probucol, habiendo interrumpido la administración de cualquier medicamento hipocolesterolemiante durante por lo menos un mes antes del tratamiento.

Después de una colecistografía oral, efectuada con la finalidad de excluir la presencia de cálculos biliares y de colecistopatías, se han sometido los pacientes al tratamiento de probucol a la dosis de 1 g/día durante dos meses. Se han determinado los lípidos séricos cada dos semanas de tratamiento. La bilis se ha recogido por medio de drenaje duodenal, después de una inyección de colecistoquinina, antes del inicio y al final del tratamiento.

Los ácidos biliares han sido determinados con método enzimático, el colesterol y los fosfolípidos con método colorimétrico; el grado de saturación de colesterol en la bilis se ha determinado por medio del índice litógeno de Thomas y Hoffmann.

La composición de los ácidos biliares se ha valorado por medio de cromatografía gas-líquida, siendo analizados los metil-trimetilsilil ésteres sobre columna 1% Hi EFF 8 BP.

De acuerdo con los resultados obtenidos parece que las modificaciones de la composición molar de los lípidos biliares producidas por el probucol son notablemente diferentes respecto a las observadas después de la administración de clofibrato.

El clofibrato provoca un aumento de la concentración de colesterol biliar y una disminución de los ácidos biliares con el consecuente aumento de la litogenicidad de la bilis por supersaturación de la bilis con colesterol. Por el contrario, después de la administración de probucol se observa una disminución del colesterol biliar y un aumento de los ácidos biliares con la consecuente disminución del índice litógeno.

Las modificaciones de la composición de los ácidos biliares observadas después de tratamiento con probucol, resultan de modesta importancia y no constantes.

EFECTOS DEL PROBUCOL SOBRE LA ABSORCION INTESTINAL DEL CALCIO Y TRATAMIENTO CRONICO CON ANTICOAGULANTES EN PACIENTES CON HIPERCOLESTEROLEMIA ASOCIADA CON AFECCIONES CARDIOVASCULARES

A. Rapado and M. Díaz-Curiel

Veinte pacientes afectados de hipercolesterolemia de tipo IIa han sido tratados durante un período medio de 14 meses con probucol a dosis variables entre 0.5 y 1.5 g/día adicionado a una dieta con bajo contenido de colesterol y de ácidos grasos saturados. El tratamiento ha significativamente reducido el colesterol sérico (-31%, $p < 0.01$) y no ha modificado el nivel de los triglicéridos.

El efecto del probucol sobre el metabolismo del calcio/vitamina D ha sido estudiado de acuerdo con su acción sobre la absorción intestinal de ^{47}Ca. La actividad sobre la vitamina K se ha determinado por medio del control del tiempo di protrombina a pacientes sometidos a tratamiento crónico con anticoagulantes.

No se han observado interacciones entre los medicamentos. Muy interesante ha resultado el efecto del probucol en una niña de 12 años de edad, homocigótica por hiperlipoproteinemia de tipo IIa, que durante el tratamiento con colestramina había presentado signos bioquímicos de raquitismo con la necesidad de una intensa terapéutica específica. En esta paciente el probucol ha reducido significativamente la tasa de colesterol sérico sin haberse producido modificaciones de la absorción intestinal de ^{47}Ca y sin ningún síntoma bioquímico de raquitismo.

PROBUCOL: VALORACION DEL EFECTO SOBRE LOS LIPIDOS SERICOS Y LAS LIPOPROTEINAS

J. Rouffy, B. Chanu, R. Bakir, and J. Goy-Loeper

El efecto del probucol — 1 g/día — sobre los lípidos y las lipoproteínas séricas se ha estudiado en pacientes afectados de hiperlipoproteinemia esencial de tipo IIa y IIb resistentes a la dieta.

Algunos de ellos habían sido previamente tratados sin resultados satisfactorios con colestiramina, colfibrato y procetofen.

La duración del tratamiento ha resultado de 1 mes para 34 pacientes (T_1); desde 3 hasta 6 meses en 16 (T_2); desde 6 meses hasta un año en 12 (T_3) y de más de 1 año en 4 (T_4). Al final de los distintos períodos de tratamiento examinados, con la excepción del T_3, se ha observado una disminución significativa de los lípidos séricos totales (desde el 8 hasta el 19%), del colesterol total (desde el 8 hasta el 12%) y del LDL-colesterol (desde el 9 hasta el 15%), además de un significativo aumento de la relación HDL-CH/LDL-CH + VDL-CH.

No se han observado interacciones con anticoagulantes. Este estudio ha demostrado que el probucol es un medicamento eficaz para obtener la disminución de los lípidos séricos totales, del colesterol total y del colesterol de las lipoproteínas de baja densidad que es la fracción lipoproteica más aterogénica.

Otro favorable resultado debido al empleo del probucol es el aumento de la relación HDL-CH/LDL-CH + VLDL-CH con la consecuente mejoría del índice aterogénico.

La tolerancia del medicamento ha resultado excelente desde el punto de vista clínico y de laboratorio.

EL PROBUCOL EN EL TRATAMIENTO DE LA HIPERCOLESTEROLEMIA EN PACIENTES CON AFECCIONES CARDIOVASCULARES

L. Scebat and J. Renais

El probucol (500 mg b.i.d.) adicionado a una dieta con bajo contenido lipídico ha sido administrado durante un período variable entre 12 y 46 meses a 33 pacientes con afecciones cardiovasculares de naturaleza aterosclerótica y con hipercolesterolemia de tipo IIa (11 pacientes), IIb más III (21 pacientes) y IV (1 paciente).

En conjunto el tratamiento ha producido una disminución del colesterol desde una concentración media de 329.5 hasta 281.1 mg/dl (– 14.5%, p < 0.001). En particular 12 pacientes se mostraron resistentes al tratamiento (disminución del colesterol ≤ 10%) mientras 20 pacientes (62.5%) respondieron al tratamiento con dieta + probucol. En 3 casos se ha observado una disminución del efecto hipocolesterolemiante del medicamento después del 6° mes. El resultado logrado en el primer año se ha mantenido en 15 pacientes (46.8%).

El efecto del probucol sobre el colesterol sérico ha resultado similar tanto en los pacientes afectados de hipercolesterolemia esencial (tipo IIa) como en los pacientes afectados de hiperlipemia mixta (tipo IIb + III). No ha habido interacción entre el probucol y los demás medicamentos normalmente empleados en las afecciones cardiovasculares, principalmente las substancias antivitaminas K y los diuréticos.

No se han observado modificaciones de las pruebas de funcionalidad hepática y renal, de la glicemia y del examen hematológico. El peso corporal ha quedado prácticamente sin variaciones.

El electrocardiograma no ha resultado modificado por el tratamiento. Tres pacientes presentaron episodios de diarrea que no alteró el tratamiento en dos sujetos, mientras en el tercero motivó la interrupción del tratamiento durante la segunda semana.

EFECTO DEL PROBUCOL EN PACIENTES HIPERCOLESTEROLEMICOS RESISTENTES AL TRATAMIENTO DE OTROS HIPOLIPIDEMICOS

S. Stefanović and L. Vučić

Se ha estudiado en 15 pacientes la acción del probucol sobre la hipercolesterolemia: 11 con hiperlipoproteinemia de tipo IIa y 4 de tipo IIb. En estos pacientes la hipercolesterolemia se había diagnosticado desde 1 hasta los 20 años precedentes al inicio de la investigación: la duración media era de 7 años. Se habían tratado todos los pacientes, sin éxito, primero con dieta, luego con dieta y clofibrato con la adición en unos casos de colestiramina o fosfatidilcolina.

Las concentraciones de colesterol precedentes a la administración de probucol oscilaban entre 306 y 565 mg/dl ($\overline{X}$: 385 mg/dl). Todos los pacientes fueron sometidos al tratamiento de 1 g de probucol/día durante un período de 3 meses.

Se efectuaron controles al final de cada mes. Al término del tratamiento en todos los pacientes, excepto uno, los valores de colesterol estaban incluidos en los límites normales de acuerdo con los respectivos grupos de edad, esto es, entre 214 y 280 mg/dl ($\overline{X}$: 229 mg/dl).

Durante el tratamiento con probucol no se observaron efectos colaterales clínicamente evidentes o anomalías en los exámenes de laboratorio y al mismo tiempo no se han citado trastornos de índole subjetiva.

SUBJECT INDEX

Subject Index